The Push
to Prescribe

The Push
to Prescribe

Women and Canadian Drug Policy

Edited by
Anne Rochon Ford and Diane Saibil

A project of the
Steering Committee of Women and Health Protection

Anne Rochon Ford, co-ordinator
Sharon Batt
Ken Bassett
Madeline Boscoe
Colleen Fuller
Joel Lexchin
Abby Lippman
Barbara Mintzes
Laura Shea

Women's Press
Toronto

The Push to Prescribe: Women and Canadian Drug Policy
Edited by Anne Rochon Ford and Diane Saibil

Published by
Women's Press, an imprint of Canadian Scholars' Press Inc.
180 Bloor Street West, Suite 801
Toronto, Ontario
M5S 2V6

www.womenspress.ca

Canadian Scholars' Press Inc./Women's Press gratefully acknowledges financial support for our publishing activities from the Government of Canada through the Book Publishing Industry Development Program (BPIDP) and the Government of Ontario through the Ontario Book Publishing Tax Credit Program.

Women and Health Protection gratefully acknowledges the financial support of Health Canada, which provided an infrastructure within which this work was completed.

Library and Archives Canada Cataloguing in Publication

The push to prescribe : women and Canadian drug policy / edited by Anne Rochon Ford and Diane Saibil.

A project of the Steering Committee of Women and Health Protection, Anne Rochon Ford ... et al.
Includes bibliographical references and index.
ISBN 978-0-88961-478-9

1. Women—Health and hygiene—Canada. 2. Women—Drug use—Canada.
3. Pharmaceutical policy—Canada. I. Ford, Anne Rochon II. Saibil, Diane
III. Women and Health Protection (Orgnization). Steering Committee

RA401.C3P87 2009   362.17'820820971   C2009-902170-6

Design and layout: Brad Horning and Stewart Moracen
Cover design: John Kicksee/KIX BY DESIGN

09 10 11 12 13   5 4 3 2 1

Printed and bound in Canada by Marquis Book Printing Inc.

Canada

This book is dedicated to Barbara Seaman (1935–2008) and
Ruth Cooperstock (1928–1985), two pioneering women
who devoted their life's work to issues of women's health and drug safety.
They helped clear the path on which we continue to travel.

We further dedicate this book to all those individuals
whose lives were taken or unnecessarily harmed as a result of
faulty drug regulation and oversight, and to their families
who live with that legacy. Such damage and loss should never have been,
and must never be again.

Table of Contents

———◆·✦·◆———

Foreword

---◆·◆·◆·◆---

Nancy Olivieri

Many prescription drugs may enhance women's health and lives. However, a system in which Canadians can rely on the pharmaceutical industry, regulators at Health Canada, or their personal physicians to license and prescribe safe and effective drugs does not exist. As articulated so clearly in *The Push to Prescribe*, the pharmaceutical industry has gained unprecedented control over the evaluation, regulation, and promotion of its own products. How does this affect the development and promotion of drugs to women?

To explore this question, it may be worthwhile to review the process through which drugs have reached the market over the last two decades. This process is now characterized by serious conflicts of interest at every level. In the decade leading up to 2003, the U.S. pharmaceutical and biotech industries tripled their investment in drug research, while the proportion of public contributions to that research remained unchanged. This reality is critical to an understanding of why the medical literature today arguably represents not much more than a series of documents franchised by the pharmaceutical industry. Industry-funded studies are up to five times more likely to recommend a new, expensive, and often incompletely studied experimental drug than are studies supported by non-profit or public funding. Over the same decade, the experts who oversee the testing of new drugs have become heavily dependent on the pharmaceutical industry. One in four clinical researchers accepts industry support to conduct research, nearly half accept "non-research" industry gifts, and one in three maintain "personal financial ties," including equity in the company conducting research, with the pharmaceutical industry. These gifts help shape a research agenda before any findings are published—or not—in medical journals. Thus, the industry can control what scientific problems and drugs are studied, how trials are designed, who is or is not enrolled in those trials, whether and how findings are published, and who disseminates the results.

Among the most egregious examples of "shaping" the medical literature was a recent exposure of SSRI drug studies in adults, in which nearly one-third of studies submitted to the FDA were found not to have been published at all. However, what was interesting was which studies didn't make it to publication and, therefore, to the attention of the average physician. Of studies emphasizing these drugs' positive aspects, nearly all (97 percent) were published; of those reporting negative or questionable findings, 10 percent were published accurately. Astonishingly, the remaining negative or questionable studies were altered to convey a "positive" outcome. In summary, of the SSRI drug trials read by the average physician (who, after all, is unlikely to search the FDA website for unpublished studies about a drug), 94 percent promoted positive aspects of the drugs, but only 51 percent were truly positive. There are few more striking examples of the erosion of the "evidence base" of medicine in this era.

It is clear from such examples that the average physician may receive only partial information about many drugs—information that, if known, might affect his or her readiness to prescribe. Simply stated, doctors can evaluate neither the effectiveness nor the safety of many new drugs they prescribe, and this is not solely a result of pharmaceutical industry influence. Surveys of both individual investigators and academic institutions report that there is widespread acceptance of provisions that permit corporate sponsors of research to restrict, and to influence in other ways, the publication of research data.

As discussed in *The Push to Prescribe*, this capture of clinical researchers is critical to women's health: we learn how industry's influence in clinical trials, including what therapeutic approaches are studied and how they are studied, disproportionately affect women. In industry-sponsored trials, for example, one approach used to prevent adverse effects coming to light is to evaluate the drug over a minimum exposure before seeking regulatory approval. While many adverse effects of drugs may not surface during brief exposures, a drug approved after short-term trials is often subsequently prescribed over decades. All this is critical to the health of women, who are prescribed more drugs than men, and over longer lives.

And yet women's diversity, as we learn in *The Push to Prescribe*, is underrepresented in clinical trials. Many trials that do enrol women underreport gender-disaggregated data—most critically, safety data. But once a drug is approved, even if studied primarily or exclusively in men and perhaps not analyzed for adverse effects in women at all, recommendations are usually promoted for both genders, with no acknowledgement of the biological differences that may critically affect drug efficacy and safety. The widely adopted American guidelines promoting statin drugs, for example, to both genders cite clinical studies that included few or, in some studies, no women. Compounding the problem is the practice of employing industry-funded "guideline writers" to author treatment recommendations. (In the case of statins, for example, enthusiastic guidelines were written, with a single exception, by "experts" funded by statin manufacturers.) If a practitioner is still not convinced of the benefits of a new drug, industry-funded "key opinion leaders" can be depended upon to promote its alleged merits in industry-sponsored "scientific" meetings.

Furthermore, as examined in *The Push to Prescribe*, what is studied in industry clinical trials arises from a "neomedicalization" attitude that treats natural experiences as "illnesses" needing drugs, and that increasingly targets women. A blatant example is the transformation of menopause to a disease, leading to the medical profession's faith in estrogen therapy. Another example is the disingenuously expanded definition of osteoporosis, so that the majority of women, by a certain age, will "require" treatment for "thin bones."

It follows that advertising practices promoting *diseases* to women operate in parallel with those promoting *drugs*—a pill for every "ill." As noted in *The Push to Prescribe*, direct-to-consumer advertising, although illegal in Canada, is widely encountered in this country. Reading this chapter, I was reminded of a favourite cartoon—the one in which a TV ad man, mimicking the seemingly unending assault of TV ads for drugs, suggests, "Ask your doctor if playing into the hands of the pharmaceutical industry is right for you."

Drug advertising disproportionately targets women, often under the guise of offering them "choices" framed in "feminist" or "empowering" language. Direct-to-consumer advertising of the SSRIs, among the most widely advertised drugs of any era, have helped transform the often socially created condition of mild depression to a market opportunity that is founded and funded upon women's perceived ill health. *The Push to Prescribe* describes how SSRI advertising depicts women more frequently than men, often in passive roles that seem counterintuitive to the "empowerment" these drugs purportedly promise. There is no doubt that this advertising is effective. Women are diagnosed with depression more often than men, and are the recipients of twice as many prescriptions for SSRIs as men, placing huge numbers at risk of the potential lack of efficacy and harm previously concealed from the public.

The Push to Prescribe also focuses its critical analysis on our pharmaceutical industry-supported Canadian drug approval process, including its requirements for reporting of adverse drug reactions. As detailed, Canadian drug approval relies upon lack of transparency, indeed secrecy. Individuals of both genders are harmed by regulatory secrecy, but there is evidence that it disproportionately affects women. One might be surprised to learn, for example, that of 10 drugs recalled recently in the U.S. because of safety issues, eight were substances that had posed greater risks for women than for men. Moreover, a gap—more accurately, the absence—of an effective post-marketing surveillance system (the reporting of adverse drug reactions *after* a drug is licensed) more significantly affects women, who are up to 75 percent more likely than men to develop an adverse drug reaction.

Canadians owe a great deal to the authors of *The Push to Prescribe* and to Women and Health Protection. Every Canadian who reads this book will realize that if we wish to reap the benefits of drug advances into healthy old age, we must, to paraphrase Paine, undergo the fatigue of supporting a drug development and regulatory system in which the precautionary principle is defended. Irresponsible study and promotion of prescription drugs, especially for women, has a bleak history. It is fitting that women, to whom drugs are heavily promoted individually and as a target group, continue in this book to be at the forefront of the battle for safer regulation and transparency.

Preface

———◦·×·◦———

Women and Health Protection (WHP) is a national working group mandated to provide research-based policy advice on the safety of prescription medicines and medical devices used by women. The group, founded in 1998 with funding from the Centres of Excellence for Women's Health Program of Health Canada, comprises university-based researchers, consumers, women's health activists, community groups, and health practitioners.

WHP was launched at a time when Canadian policy was being driven by a worldwide process of deregulation aimed at promoting global trade. Many of those following the proposed policy changes were concerned that the existing system of regulatory protection, established to maximize the safety of pharmaceutical products, might be weakened, if not completely dismantled. These safety regulations, recognized by many for their importance, had been developed over the course of several decades in response to drug disasters that specifically affected women. Therefore, when the federal government called for reactions to proposed regulatory changes, individuals and organizations, who shared a desire to ensure that Health Canada was considering the full implications for women's health in all decisions regarding medications and devices, came together to form a network.

WHP has kept a close watch over proposed and actual changes in the federal health protection legislation for the past decade. Over the years, we have explored in detail issues related to the development, regulation, promotion, and monitoring of prescription drugs and medical devices as they are produced for, marketed to, and used by women.

The group has commissioned research and papers on a range of topics that focus on women and pharmaceuticals. The collected writings of Women and Health Protection, most of which have been posted on the WHP website (www.whp-apsf. ca), represent a unique and invaluable body of work in the areas of health policy and women's studies. WHP's reviews have examined Canadian drug regulation filtered through a lens of sex and gender. By recognizing that women are often the first to experience the harmful effects of lax regulations, WHP has studied and exposed a range of broad pharmaceutical policy issues.

Women's use of prescription drugs and devices is ever-increasing—and there is a tendency to assume that our government's drug regulatory system will protect us from potential negative health effects of this increased consumption. The work compiled in this book rigorously analyzes both our drug use and our assumptions about the effectiveness of government regulations. Taken together, the chapters present a critical view of the overselling and overuse of pharmaceuticals and reveal the myths that suggest that the "more drug choices … the better" and that "substituting industry regulation for government regulation is better for our health."

There is a long history of women in Canada being given unsafe drugs and devices. And there is an equally long history of women organizing around health issues, of women pushing back and trying to effect change. In the years that followed the revelation of harms created when pregnant women were given thalidomide and diethylstilbestrol (DES), clinicians, activists, and researchers mobilized in Canada and elsewhere to pressure governments for tighter controls on drug approvals, for better reporting and monitoring of adverse drug reactions, and for improved enforcement of measures to prevent harms caused by overprescribing. They conducted research, wrote public information pamphlets, and formed support networks for others harmed by faulty drugs and devices, always linking their work to that of the larger women's and social justice movements.

Women and Health Protection is one part of that history of activism around policy development at the intersection of pharmaceuticals, women's health, and health protection. The chapters herein update and highlight the principle themes and lessons learned from our many years of research and writings on these issues. We believe that this compilation will fill a significant gap in the published material available in this field.

The WHP Steering Committee developed the concept for this volume, decided on its contents, and reviewed the early and final drafts of the manuscript, with members providing critical and substantive content to each of the chapters. Diane Saibil edited the manuscript and was responsible for overall coordination of the project. Anne Rochon Ford, coordinator of Women and Health Protection, served as liaison between the group and the publisher and provided support to the project throughout.

Acknowledgements

The Steering Committee of Women and Health Protection would like to thank the larger community of "Biojesters," that group of academics, activists, and clinicians across Canada and abroad who make up our listserv, Biojest. Discussions on the list have provided an endless source of information, thoughtful questioning, and friendly debate about many of the issues in this book. In particular, we note the help of Alan Cassels and Terence Young in seeking particular references at the 11th hour.

Among the individuals who were not part of the Steering Committee but who played a part in the preparation of this volume, thanks go to Ann Silversides for her chapter on transparency, and to Harriet Rosenberg, Danielle Allard, and Linda Furlini, who contributed their experiences and knowledge by providing case studies to supplement the text.

A huge thank-you goes to Susan White, of the Canadian Women's Health Network, for her tireless and thorough work in reviewing the manuscript and ensuring the accuracy of the references.

The Steering Committee would like to personally thank Diane Saibil, who, above all others, knew how to keep her eye on the goal. Her exceptional organizational skills and patience were greatly needed to usher us through this process.

Thanks are also due to Megan Mueller, who, on behalf of Women's Press, welcomed this project from the outset and supported it throughout with great enthusiasm and patience.

And finally, we wish to acknowledge the financial support of the Bureau of Women's Health and Gender Analysis and its many staff, who, over the years, have brokered funding that supported the infrastructure within which we have been able to carry out this work. In particular, we are grateful to Sari Tudiver, who always believed in the value of what we were doing and did her utmost to help move some of our work through the corridors of Health Canada.

Disclaimer

Women and Health Protection Steering Committee
November 2008

Chapter 1

Introduction

———◆———

The Steering Committee
of Women and Health Protection

The ad in a popular Canadian women's magazine reads: "What would you do with a few pounds less? … Ask your doctor about Julie's story…. Medical treatments are available."

Advertisements such as this have become part of our environment in Canada, and the products advertised are hot topics of discussion in magazines, on television and radio, and even in films. The pharmaceutical industry itself has become the focus of bestselling books, both fiction and non-fiction, government committee hearings in North America and abroad, and a range of scholarly treatises. This ever-present attention to the pharmaceutical industry reflects the extent to which prescription medicines—including how they are produced, regulated, marketed, and used—have infiltrated many aspects of everyday life. The nature and extent of this infiltration, and how this has special meaning for women, are at the core of this collection of papers.

An underlying assumption in the chapters that follow is that how knowledge is made, who is included and excluded in creating knowledge, and whether particular pieces of knowledge have legitimacy are fundamental concerns for feminists. We take for granted that the production of knowledge is inextricably tied to how power, control, and privilege are distributed in a society. And, in consequence, we explore how industry, government, academic researchers, and women's groups—separately and interconnectedly—produce knowledge about medical drugs and devices and about women's use of these products.

We hope that those with an interest in health policy issues as they relate to prescription drugs and women's health will find the material in this book relevant and informative.

Historical Context

Canadian feminists have a long history of activism and collective action on issues related to women's health in general and, more specifically, on those issues concerning women in relation to medical drugs and devices. Much of this activity has focused on public education, public policy analysis, scientific research, and raising public awareness about women's experiences. The individual and collective expertise of women in the area of health protection—preventing disease and other causes of disability—is substantial and has informed efforts to influence government health policy decisions, including decisions about drug regulation.

Personal experiences inform and strengthen women's analysis of public policy, including those policies that address the activities of the private sector. During the 1970s and 1980s, these experiences formed a backdrop to a rising interest among Canadian feminists in the links among health, sex, and gender, and supported an emerging critique of the medical industry and of the medicalization of many of the social conditions confronting women. Women began to organize and promote changes in the way medicine was practised. They sought to diminish the increasing reach of medicine where it was inappropriate, but also argued that real problems that were experienced differently (e.g., heart disease), mainly (e.g., autoimmune disorders), or exclusively (e.g., breast cancer, endometriosis) by women were frequently ignored or minimized in the mainstream practice of medicine. As well, relationships between the medical profession and the pharmaceutical industry came under scrutiny and continue to be an important focus of the women's health movement.

An early example highlighting the importance of women's personal experiences in understanding drug regulation and safety issues centres on the drug diethylstilbestrol (DES), a synthetic hormone developed in 1938 and prescribed until 1971 to an estimated 200,000–400,000 Canadian women to prevent miscarriage.

In 1971, when researchers found a link to cancer in women exposed to the drug in the womb, Health Canada banned its use in pregnancy, but failed to warn exposed women about the risks. The concern "not to alarm the public" was not only paternalistic; it meant that exposed women failed to get needed health care. Women exposed to DES while they were still in the womb need special gynaecological exams because they face risks of a rare form of vaginal cancer. They are also more likely to have reduced fertility and complications in pregnancy. The problems of such women and those of their mothers, who took DES while pregnant and who face higher risks of breast cancer, can be better managed if they and their health care providers know they were exposed.

Women exposed to DES created DES Action groups in Canada, the U.S., and several other Western countries to provide information, to stimulate needed research, and to support the needs of the DES-exposed. The groups also worked to improve health protection laws in their respective countries.

Building on this base, and concerned that regulators and politicians were not addressing some of the key issues related to the health protection of women, women's health activists and women harmed by a range of drugs and devices followed the example of DES Action groups worldwide and formed networks for change. These networks also had roots in Canadian activism to obtain safe, affordable, and accessible birth control, including efforts to remove laws banning the distribution of birth control devices, or even information about contraceptives—efforts that continued until 1969 when, after decades of organizing, the statute banning contraceptives was finally repealed (Library and Archives Canada, 2008).[1]

The Story of the Dalkon Shield

Two years after the repeal of the statute banning contraceptives, the Dalkon Shield IUD appeared on the market. The story of the Dalkon Shield—dubbed "the IUD that gave the device a bad name" by the Toronto Women's Health Network (2002)—incorporates some of the main themes that have characterized the work of women's health activists over the past four decades: politics, ethics, and safety. At the time the Dalkon Shield was approved, the Health Protection Branch (that branch of Health Canada responsible for the regulation of drugs, today called the Health Products and Food Branch) lacked the regulatory authority to ensure that contraceptive (or any) devices were safe and effective. In fact, at the time the Dalkon Shield was approved, medical devices—unlike drugs—required no pre-market testing at all.

As the controversy over the Dalkon Shield was heating up, the Health Protection Branch moved to create the Bureau of Medical Devices. One of its first actions was to issue a warning to Canadian women to have the Dalkon Shield removed regardless of whether they had noticed problems with it. The Branch also drafted amendments to the *Food and Drugs Act* to require manufacturers to prove the safety of medical devices before market authorization was granted (Regush, 1992). But it did not immediately impose a recall of the Dalkon Shield, which remained on the Canadian market until 1985, five years after it was removed from shelves in the United States.

The lack of an adequate regulatory intervention led many women in Canada and around the world to focus on legal remedies. It was estimated that up to 123,000 Canadian women were fitted with the Dalkon Shield between 1971 and 1974 ("U.S. Court Frees $2.5 Billion," 1989). Women across the country collected stories of adverse reactions, largely in support of a lawsuit, and created public awareness campaigns highlighting the reported risks associated with the Dalkon Shield. Women harmed by the Dalkon Shield headed for the courts and both the legal system and the media were effectively used by health activists to alert women to the growing number of lawsuits and to the problems being revealed about the contraceptive device. "I saw them holding up a picture of a Dalkon Shield on CBC television," one woman told the *Montreal Gazette* in 1987. "I didn't even know what it was called, but I recognized it. It was a relief for me because it suddenly made sense. I knew that all my trouble started when it was put in. But no one had ever made the connection" (Kalbfuss, 1987).

A network of activists from across the country brought a wealth of knowledge and expertise to the issue, and support to the women coming forward with complaints about the problems associated with the Dalkon Shield. The interaction among women who had suffered the ill effects of the device and those who were developing a sophisticated analysis of the health protection system in Canada was beneficial to both groups.

The efforts of these women, coupled with heavy media coverage of the legal and political battles surrounding the Dalkon Shield, emphasized the failure of both the regulatory and legal systems to protect women from harmful devices and drugs. What also emerged during this time were revelations about the questionable marketing practices of the manufacturers of some drugs and devices in the form of sexist advertising to doctors and unbridled promotion of products whose safety was in question. Although the 7,000 members of Dalkon Shield Action Canada failed to win their case in court, the women's health movement had gained valuable experience in the broad arena of health protection, further strengthening the foundation on which the Canadian Women's Health Network—and Women and Health Protection— would be built.

Another Milestone: The Royal Commission on New Reproductive Technologies

Following the creation of the first "test tube baby" in 1978, there were rapid developments in the field of new reproductive technologies. A coalition of feminist health activists (the Coalition for a Royal Commission on New Reproductive Technologies) formed to pressure the Canadian government to address the lack of regulation in Canada relating to these technologies. In October 1989, in direct response to extensive lobbying by the coalition, the Royal Commission was established with Professor Patricia Baird, a British Columbia-based academic paediatrician and medical geneticist, at its head.

The commission's final report, entitled *Proceed with Care,* was delivered after several years of delay and much greater expense than anticipated in November 1993. It contained 293 recommendations. Unfortunately, follow-up to the report has proceeded at a snail's pace and has not adequately addressed the concerns of the commission's proponents. Following numerous thwarted attempts, the *Assisted Human Reproduction Act* was finally passed in March 2004, banning, among other things, human cloning, "rent-a-womb" contracts, and the sale of human eggs and sperm. The Act also created an agency to regulate those activities that were not banned. However, as of this writing, there is still no central collection of data to allow estimates of safety and effectiveness of the procedures used; there is no full-scale effort to deal with the causes of infertility; the reproductive technology "business" continues at an ever accelerating pace; there is widespread "reproductive tourism"; and there are still no laws forbidding anonymity of donors, thus leaving the demands of the activists over the past quarter-century mostly unmet.[2]

A Tradition of Collective Action for Collective Rights

The mobilization that took place to inform women about the Dalkon Shield, to challenge the Health Protection Branch of Health Canada, and to lobby for the creation of the Royal Commission, among other things, is reflected today in ongoing questioning and activism regarding the safety and appropriateness of a host of drugs and devices, including antidepressants, osteoporosis drugs, statins, silicone breast implants, and the long-acting injectable contraceptive Depo-Provera (depot medroxyprogesterone acetate [DMPA]). This work is being done by a combination of women's health researchers and policy analysts, and women who have been directly affected—often negatively—by these products.

Box 1.1: The Ongoing Saga of Depo-Provera

The multi-decade story of Depo-Provera, an injectable contraceptive administered once every three months, has served as a bellwether of key trends in the history of the movement for safe pharmaceuticals for women.

Depo-Provera is a long-acting, synthetic hormone manufactured by Pfizer, previously Upjohn Canada. It was first approved for the treatment of endometriosis and threatened or habitual miscarriage in 1960. In 1974, it was shown to be ineffective for these purposes, but it was found to be successful as a form of contraception when early research for other purposes revealed that the drug caused women to stop menstruating.

In 1985, news that Depo-Provera was about to be approved as a contraceptive triggered considerable protest from Canadian women's health and social justice groups. The Canadian Coalition on Depo-Provera was formed, comprising 80 groups representing health professionals, disability advocates, international non-governmental organizations, women's health advocates, and representatives from Aboriginal communities. The coalition maintained that not enough was known about the drug to support its approval as a contraceptive. At a series of cross-Canada meetings on fertility control in 1986, women with disabilities, and Aboriginal women provided compelling personal testimonies about their concerns based on their own experiences with the drug. They talked about being given Depo-Provera without their consent, about the negative impact the drug had on their sexuality and body image, and about being assured that there were absolutely no harmful effects when, in fact, some experienced circulatory problems, weight gain, irregular bleeding, and headaches.

Despite ongoing opposition from women's groups, Health Canada approved Depo-Provera for birth control in 1997. Then, in 2004, the U.S. Food and Drug Administration issued a black box warning, the strongest safety warning the FDA can issue, "as a result of the drug manufacturer's and FDA's analysis of data that clarified the drug's long-term effects on bone density" (Food and Drug Administration, 2004, para. 5). This was followed, in 2005, by a Health Canada warning that Depo-Provera "has been associated with loss of bone mineral density (BMD) which may not be completely reversible. Loss of bone mineral density," it continued, "is greater with increasing duration of use" (Health Canada, 2005, para. 5). Other reported side effects included increased susceptibility to sexually transmitted infections (chlamydia and gonorrhoea), menstrual irregularities, abdominal pain or discomfort, and weight gain.

After the Health Canada advisory was issued, Dr. Lorri Puil, of the Therapeutics Initiative at the University of British Columbia, searched the literature up to March 2006 for published studies that examined the relation between Depo-Provera use and bone health. Puil found studies clearly indicating that women using Depo-Provera may experience a significant loss of bone mineral density, something that may contribute to increased incidence and severity of certain types of fractures. She also found that women aged 18–25 years were not included in the studies that led to Health Canada's warning. Assessing effects on this age group is important because peak bone mass may not be reached before a woman turns 30.

This systematic review of the evidence identified a need for clinical outcome data. Puil (2006) notes that: "Postmarketing data have included rare reports of fractures in DMPA users aged 16 to 45 years (Depo-Provera Product Monograph, June 30, 2005). This information has been requested from the FDA but cannot be used to calculate incidence rates due to the voluntary nature of reporting and the unknown denominators (total population exposed)" (p. 4). She also states that "No conclusions can be drawn about the risk associated with DMPA exposure without the appropriate studies that assess fracture occurrence in exposed and unexposed women or adolescents or validation of the surrogate marker BMD in these age groups" (Puil, 2006, p. 9). Such studies should include long-term risk assessment.

Advertising campaigns by the manufacturer of Depo-Provera typically portray it as a convenient, hassle-free method of birth control. In North America, it is a popular method among girls and women who do not tolerate estrogen-based contraceptives. Even before its approval as a contraceptive, Depo-Provera was promoted by family planning programs and population control agencies, mainly in the so-called "developing" countries, because it was identified as a highly effective, provider-controlled technology that promised to drive down birth rates among poor women. But women in these countries—where access to local health care facilities is often inadequate or non-existent, and the right to informed consent is often overlooked—have indicated that they want user-controlled methods of contraception without major side effects (Canadian Women's Health Network, 2004; Sarojini & Murthy, 2005).

In the industrialized world, Depo-Provera is disproportionately prescribed to society's most marginalized and disadvantaged: Aboriginal women, women with disabilities, incarcerated women, girls and women in long-term care facilities, women with drug and alcohol addiction problems, poor women, women of colour, and teenagers (Bunkle, 1993; DisAbled Women's Network Ontario, n.d.; Littlecrow-Russell, 2000; Roberts, 1998; Smith, 2003; Tait, 2000; Women's Health Interaction & Inter Pares, 1995). And recipients are often not fully informed of the side effects and potential health risks of the drug. The patterns are telling; in the United Kingdom Depo-Provera is used most often by Asian and West Indian women, in Australia by Aboriginal women, and in New Zealand by Maori and Pacific Island women (Women's Health Action, 2005).

Unfortunately, there are no data on Depo-Provera utilization in Canada by region or subpopulation. However, it is known that Depo-Provera was administered to women with disabilities long before it was officially approved for contraceptive use. According to DAWN Ontario (DisAbled Women's Network Ontario, n.d.), "physicians and institutional staff have administered Depo-Provera to women with mental or physical disabilities, rarely informing them of the drug's side effects. Some disabled girls as young as 12 have been given the drug ..." (para. 10) (see also

Zarfasm, Fyfe & Gorodzinsky, 1981). For the convenience of caregivers, girls and women in some long-term care institutions are given Depo-Provera to stop periods for "hygienic reasons" (whether or not they are sexually active), and to prevent pregnancies. Such practices raise ethical issues about informed consent and the use of Depo-Provera as a form of (temporary) sterilization.

Although detailed documentation is not available, there is growing evidence that Depo-Provera is prescribed disproportionately to Aboriginal women and teenagers in Canada. A November 2005 *Maclean's* story on the overprescribing of Depo-Provera as birth control to Native women (Hawaleshka, 2005) referred to a survey of 25 Aboriginal women and teenagers on Vancouver Island, which found that 50 percent were using Depo-Provera. Many of the users reported that they had not been informed of the health risks associated with the drug. Whereas 2 percent of all Canadian women using contraceptives use Depo-Provera, it is estimated that 10–20 percent of Aboriginal women using contraceptives use Depo-Provera (Hawaleshka, 2005).

This is particularly worrying in light of statistics from Manitoba indicating that Aboriginal women and men have more than twice the rate of hip fractures compared with non-Aboriginal Manitobans. Preliminary data from the First Nations Bone Health Study suggests that there may be a high incidence of osteoporosis in Aboriginal women (Leslie, Metge, Weiler, Young, Yuen et al., 2002).

The evidence currently available has not established that Depo-Provera is a safe drug, yet it has been prescribed for use by women for close to 50 years and continues to be prescribed in Canada for long-term contraceptive use by girls and women. And, there is evidence that it is those girls and women on the margins of our society who are most likely to receive this prescription.

Source: Adapted from Shea, L. (2007). *Reflections on Depo Provera: Contributions to improving drug regulation in Canada.* Toronto: Women and Health Protection.

Another significant feature of the Canadian women's health movement has been the struggle for resources. The pharmaceutical industry has extremely ample resources available to promote their point of view. To be able to represent women's interests, women's groups have often had to make the pursuit of core funding from the public purse a central part of their agenda. Groups such as Women and Health Protection and the Canadian Women's Health Network are a legacy of this part of the struggle.

There is strong evidence that collective action by independent community-based groups of women has been critical to health protection for women, as well as for their children and communities (Armstrong, Lippman & Sky, 1997).[3] Efforts in Canada have been distinguished by a commitment within the women's health community to collective rights as opposed to an individual rights framework. A strong and recurring theme, articulated by women's health activists, has been a precautionary approach to drug safety and the use of medical devices, a theme that is reaffirmed throughout this volume (see, in particular, Chapter 3). This approach is also articulated in numerous government documents, but, unfortunately, rarely put into practice.

Today's Neo-liberal Context

The authors of these chapters explicitly recognize that the distribution of economic and political privilege is a strong determinant, both directly and indirectly, of women's health. These societal and social realities are constant and forceful reminders that women have multiple identities beyond gender, defined by variables such as class, race, sexual identity, age, ability, immigrant status, or geography, and that these occur in many differing combinations. Women, as a result, experience risks to health, moderated by the effects of the fault lines in society along which power is distributed and resources allocated to and among people in complex and entangled ways.

Many of these fault lines have deepened following the erosion of the strong social safety nets and policies based on collective rights developed during the post-World War II period. In their place are increased privatization of health and social services, competition over public funding, and global harmonization of economic and trade policies that leave individual women to fend for themselves. Much of this ideological shift in Canadian society, as elsewhere, is characterized by neo-liberal restructuring (see box), and the latter has been particularly severe for women.

Box 1.2: Neo-liberalism Defined

Neo-liberal policies put the emphasis on economic growth and free market forces, favour deregulation, and minimize government's role in social programs. These policies encourage the consumer orientation that dominates contemporary North American society.

In fact, the feminization of poverty in Canada and around the globe has been a growing phenomenon, one with particular relevance to women's health and the various measures proposed to deal with illness and disease. Despite the existence of medicare in Canada, impoverished people are more likely to experience illness and to have less access to health services compared to those with higher incomes. Income, education, gender, race, where one lives, as well as one's culture and social environment, and societal structures for dealing with such things as employment, housing, immigration, and racism are all determinants of health, both singly and together.

When Choice Is Not Really Choice

Feminist concerns with a neo-liberal orientation toward health and health risks centre on the fact that this orientation individualizes and depoliticizes health. Managing health and health risks is framed, simplistically, as individual choice. In this scenario, making the wrong choice can be construed as the reason an individual becomes ill. However, the ability of individuals to exercise choice, as well as the choices that are available, are strongly and necessarily influenced by the determinants of health mentioned above. In this paradigm, concepts such as choice and empowerment, language used by feminists to describe specific goals, are co-opted and distorted to mean personal responsibility for preventing or managing disease. The underlying neo-liberal message is that women can—and should—minimize their risk of disease by changing their lifestyle or choosing to take a pill. This undermines a collective approach to prevention. Feminists continue to challenge this model of individual responsibility in view of the evidence that options, and the ability to select among them, are seriously constrained by social policies and societal structures that underlie the determinants of health and well-being.

It may also be worth considering if the marketing strategies of the biomedical and pharmaceutical industries should themselves be recognized as determinants of—if not actual risks to—women's health. Since the late 1980s, the pharmaceutical industry has won significant victories, including a relaxation of regulatory standards around the introduction of new drugs and their monitoring once they are on the market, as well as the extension of patent protection on new brand-name drugs. The former are part of an ongoing international effort to harmonize regulatory standards to fit the industry's requirements. The latter is in line with international treaties such as the North American Free Trade Agreement and with the Trade-Related Aspects of Intellectual Property Rights (TRIPs) agreement to establish a global regime supporting extended monopoly protection for the drug industry, as well as other industries, through increased protection for so-called "intellectual property" rights. While these rights are, in themselves, subjects of debate, of no less concern is how they are increasingly pitted against the public interest, including collective rights, such as access to essential medications, and how these conflicts may further disadvantage women's health.

Sex, Gender, Diversity, and Their Intersections

In this book, we write of "women" and emphasize their "gendered" roles. However, we must caution our readers about the need to avoid assuming there is any "one" or "essential" woman and of the importance of recognizing the fluidity of gender itself, as well as of the traditional ways in which "sex" and "gender" are distinguished (see box below for one approach).

Box 1.3: Sex and Gender Defined

"Sex" usually refers to the biological, anatomical, and physiological characteristics that distinguish females and males. "Gender" refers to the various socially constructed roles, expectations, and relationships that society differentially ascribes to males and females across their lifespans, and that intersect with other social and culturally determined factors such as race and ethnicity, ability, sexual orientation, etc. Both sex and gender are determinants of health; their interactions and diverse expressions help explain some of the gendered patterns of disease and health care we observe. Thus, we find that some diseases/conditions are unique to almost all women; some are more prevalent in certain women than men, and even when men and women have the same diagnosis, the care they receive may differ based on gender or other individual and group characteristics. To promote and protect women's health, we need to understand fully the influences of biology and of gender, and to assess, as well, differences among women that reflect their varying experiences (Bartlett, Doyal, Ebrahim, Davey, Bachmann et al., 2005) in contexts where power differentials underlie health disparities.

Gender-based analysis (GBA) describes a process that assesses the different impacts of proposed and existing policies, programs and legislation on women and men (Williams, 1999). In 1995, the Canadian government adopted a policy that required federal departments and agencies to apply GBA to all future policies and legislation (Williams, 1999). Within Health Canada's practice of gender-based analysis, sex refers to biological characteristics such as anatomy and physiology. The existence of sex-specific conditions, such as endometriosis among women, is acknowledged, as are the biological differences between women and men that may strongly influence both different responses to the same treatments and the need for different treatments to obtain the same responses. Within this policy, and by contrast with sex, gender refers to the range of socially determined characteristics that reflect differential attitudes, values, relative power, and other societal expectations and assumptions about women and men.

While traditional GBA acknowledges that sex and gender interact with the social and structural determinants of health—such as income, education, and inequality—as well as with each other, it also recognizes how impossible it is to neatly distinguish between the two concepts. In fact, and perhaps too often, both terms may be conflated or used inappropriately. As Olena Hankivsky and colleagues (2007) note, "there exists an inherent difficulty in understanding where 'sex' stops and where 'gender' begins. 'Sex' is in a constant state of negotiation and gender is also a contested category" (p. 155).

Recognizing the complexities involved, the Canadian Research Institute for the Advancement of Women (CRIAW) offers the following critique of gender-based analysis:

> While GBA has brought greater awareness of women's inequality relative to men, a "gender only" lens that primarily looks at differential gender impacts or discrimination between women and men fails to account for the complexity of women's lives. Prioritizing one identity entry point (i.e., gender) or one relation of power (i.e., patriarchy) to the exclusion of others (i.e., race, class) misrepresents the full diversity of women's lived realities. (CRIAW, 2006, p. 5)

CRIAW goes on to define their emerging "intersectional" approach as a framework that "attempt[s] to understand how multiple forces work together and interact to reinforce conditions of inequality and social exclusion" (CRIAW, 2006, p. 5). The authors of this volume's chapters are well aware of the difficulties in—perhaps even the futility of—setting up some boundary lines that would say, for example, this relates to "sex" and this to "gender." We understand that there is no core feature that expresses "woman-ness," but rather that women's multiple and layered identities are a reflection of their social relationships within a (still) sexist society that is also divided by race and class—some of the issues addressed by an intersectional approach. At the same time, to maintain our focus on the main subject matter of this book—the drugs and devices made available by industry and government, marketed through the media, and eventually sold to or purchased by individuals—we have stopped short of what a full intersectional analysis would require, a delving into a full analysis of women's lived experiences of their own health, of the health of their families, or their health practices.

What You Will Find in This Book

The chapters that follow highlight and illustrate some of the broader issues that arise in an exploration of how health protection policies have an impact on women with respect to pharmaceuticals. Among these issues are the right to informed consent, the right to know, and the co-optation of language: what words such as "choice" and "empowerment" mean in the real world, a world in which biology *and* social relations *and* structural determinants of society matter greatly.

The book is divided into two main sections, each of which begins with a brief overview of the linked chapters therein. The first section focuses on the social, cultural, political, and physical environment in which drugs are prescribed to women, while the second addresses the regulatory environment within which women obtain approved drugs and medical devices in Canada. The material presented is based in public policy research as well as an understanding of the pharmaceutical industry. Although public policy is obviously a moving target, we believe that observations and analysis of particular public policy trends and events can shed light on the development and application of public policy about prescription drugs in a more general way. The specifics may evolve and change, but the analyses and observations about how to interpret the process and what questions to ask remain valid.

A Final Word

Once upon a time, drug manufacturers produced and marketed mainly medicines and devices. As many authors have pointed out recently, the industry now also creates and markets diseases themselves (Cassels & Moynihan, 2005). As a result, not only may pharmaceutical products treat some truly serious diseases for which cures remain elusive, but they may also be taken by healthy women and thereby cause serious problems that need not ever have happened at all. This surge in the use of drug therapy to treat a myriad of minor, even questionable, medical conditions and diseases, such as premenstrual dysphoric disorder, is contributing to an increase in harmful side effects, some causing hospitalization and even death. Conditions such as restless legs may seriously affect a very small portion of the population that may benefit from drug treatment, but aggressive marketing has turned twitchy legs into a chronic disease suffered by large numbers of people, thus creating a potentially large world market for drug manufacturers (Woloshin & Schwartz, 2006).

It is our hope that the material that follows will provide our readers with an understanding of the health policy issues addressed so that they can begin to pose and answer questions about whether and how government can regulate drugs, devices, and industry in a precautionary way, the only way that will fully protect and promote women's health.

Notes

1. The law that legalized birth control in Canada also provided access, with a hospital committee's approval, to abortion.
2. Much of the history of the Royal Commission, including the growing disillusion with and disappointment in its work by many of the women who had initially lobbied for its creation, as well as the background to lawsuits against the commission by some of its original members, have been documented in a two-volume collection, *Misconceptions* (Basen, Eichler & Lippman, 1993).
3. It is not that these issues are of no concern to men; they are and should be. But for women, they take on multidimensional aspects that touch on our collective and individual health. Because women often act as the health care gatekeepers for the family, the dispensers of and the knowledge keepers about pills and remedies, their relationship with the world of medicine has a direct impact on their communities and their families.

Part I

The Push to Prescribe
Who Defines What Drugs We Need and How Do They Do It?

———◆◆◆◆———

We live in a culture in which medicinal drugs are ubiquitous and widely accepted. Moreover, the prescribing of these products for women takes place within particular social, cultural, and political environments. The chapters in this section consider how the current Canadian society and government view medicines, and how these views have been, and continue to be, shaped. Understanding this context in which drug prescribing and drug taking occur is essential to an informed examination of Canadian public policy as it relates to the regulation of medicines.

The development, manufacturing, and selling of prescription drugs is a multibillion-dollar industry dominated by large corporations that exist to be profitable. This industry is viewed by many, especially those in government, as a key economic sector. The chapters in this section describe the impact of the pharmaceutical industry on the general public, and on women in particular, and point to some of the implications for women's health.

In Chapter 2, Barbara Mintzes describes the world of direct-to-consumer advertising, covering its legal status in Canada, the impact on Canadians of its legal status in the U.S., and its particular targeting of women. She reveals some of the mythology that has developed about direct-to-consumer advertising being educational and empowering. Barbara is an assistant professor with the Therapeutics Initiative at the University of British Columbia. She has a long history as a researcher, writer, and activist in women's health and pharmaceutical issues.

Chapter 3, by Sharon Batt and Abby Lippman, examines how our contemporary neo-liberal political culture supports and promotes not only the medicalization of women's lives, but also a phenomenon referred to as neomedicalization, whereby "risk" is medicalized to promote increased use of medicines by healthy people, purportedly to reduce their chances of becoming ill. Sharon is a doctoral candidate in bioethics at Dalhousie University. A founder of Breast Cancer Action Montreal and author of *Patient No More: The Politics of Breast Cancer*, Sharon is a researcher and writer with many years of activism in the areas of breast cancer and environmental health. Abby Lippman is a professor of epidemiology at McGill University and past chair of the Canadian Women's Health Network. She has worked successfully to combine her academic and activist lives for several decades.

In Chapter 4, Sharon Batt looks at the ways in which government consultations on drug policy are structured and the extent to which funding sources may influence the types of "public" input and advice the government receives as it develops policies and legislation to regulate medical drugs.

Chapter 2

"Ask Your Doctor"
Women and Direct-to-Consumer Advertising

—◦◦◦◦—

Barbara Mintzes

Introduction

At a bus shelter, a billboard features a photo of a young woman with the slogan, "Express yourself," accompanied by the package and brand name of a birth control pill. On television, older women twinkle with glee as they suggest asking your doctor about Celebrex (celecoxib), an arthritis drug. On the newsstands, U.S. women's magazines carry advertisement after advertisement for medicines.

Canadians are often surprised to hear that advertising of prescription drugs to the public is illegal because we see so much of it. These ads have much in common with other advertising, both in the way the product and messages are presented, and the use of a range of techniques to create an emotional connection between the viewer and the advertised brand. They also include broader social messages about health, disease, gender roles, and the use of medicines. There is no suggestion that a health problem may be minor or self-limiting and a medicine a poor solution, or that there is any need for caution in deciding whether or not to use a medicinal drug.

Direct-to-consumer advertising of prescription drugs (DTCA) is legal in two countries, the U.S. and New Zealand. Elsewhere it is prohibited as a health protection measure. The growth of this type of advertising is relatively new: in the U.S. the first DTCA for prescription drugs dates to the early 1980s, but DTCA did not take off until the 1990s, and TV ads did not become widespread until 1998, after a shift in U.S. regulatory policy.

Canada's federal *Food and Drugs Act* prohibits prescription drug advertising to the public, with the exception of "name, price, and quantity," a provision introduced in 1975 to allow comparative price advertising. However, enforcement of the law is limited, with no restrictions imposed on cross-border U.S. advertising, and limited regulatory response to the increasing volume of "made-in-Canada" advertising. This "made-in-Canada" advertising of questionable legality includes two types of ads. Branded "reminder ads" state the name of the product, but not what it is for. "Disease-oriented" ads talk about a condition and do not mention a brand name, but push viewers to "ask their doctor" about a new treatment. Much of the recent advertising that skirts the limits of the law—and beyond—has targeted women. Even some advertisements for products intended for men—such as those for erectile dysfunction—are strategically placed in magazines read primarily by women.

Advertising of prescription medicines can stimulate unnecessary and inappropriate use, leading to greater risks of harmful drug reactions and increased drug costs. This potential for harm is relevant both to women and men. However, there is reason to be concerned that women are especially vulnerable to harm from prescription drug advertising both for social and biological reasons. This chapter begins with an overview of the policy discussions on DTCA, especially in terms of effects on women, and then discusses case studies of specific types of drugs.

Why Is DTCA Prohibited in Canada?

In Canada, as in other countries that prohibit DTCA, the ban on advertising of prescription medicines to the public is a health protection measure linked to prescription-only status. Some medicines require a prescription because they have more serious harmful effects, because we have inadequate knowledge of harmful effects, or because these medicines treat complex or serious health problems that cannot easily be self-diagnosed and managed. A second rationale for restrictions on DTCA is the heightened vulnerability of people who are seriously ill. A person who is in pain, who faces a grim diagnosis, or who is caring for a seriously ill child differs in a fundamental way from someone who is shopping for a new pair of jeans.

The intent of the prohibition of DTCA was "to protect the purchasing consumer against injury to health and against deception" (House of Commons, 1939, cited in Health Canada, 2007, p. 6). From a business perspective, however, the pharmaceutical industry is highly competitive and companies are under pressure to garner market share and expand sales. At the heart of the discussions about DTCA is whether prescription drugs should be viewed as consumer products or medical treatments.

Why DTCA Is of Special Concern to Women

Many of the concerns about DTCA's effects on health and drug costs are not specific to women. DTCA can drive up drug costs because the drugs that are advertised tend to be expensive new drugs; often there are cheaper alternatives available that are just as effective. Additionally, it is a cost driver if it leads to more medicine use. However, there are two main reasons for women to be especially concerned about harm from DTCA: targeting of women in advertising, and extra vulnerability to harm from unnecessary or inappropriate medicine use.

Advertisers tend to focus their spending where they know the returns will be good. Because television, radio, magazines, and billboards reach the mostly healthy general population, most DTCA is for drugs for relatively mild problems and for common chronic conditions that are treated by family doctors. Women visit family doctors more often, making up around two-thirds of primary care patients. This is probably why there are so many ads for medicines in women's magazines and on daytime television (Bell, Kravitz & Wilkes 2000; Brownfield, Bernhardt, Phan, Williams & Parker, 2004). Women also live longer on average than men, but have more years of disability. Some of the most common chronic diseases associated with long-term medicine use, such as arthritis and asthma, are reported more often in women than men. These diseases represent large markets for drug manufacturers.

There are sometimes biological reasons for the greater vulnerability of women on average to certain types of harmful drug reactions. Many drug effects are dose-related. The average woman is smaller than the average man and so, at standard drug doses, receives a higher dose per body weight. Women are also more vulnerable to certain types of abnormal heart rhythms caused by drugs (Correa-de-Araujo, 2005). When a drug first comes to market, knowledge of uncommon or longer-term harmful effects is inadequate, and usually no analyses will have been carried out to see whether effectiveness or safety differs between women and men, despite the existence of regulations (U.S.) or guidelines (Canada) for sex-disaggregated analyses of clinical trial data. Sex-specific adverse effects or limited effectiveness are therefore not necessarily known. We also know the least about the safety of new drugs because they are tested on a relatively small number of people, and usually on a restricted type of patient (for example, excluding the elderly or those with other serious health problems; see Chapter 5 for more detail about clinical trials of drugs. But it is, of course, the newest drugs that are most heavily advertised.

Box 2.1: What Are the Specific Concerns about Harm to Women from DTCA?

- Unnecessary medicalization of normal life stages and events, such as pregnancy
- Promotion of inappropriate medicine use for mild health problems
- Harm from unnecessary exposure to medicines, including polypharmacy (use of many medicines at once), and exposures during pregnancy and breastfeeding
- Rapid growth in drug costs will overwhelm health care budgets, leading governments to cut services or shift costs to the public, which will harm women disproportionately because women use more health services than men
- Promotion of individual drug solutions for social problems, including those linked to gender inequality, such as depression among single mothers living in poverty
- Negative stereotyped images of women in advertising

There are also social reasons for women's vulnerability to harm from advertising: DTCA plays on gender stereotypes and contributes to the unnecessary medicalization of normal aspects of women's lives, such as menstruation and menopause, and overprescribing of psychotropic drugs such as antidepressants and tranquilizers. Women are diagnosed with psychiatric problems such as depression and anxiety more often than men (Piccinelli & Wilkinson, 2000).

As a cost driver, DTCA puts a significant strain on publicly provided health care services. This may lead to differential harm to women because women use more health care and make up the majority of those without drug and health benefits and who live in poverty. If unsustainable increases in drug costs lead provincial governments to shift more health care costs onto the public through copayment or delisting of services, those least able to pay will bear the largest financial burden.

Strong Pressure for Change

With the growth of DTCA and evidence of its profitability, countries in which the practice is prohibited have been under intense pressure to change their laws. In Canada, there have been three major national consultations about introduction of DTCA since 1996, none of which has resulted in new legislation. There were negative media reports each time and this lack of tabled legislation may reflect the political sensitivity of the issue. However, enforcement of the law has become increasingly limited (Gardner et al., 2003).

Additionally, in the spring of 2008, extensive amendments to the *Food and Drugs Act* were proposed for the first time, in Bill C-51. Bill C-51 included two changes related to DTCA. The existing barrier to prescription drug advertising that was in the Act—rather than in the accompanying regulations—was to be deleted. This barrier is a prohibition of advertising to the public of any products for listed serious diseases (Section 3 and Schedule A of the act). Because most prescription-only medicines prevent or treat serious diseases, Section 3 and Schedule A create a barrier, in law, to the introduction of prescription drug advertising to the public.

A new clause in Bill C-51 stated that advertising of prescription drugs was to be prohibited *unless authorized by the regulations*. This would have allowed any and all forms of DTCA to be introduced in Canada solely through regulations, which involves only the Cabinet and not a full parliamentary vote. By July 2008, it was not as yet clear whether these provisions in the bill would stand as proposed or be amended.

Ontario Court Case on DTCA: 2005–2008

In December 2005, one of Canada's largest media companies, CanWest MediaWorks, filed a legal action in the Ontario Superior Court challenging the *Food and Drugs Act* prohibition of DTCA. CanWest's claim is that the law prohibiting DTCA infringes on its freedom of expression because it cannot run advertisements for prescription drugs in its newspapers, on television, or in other media. As we go to press, Health Canada is defending the law on public health grounds. In addition, a public interest coalition of unions and non-profit groups successfully obtained standing in court in support of the law. Included in the coalition are the Canadian Federation of Nurses Unions; Canadian Union of Public Employees; the Canadian Health Coalition; Women and Health Protection; the Communications, Energy, and Paperworkers Union of Canada; the Society for Diabetic Rights; the Medical Reform Group; and Terence Young for Drug Safety Canada. (Terence Young is the father of Vanessa Young, who died at the age of 15 after taking Propulsid [cisapride] for an unapproved use. This drug was advertised to the public in the U.S.)

The coalition was granted standing in the case in order to address two key issues, one of which is whether women are especially vulnerable to harm from DTCA. The second is the effect of DTCA on employee health benefits.

Marketing to Women as a Way to Increase Advertising Effectiveness

Marketers have stressed the benefits of targeting women in DTCA. For example, in an article in *The Business Review*, Handlin (2007) argues that medicines' advertising can be made more effective by targeting women more often, even in products intended for use by both sexes. Her main reasons are that women are more often the "health care gatekeepers" for their families, that they seek more health information on the Internet, read more mass-media magazines, and tend to watch more television than men. Women also pay more attention to DTCA and are more concerned about their health. In a New Zealand survey, for example, 29 percent of women had used a magazine or newspaper ad as a source of health information as compared with 15 percent of men (Toop et al., 2003).

Handlin points out that women respond positively to messages suggesting that they can help others by recommending an advertised medicine. She also suggests depicting women directly in ads, which can "speak subliminally to certain deep-seated psychological needs that help motivate buying behaviour … such as the need for self-actualization, for social acceptance, or for attractiveness to the opposite sex" (Handlin, 2007, p. 35).

Emotional Appeals: Medicines Lead to Control over One's Life

A content analysis of the persuasive and informational messages in a systematic sample of U.S. television ads for prescription drugs (Frosch, Krueger & Hornik, 2007) found that nearly all included emotional appeals. Most often this was a portrayal of the use of a medicine as a way of gaining more control over one's life. Eight out of 10 of the ads also portrayed medicine use as a way of obtaining social approval. For example, in one advertisement for a drug for acid reflux (heartburn), Nexium (esomeprazole), the wife/mother starts to talk with her family as she drinks a glass of orange juice and the husband smiles at her as she begins to participate in the meal. Another ad for a sleeping pill, Ambien (zolpidem), shows co-workers being interested in a woman photographer's activities, presumably after she is able to focus better on her work because she has slept after taking this sleeping pill.

The analysis of Frosch et al. (2007) highlights the social content of these television commercials and the use of emotional appeals that have little to do with the clinical effects of the medicines they are advertising. The ads also often included messages that lifestyle change on its own may not solve the problem. Loss of control because of a medical problem was often depicted in a way that extended beyond the medical sphere, "and often included an inability to participate in social, leisure, or work activities" (Frosch et al., 2007). Conversely, taking a medicine was always depicted as a way to regain complete control. As the authors point out, this is at odds with clinical trial evidence, which tends to show a much more modest effect.

An Antidote to Medical Paternalism?

Ads for prescription drugs resonate closely with the claimed benefits of DTCA. DTCA has been posited as an antidote to medical paternalism. Until recently, most doctors were men, and there are many examples of paternalistic practices in the medical literature, ranging from unnecessary hysterectomies or overprescribing of psychiatric drugs to undertreatment of women with heart disease. Main (2008) discusses "the prospect for empowering patients' involvement in their own health care," adding that "DTC advertising can facilitate and foster a more open flow of communication between patients and their physicians" (p. 246), thus enabling a more active role for patients in health care decisions. A second related claim is that DTCA plays an educational role in raising awareness of health problems and available treatments.

To test the claim that DTCA is educational, Robert Bell and colleagues (Bell, Wilkes & Kravitz, 2000) analyzed 10 years' worth of magazine ads in the U.S. in order to see how often they contained key information needed for shared informed treatment choices. Except for the name of the condition and one or more symptoms,

Table 2.1: Educational Content in 10 Years of U.S. Print Advertising

Does the Ad Mention?	320 Ads in 18 U.S. Magazines, 1989–1998
Treated condition:	
• *The name of the condition*	*Yes, in 96% of ads*
• *Any symptoms*	*Yes, in 60% of ads*
• Any myth or misconceptions debunked	No, in 91% of ads
• How common the disease or condition is	No, in 88% of ads
• Any causes or risk factors	No, in 73% of ads
Drug treatment:	
• The likelihood of treatment success	No, in 91% of ads
• On average, how long one needs to take the drug	No, in 89% of ads
• How long it takes the drug to start to work	No, in 80% of ads
• Other helpful activities, like exercise or diet	No, in 76% of ads
• Any other possible treatments	No, in 71% of ads
• How the drug works	No, in 64% of ads

Source: Adapted from Bell, R.A., Wilkes, M.S. & Kravitz, R.L. (2000). The educational value of consumer-targeted prescription drug print advertising. *Journal of Family Practice*, 49(12), 1092–1098.

basic required information was usually missing (Table 2.1). In a second analysis of the same large set of magazine ads, Bell and colleagues (Bell, Kravitz & Wilkes, 2000) report that women were more than twice as likely as men to be targeted in ads for products used by both sexes.

The absence of information on the likelihood of treatment success is often linked to images and headlines that hint that the product is highly effective. Woloshin, Schwartz, Tremmel, and Welch (2001) analyzed a sample of 67 ads from 1998–1999 magazines. Women's magazines had many more ads for medicines than gender-neutral or men's magazines. The benefits of these medicines were usually described in a vague, general way, with phrases such as "clinically proven," testimonials and appeals to widespread use, such as, "more than 1,000,000 people have begun using Rezulin to help manage diabetes" (p. 1144).

Misplaced Faith in Regulation

The Rezulin (troglitazone) example highlights the safety concerns about DTCA. Rezulin was eventually withdrawn from the U.S. market following nearly 400 reports of deaths in which this drug was the suspected cause (Willman, 2000). U.S. Food and Drug Administration (FDA) surveys of random samples of the U.S. public in 1999 and 2002 found that around a quarter believed that only the safest drugs were advertised on U.S. television (Aikin, Swasy & Braman, 2004).

More recently, one of the most heavily advertised drugs, the arthritis drug Vioxx (rofecoxib), was withdrawn from the market in 2004 because of increased risks of heart attacks and strokes. Vioxx was no more effective, albeit more expensive, than other arthritis drugs; advertising to the public played a large part in promoting its widespread use. Graham et al. (2005) estimated that between 88,000 and 140,000 Americans had heart attacks because of Vioxx use during its five years on the market. In Canada, in 2001, two-thirds of prescriptions for anti-inflammatory drugs were for women and the most commonly prescribed drug was Vioxx (IMS Health, 2002).

In 2007, another heavily advertised drug, Zelnorm (tegaserod), was withdrawn from the market because of cardiac risks. Mainly marketed for irritable bowel syndrome (IBS) in women, Zelnorm television ads featured women who bared their bellies to reveal text advertising messages. Women of many different ages and colours were depicted, suggesting widespread use. The impression was of a highly effective product, whereas a systematic review of studies testing the drug's effectiveness found that effects on symptoms were so modest that their clinical relevance was unclear (Evans, Clark, Moore & Whorwell, 2007).

Overactive Bladder or Overactive Marketing?

In some cases, there are questions about the benefits of a whole class of heavily marketed drugs. For example, drugs for overactive bladder in women result in around

Table 2.2: A Few Examples of Problematic Ad Campaigns Targeting Women*		
Sample Advertisement	Main Message	The Problems
Celebrex TV ads 2006–2007 (Canada)	This medicine helps older people be active, cheerful, and full of life.	Celebrex (celecoxib) is no more effective than other similar drugs for arthritis, and is associated with serious risks of heart disease. Health Canada put out a safety advisory telling doctors to prescribe it only if needed, at the lowest possible dose for the shortest possible time. This ad aims to stimulate many more prescriptions.
Alesse billboard ad (Canada)	Express yourself.	The message promotes identification with a brand as a source of self-expression and identity for young women. This pill has the same ingredients as equally effective cheaper products.
Nexium magazine ad (U.S.)	A more serious problem, erosion of the esophagus, may lurk behind common heartburn.	Most heartburn is minor; this is classic fear-mongering. Nexium is more expensive than equally effective alternatives. This class of drugs is overprescribed. Long-term use is linked to a higher risk of serious infections in hospital (Forgacs & Loganayagam, 2008).
Topamax magazine ad (U.S.)	You can avoid the risk of a migraine by taking this drug.	Stereotyped portrayal of women as the weaker sex, unable to perform at work without help—from a man or a pill. Promotes an unrealistic image of effectiveness in a drug with serious risks. The ad suggests that anyone with migraines might benefit from a drug for prevention, regardless of how often or how severe those migraines are.
Bipolar disorder ad (U.S.)	You may not have depression; you may have bipolar disorder.	The ad fails to distinguish between a serious psychiatric condition, and the normal human range of emotions. These ads target young women previously treated for depression, removing any social or personal context from emotional reactions. Cultural norms that encourage women to invalidate their own needs and experiences contribute to higher rates of diagnosis of mood disorders (Schreiber, 2001).

* All of these advertisements were collected in Canada. North American editions of U.S. magazines sold in Canada contain U.S. DTCA that is illegal in Canada. Similarly, U.S. TV ads reach Canadians via satellite and cable TV.

one fewer episode of incontinence every two days compared with a placebo (or "sugar pill") (Therapeutics Initiative, 2005). However, over a 12-week period, around 3 percent more women on the drug than on placebo experienced a serious adverse event (an event that leads to hospitalization or prolongs hospital stay or is life-threatening) (Therapeutics Initiative, 2005).

The 2006 advertisement from a U.S women's magazine (Figure 2.1) presents a very different impression, that of 100 percent relief. Note, as well, the text telling women that overactive bladder is "a real medical condition" that needs to be treated, and that symptoms "may" (or may not) include incontinence. In an article in *Pharmaceutical Executive*, Parry (2007) discusses this as an example of "Branding a disease" by transforming "the archaic and demeaning idea of 'incontinence' into the more positively accepted 'overactive bladder'" (p. 2). Parry describes this campaign as eliminating the stigma associated with incontinence and making women more comfortable identifying themselves with the newly named condition, and doctors more likely to treat it with drugs. Gone are suggestions to drink less or make sure there is a toilet close by.

Is this empowerment or manipulation? Overlooked in this defence of overactive bladder as a more woman-friendly term is the difference between urge incontinence (the inability to prevent urine from leaking), which is undeniably distressing, and the need to go to the toilet eight or more times a day, at worst an inconvenience. Overlooked as well is some evidence that non-drug approaches such as bladder training and pelvic floor exercises are at least as effective as drugs, without the same potential for harm. And, there is no mention of the need to balance the likelihood of potential benefit against the likelihood of harm from medicine use. The smaller the likely benefit, the greater the likelihood that harm will outweigh benefit.

Challenging Social Stigmas?

Can advertisers play a useful role in challenging social stigmas related to specific health conditions? The problem is one of conflicting interests and priorities. Because a drug company has an interest in expanding the boundaries of treatable disease in order to maximize sales, the tendency is always to define a disease more broadly in order to sell more medicines. A second tendency is to define the problem as individual or biochemical and as something that can be overcome through drug treatment.

One example often cited as challenging social stigmas is advertising for Viagra (sildenafil) for men with impotence or, as it has been rebranded, erectile dysfunction (ED). However, these ad campaigns rapidly positioned the product as being useful for a much broader range of men than those in whom it was originally tested. Lexchin (2006) points out that Pfizer carried out a systematic strategy in its advertising and on its website to position Viagra as a lifestyle product for younger and younger men. "The message ... is that everyone, whatever their age, at one time or another, can

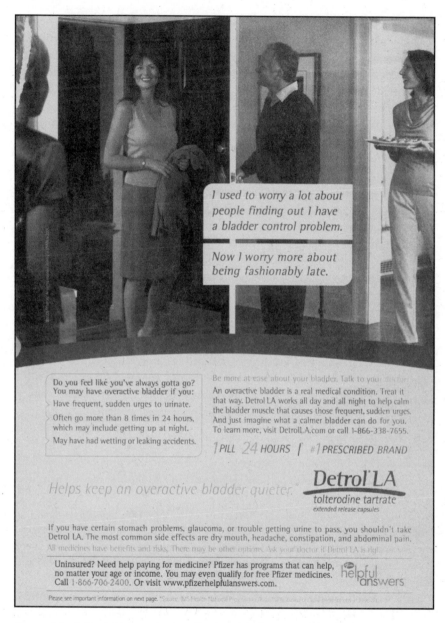

Figure 2.1: A Detrol advertisement that appeared in *Prevention Magazine*, February 2006

use a little enhancement; and any deviation from perfect erectile function means a diagnosis of ED and treatment with Viagra" (p. 431). Not only is Viagra's effectiveness exaggerated, but the advertising campaigns promote stereotyped images of sexuality and carefully avoid any suggestion that the problem may be social or emotional, having to do with the relationship with a sexual partner, rather than being physical in origin.

A similar process has occurred with the marketing of "female sexual dysfunction" as a condition. Investigative journalist Ray Moynihan (2003) traced the way the manufacturer of a testosterone patch for women funded research and consensus conferences to define this new "dysfunction." Missing from the picture was the idea that sexual difficulties may reflect relationship problems or previous life experiences. Instead, a narrow, performance-oriented image of sexuality was promoted.

Similarly, a stereotyped view of women is featured in the Canadian "I am Julie" ad campaign for the obesity drug Xenical (orlistat) (see Figure 2.2). This is a kind of DTCA called "disease-oriented" or "help-seeking" ads. Companies tend to use these types of ads if their product has a large share of a market for a specific condition, since any increase in prescribing for the disease in question will overwhelmingly be to the specific company's benefit. Often the campaign aimed at the public is accompanied by advertising and free samples for doctors. These ads do not mention the brand name, but suggest instead to "ask your doctor" about a treatment.

Xenical is not approved for the uses pictured in these ads, in which women of normal weight want to lose a few pounds. It is only approved for weight loss if a person is obese or is very overweight and has risk factors for heart disease. Xenical is expensive and not very effective, leading to, on average, a difference of 3 kg (6.5 lbs) between drug and placebo in clinical trials after one year. It also commonly leads to unpleasant side effects like oily diarrhea and anal leakage. Not only do these advertisements misrepresent the effects of drug treatment, they promote and reinforce the idea of a single ideal slim body image for women and the idea that women's lives will somehow begin "5 pounds from now."

Many of the claims made in support of DTCA borrow feminist language of empowerment and choice. This obscures not only some of the highly stereotyped sex roles in advertising, but also the lack of information on effectiveness, safety, convenience, or costs of advertised medicines compared with available drug or non-drug alternatives.

It is worth contrasting these claims with the advertisements described above. A misleading impression of the potential benefits and harmful effects of medicines does not enhance personal autonomy or choice. Similarly, early recognition of mild and transient symptoms that do not really need treatment is not necessarily going to lead to better health. Legitimization of women's health concerns is important. However, as is described in the Nexium (esomeprazole) example in Table 2.2, sometimes marketers deliberately fuel anxiety about future ill health in order to sell a product.

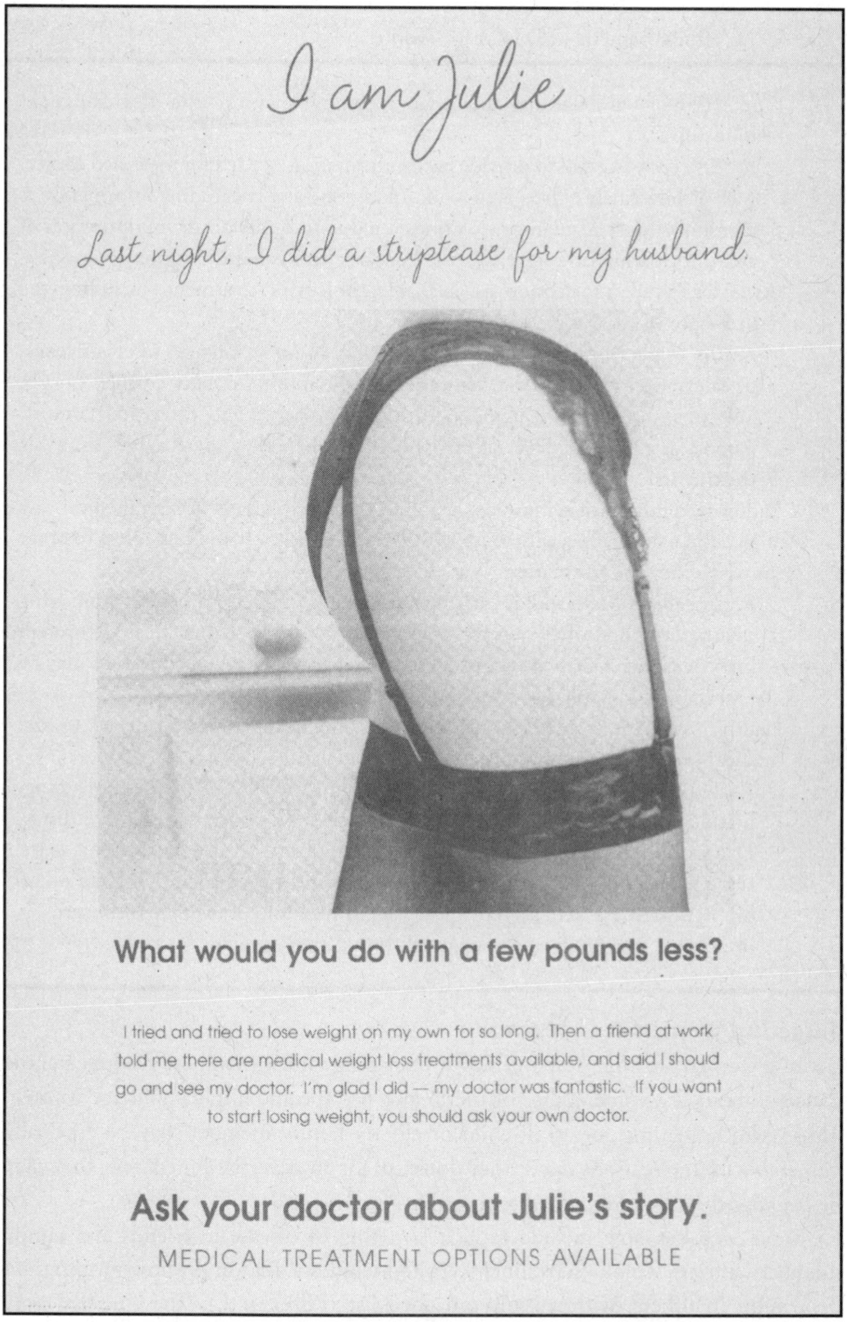

Figure 2.2: A Xenical advertisement that appeared in the *Globe and Mail*, March 9, 2004

Box 2.2: Claimed Benefits of DTCA for Women

- Empowerment and greater personal autonomy within the doctor-patient relationship

    Reality check: Ads fail to provide basic information needed for informed choice, such as how likely a drug is to work. Inaccurate and misleading information is common. Most regulatory violations are due to omission or minimization of risk information or exaggeration of benefits. This is hardly empowering.

- Better access to information on available choices of treatment, including the newest state-of-the-art drug treatments

    Reality check: Most new drugs offer minimal to no advantages in effectiveness or safety over existing treatment alternatives, and are usually costlier. DTCA fails to inform women about non-drug approaches and drugs that are off-patent, as these are never advertised, even when they are the best available treatments.

- Earlier recognition of symptoms, enabling women to access needed medical care at an earlier stage, especially those with limited education and less access to other sources of health information

    Reality check: Many mild, early symptoms are unlikely to benefit from drug treatment. They often resolve on their own or are better treated through lifestyle changes such as diet or exercise. Those with limited education may be especially vulnerable to advertising hype.

- Legitimization of women's health concerns, including those dismissed by the medical profession as unimportant

    Reality check: One of the major concerns about DTCA is disease-mongering, broadening the boundaries of treatable disease in order to sell more drugs. DTCA only legitimizes concerns for which advertised drug treatments exist. Other concerns—for example, about social and personal life problems—are often misrepresented as biological. Legitimization of women's concerns is important, but needs to be separated from a sales agenda.

Targeting Women as Caregivers

Because women are often responsible for managing family members' health care, the concern about the vulnerability of the ill also has specific implications for women. Those who are caring for an ill child or elderly family member may be especially vulnerable to implications that if they don't ask for an advertised medicine, they may be denying their loved one the best possible care.

Some websites now include explicit targeting of disease in friends and family members. Pfizer's Zoloft (sertraline) website includes a section on how to recognize depression in others, with a symptom checklist (Pfizer, n.d.). The checklist only requires a person to have had several days of symptoms within the last two weeks. This is inconsistent with minimal psychiatric diagnostic (*Diagnostic and Statistical*

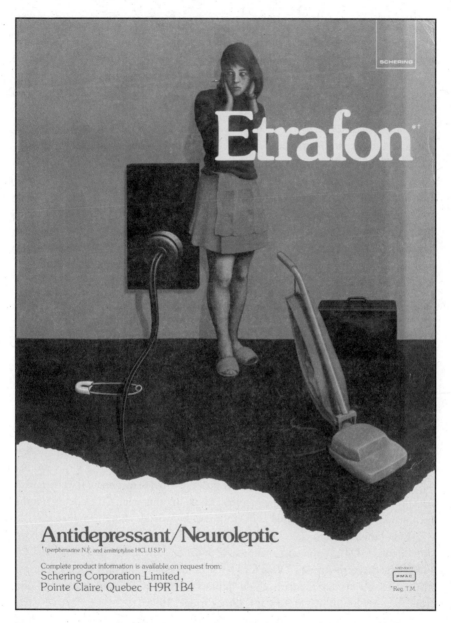

Figure 2.3: An Etrafon advertisement that appeared in *Canadian Family Physician*, May 1975

Manual, or *DSM IV*) criteria for a depression diagnosis. A hard-to-read fine print disclaimer states that the list "is intended only for the purpose of identifying symptoms of depression and is not designed to provide a diagnosis or treatment" (Pfizer, n.d.).

There have been similar messages in advertisements to physicians in medical journals (a form of prescription drug advertising that is legal in Canada as in other countries, unlike DTCA). For example, the Etrafon advertisement in the 1975 *Canadian Family Physician*, a medical journal aimed at family doctors, plays on similar emotions (see Figure 2.3). The message in advertising is often that "there is something you can do."

Medicalization of Normal Life Events

In her book *Disease-Mongers*, journalist Lynn Payer (1992) pointed out that "trying to convince essentially well people that they are sick ... is big business" (p. 5). DTCA contributes to unnecessary medicalization in two main ways: by redefining normal, healthy aspects of women's lives as medical problems, and through the offer of individual drug treatments as solutions to emotional and life problems whose origins are often social.

One of the most blatant examples of medicalization is the redefinition of menopause as a medical event, rather than a life stage. Peppin and Carty (2001) analyzed the messages conveyed through the images used in six advertisements for Premarin (conjugated estrogens*)* in the *Journal of the Society for Obstetricians and Gynaecologists of Canada* from 1989–2000. Although the promotional message had shifted from the focus on menopausal symptoms in earlier advertising to osteoporosis prevention, the ads shared a stereotypical view of menopausal women and the doctor-patient relationship. For example, in one ad the image of a man's arm in a white lab coat was used to suggest scientific authority; the attractive, well-off woman patient is listening intently, presenting an image of the compliant "good patient." In yet another advertisement, doctors are told directly that they can provide menopausal women with "the proper perspective," dispelling incorrect ideas. In other words, the doctor, not the menopausal woman, is presented as the source of knowledge about menopause.

Wide-ranging health claims that go well beyond approved product uses have been prominent in DTCA for post-menopausal hormone therapies. In 1998, the U.S. FDA judged Wyeth-Ayerst's TV ad for Premarin to be false and misleading because it made vague claims that Premarin could "protect against future health problems," and "can affect my health in a lot of ways" (Stockbridge, 1998).

Wyeth-Ayerst used celebrity endorsements from ex-supermodel Lauren Hutton and R&B and soul singer Patti LaBelle. LaBelle was featured in an "I said yes to HRT" ad campaign in 2001 and 2002, in which she is quoted as saying that, "I've been on Prempro (conjugated estrogens/medroxyprogesterone acetate) for years. I feel wonderful." The ad also highlights widespread use, citing "17 million women in the U.S. who said yes to hormone replacement therapy."

In 2002, the Women's Health Initiative (WHI), the largest randomized controlled trial of hormone replacement therapy, found that around 1 percent more women taking combined hormone treatment for five years experienced serious harm, mainly from heart attacks, stroke, blood clots, and breast cancer, as compared with women on placebo (Writing Group for the Women's Health Initiative Investigators, 2002). If the 17 million women cited in Wyeth-Ayerst's DTCA campaign took Prempro for five years, this translates to an estimated 170,000 women experiencing life-threatening harmful effects.

Box 2.3: A Pill for Every Ill—or an Ill for Every Pill?

Jennifer* first went on antidepressants at age 18 when her boyfriend left her. It was her idea: she felt bad and wanted help. Her parents agreed. They were concerned because after the breakup she was unco-operative around the house, slamming doors and yelling at her younger sister for no reason. Jennifer's doctor asked if she'd felt bad for over two weeks. She had, so the doctor prescribed an antidepressant.

The story is so familiar that it's unremarkable. We all know someone who is unhappy, unemployed, divorced, stressed out, or lonely who ends up on antidepressants. Sadness from a relationship breakup or a job layoff is an understandable human reaction. But is it really a medical problem?

There are three main concerns about taking a medicine for a normal life situation:

- The medicine may not work. An antidepressant that treats symptoms of major clinical depression may not provide relief for normal sadness after an upsetting event. This is an untested, off-label use of a medicine.**
- The decision to take a medicine is a balancing act: the probability of benefit needs to be weighed against the probability of harm. With conditions like AIDS, a heart attack, or schizophrenia, the decision is easy. Even severe side effects may be worth risking if the untreated disease is life-threatening or debilitating. However, if a person doesn't have a medical problem in the first place, a medicine won't help and no side effect, no matter how mild, is worth risking.
- Treating a life problem as medical can distract from real solutions. Jennifer wanted help and was offered a medicine as a gesture of help, but she may have needed a different kind of help to find her way in life. A person—not a medicine—can provide this kind of help.

Advertisements for prescription drugs often blur the boundaries between normal life and medical problems. Antidepressants ads don't just sell drugs. They also sell the idea that depression "may be related to the imbalance of natural chemicals between nerve cells in the brain" and that the drug "works to correct this imbalance" (Pfizer,

2004). These unproven biological explanations remove the social or personal context, even for mild problems or for distress that is clearly related to an event.

Researchers Jeffrey Lacasse and Jonathan Leo (2005) reviewed the evidence on the link between depression and brain chemistry. They found no scientific support for this theory: "There is not a single peer-reviewed article that can be accurately cited to directly support claims of serotonin deficiency in any mental disorder." When the United States Food and Drug Administration (FDA) allows companies to say in ads that depression "may be related" to a chemical imbalance, "may" is the key word. However, these ads—often accompanied by scientific-looking diagrams of chemicals and receptors—can be made to look misleadingly scientific.

Antidepressants do affect brain chemistry, but that doesn't mean depression is caused by an imbalance of brain chemicals. A beer or a glass of wine can help shy people loosen up, but nobody claims that shyness is caused by alcohol deficiency.

The same companies that create ads for Coca-Cola or Budweiser are creating these ads. The image of the happy, treated patient—like the glowing housewife in 1960s "whiter than white" detergent ads—has little to do with what the product is like, and everything to do with making it look like something you need.

Anxiety sells. Ads like this should make you pause and remember who's telling you this and why. The best cure may be a little healthy skepticism.

* pseudonym
** Medicines are approved for specific uses for which they have been tested in pre-market studies. Once on the market, they may be prescribed for any use, including unapproved or "off-label" uses. There is often inadequate evidence to support the effectiveness or safety of these "off-label" uses.

Source: Abridged and adapted from Mintzes, B. (2007). A pill for every ill—or an ill for every pill? *Visions: BC's Mental Health and Addictions Journal, 4*(2), 21–22.

Women and Statins: DTCA Misrepresents Disease Risks and Drug Effects

The advertisement reproduced in Figure 2.4, which ran in *Good Housekeeping* magazine, features a healthy, fit-looking young woman in a track suit, certainly not someone who appears to have had a previous heart attack or other heart disease. The "educational" message of this and other DTCA for cholesterol-lowering drugs is clear: if your cholesterol is high, or you have too much "bad cholesterol" and not enough "good cholesterol," it needs to be treated with a statin, in this case Crestor (rosuvastatin calcium), which AstraZeneca markets. High cholesterol is, in fact, a risk factor, not a health problem in itself. The aim of treatment is to prevent heart attack and stroke. But, for women who do not already have heart disease, exercising, quitting smoking, and maintaining a healthy diet and body weight are the most effective approaches to achieve this aim, not taking a statin (Rosenberg & Allard, 2007).

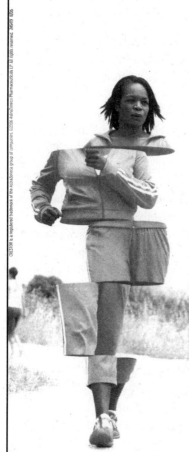
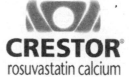

Figure 2.4: A Crestor advertisement that appeared in *Good Housekeeping*, April 2007

The message in this and other advertising for cholesterol-lowering drugs is very different from what a public health message about heart disease prevention would look like. These ads often convey the message that non-drug approaches are unlikely to be effective (Frosch et al., 2007).

The difference between an advertising message and a public health message was highlighted in the successful marketing of another new cholesterol-lowering drug, ezetimibe. In the U.S., this drug is marketed as Zetia and Vytorin. The latter is a combination product with a statin, simvastatin. There is no evidence that ezetimibe's ability to lower cholesterol levels leads to any clinical benefits and it has not been shown to prevent buildup of plaque in the arteries (Kastelein et al., 2008). The combination drug, Vytorin (ezetimibe + simvastatin), was one of the most heavily advertised drugs in the U.S. in the first few years after its launch. The DTC ads, many of which ran in women's magazines as well as on television, highlight the combo's two different actions (see Figure 2.5). They fail to tell viewers and readers what they really need to know: that cholesterol-lowering in itself is not a health benefit, and that the drug's effects on health remain unknown. The cost to the U.S. public? Beyond the potential for harm through the use of an ineffective treatment—for example, if people do not take other steps to prevent heart disease—an extra $1.5 billion per year was spent on ezetimibe (Aldhous, 2008).

From Birth Control to Menstrual Suppression

It is important for information about birth control to be accessible so that young women and men can know what methods are available to prevent pregnancy and sexually transmitted diseases. Here again, DTCA does a poor job of providing the type of information needed. Only the newest brands of hormonal birth control are advertised and no information is provided on the pros and cons of different options. In 2000, in one of the first Canadian ad campaigns for a prescription drug, Wyeth-Ayerst juxtaposed the headline "A lesson in deep dark secrets" with a young woman and the Alesse (levonorgestrel/estradiol) pill pack, suggesting that taking the birth control pill can be a woman's secret (see Figure 2.6). This message may have helped to sell birth control pills, but it is hardly a positive message for sexual health. Keeping birth control use secret is unlikely to support open communication about sex or condom use to prevent the spread of sexually transmitted diseases. It also reinforces a view that birth control is entirely a woman's responsibility.

There are many competing birth control pills on the market and it is hard for manufacturers of each new product to gain market share. Effectiveness among products is similar, and although there are some safety differences, risks of older low-dose pills containing levonorgestrel or norethindrone tend to be lower than newer products. Manufacturers have little incentive to highlight these differences in safety profile as they favour less expensive products. Instead, new delivery forms have been

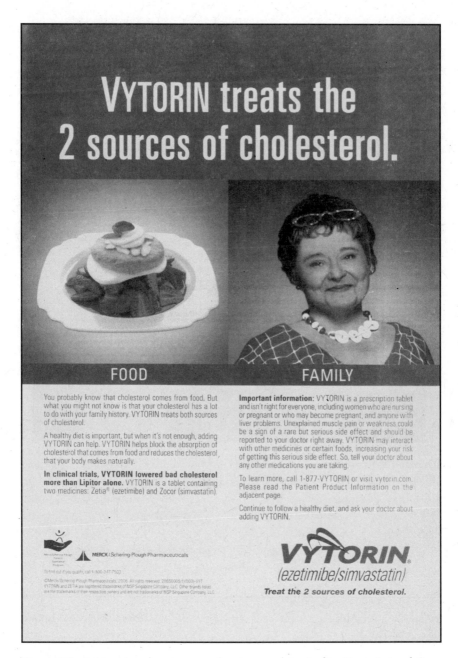

Figure 2.5: A Vytorin advertisement that appeared in *Ladies Home Journal*, June 2006

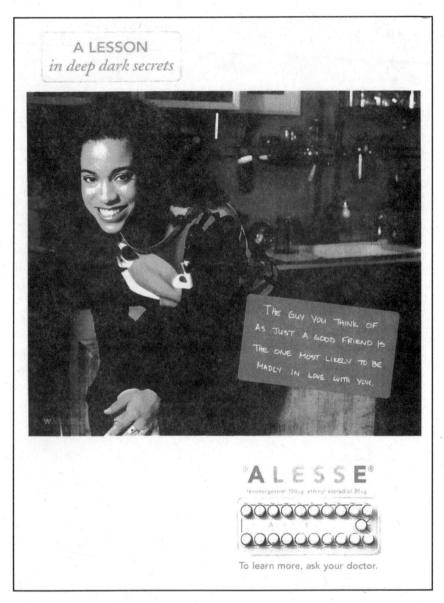

Figure 2.6: An Alesse advertisement that appeared in *Healthy Woman*, October/ November 2002

developed. One example is Seasonale, a low-dose levonorgestrel-estradiol pill that is similar to older products, except that it is packaged for continuous use for three months at a time.

The U.S. FDA found a DTCA television advertising campaign for Seasonale to contain inaccurate information because it stressed that women could have just four periods a year, but did not mention that breakthrough and irregular bleeding occurred so often on Seasonale in clinical trials that women had similar numbers of days of bleeding as with a monthly pill. The FDA also found that the advertisement minimized the serious risks associated with the use of this product (Chitale, 2004). All oral contraceptives lead to higher risks of potentially fatal blood clots (venous thromboembolism) and stroke. There is no evidence thus far that this oral contraceptive is riskier than others. However, the possibility of a higher risk from the higher annual hormone exposure (because of fewer pill-free periods, four rather than the usual 13 per year), or other differences associated with this pattern of use, has not been evaluated in the longer term. The FDA letter on this promotional violation highlights the gulf between the advertising hype and the product's documented effects.

Ads for newer combined hormonal birth control methods, such as the contraceptive patch Evra (norelgestromin/estradiol), also fail to provide the type of information users need. Evra was approved in Canada in 2003. Canada's Common Drug Review (CDR) recommended against provincial reimbursement in June 2004 after having reviewed the safety and effectiveness evidence. Although the patch is twice as expensive as birth control pills, pregnancy rates do not differ and more women experience side effects on the patch (Common Drug Review, 2004).

The CDR published its recommendation on the web, but neither the CDR itself nor other Canadian health organizations did anything to actively publicize it. In contrast, in 2004 Canadian women's magazines were full of ads for the patch (see Figure 2.7).

The headline implies that the patch is simpler to use than the pill. Patches are changed once a week; pills are taken daily. This makes no difference to pregnancy rates. If the patch were appreciably simpler, women might forget it and get pregnant more often. The idea of greater simplicity also ignores skin irritation, patches that fall off accidentally, the need to avoid saunas and hot tubs, or the extra environmental problems associated with disposal of the patch (see Chapter 9).

The higher rates of breast pain and engorgement on the patch in clinical trials were an omen of more serious problems to come. These are estrogen-related side effects. After approval, the U.S. FDA found that the patch released 60 percent more estrogen than originally believed. The estrogen dose is similar to early higher dose birth control pills. Two of three follow-up studies of users have shown double the rate of potentially fatal blood clots as modern low-dose pills. The Canadian version

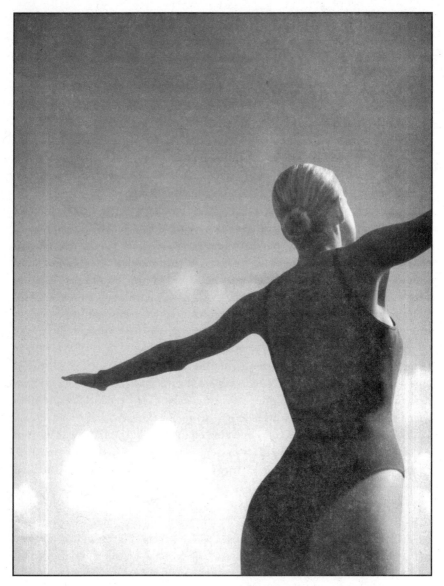

Figure 2.7: An Evra advertisement that appeared in *Verve Fashion Magazine,* Summer 2004

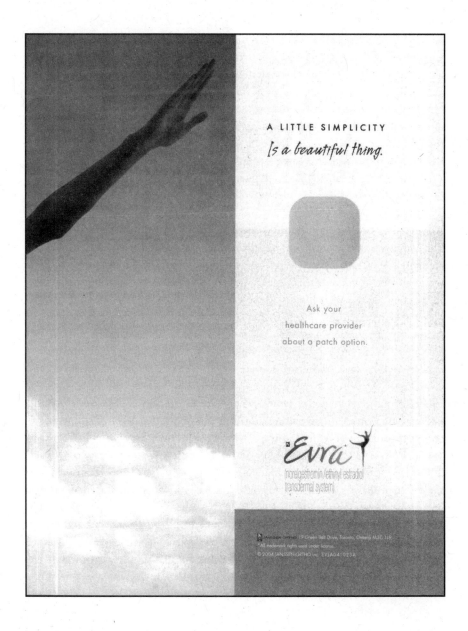

of the patch has less estrogen in it than the U.S. formulation, but it is not clear if the amount released into a woman's bloodstream differs. Health Canada issued advisories in 2005 and 2006 about the patch, stating that it was reviewing the research evidence and disseminating the U.S. warnings (Health Canada, 2006). By early 2008, two Canadian women had died while on the patch, one of heart attack and the other of pulmonary embolism, and 15 others had experienced venous thromboembolism (potentially fatal blood clots). These are voluntary adverse reaction reports in which the patch was the suspected cause (Springuel, 2008).

These examples highlight the difference between the images used to sell these newer contraceptives and the scientific evidence on their effects and safety.

Advertising of Antidepressants, Anti-anxiety Drugs, and Sedatives

The targeting of women in advertising of mood-modifying drugs, such as antidepressants, anti-anxiety drugs, and sedatives, continues a long history of more frequent prescribing of these drugs to women than men, especially in primary care. In a review of the marketing of these drugs, Lexchin (1995) points out that sex differences in prescribing rates persist after controlling for factors such as the patient's symptoms, physician diagnoses, socio-demographic status, and health service characteristics. A more recent large population survey in Norway confirms that at similar levels of emotional distress, more women than men received antidepressants (Hausken, Skurtveit, Rosvold, Bramness & Furu, 2007).

The kind of targeting of women that has occurred in DTCA mirrors earlier targeting of women in advertising aimed at physicians. Analyses of advertising of antidepressant and anti-anxiety drugs in medical journals from 1959–1975 (King, 1980), 1986–1989 (Hansen & Osborne, 1995), and 2001–2002 (Curry & O'Brien, 2006) have found that women are depicted as patients more often than men. The most recent analysis, in an Irish medical journal, compared ads for antidepressant and cardiac drugs (Curry & O'Brien, 2006). Not only were women presented as the main users of antidepressants (in 86 percent of ads featuring a patient) and men of cardiac drugs (in 92 percent), men tended to be depicted in active roles, and women in passive roles. Curry and O'Brien (2006) point out that these stereotypical images reinforce common meanings of gender and health and are likely to affect treatment decisions.

Twice as many women as men receive prescriptions for antidepressants, whether the diagnosis is depression or an anxiety disorder. Community surveys in a range of countries consistently identify more women than men as experiencing depression. However, a range of reasons, both real and artificial, contribute to these gender differences, including measurement biases that reflect differences in how men and women answer questionnaires (Wilhelm et al., 2008). Wilhelm et al. (2008) followed 170 newly trained teachers from 1978–2003 to examine depression rates of men and women with similar status and work experience. Most of the differences between the sexes disappeared after they took into account differences in memory of episodes recorded in previous surveys, which men tended to forget to mention. Most community surveys are one-time events that cannot examine sex differences in recall or reporting of past depression episodes.

One of the arguments made in favour of DTCA for antidepressants is that depression is undertreated and DTCA can help people to recognize symptoms and seek care. This ignores both the limited effectiveness of antidepressants (see below) and the fact that many people identified as having untreated depression in community surveys are reporting transient problems that are unlikely to benefit from treatment. Patten found that those identified with depression in two large Canadian community health surveys who were not treated with antidepressants had shorter episodes of depression, 11 versus 18 weeks on average compared to those with drug treatment (Patten, 2004).

Most untreated depression identified in epidemiological surveys is mild to moderate, not severe. A recent meta-analysis highlights the likely lack of benefit from antidepressant treatment. In all of the studies submitted to the U.S. FDA for four antidepressants, the drugs had an appreciable clinical benefit, as compared to placebo, for only the most severe depression (Kirsch et al., 2008). The authors looked at four of the six drugs on the U.S. market because they could get full clinical trial results for these drugs from the FDA. This study is important because it was not limited to studies the company published, which tend to be more positive. This evidence of limited effectiveness contrasts with the images in antidepressant ads (see Figure 2.8).

Antidepressants are among the medicines most commonly advertised to the U.S. public (Donohue, Cevasco & Rosenthal, 2007).

Grow, Park, and Han (2006) analyzed the symbolic messages in print DTCA for antidepressants that appeared in U.S. editions of *Reader's Digest* and *Time Magazine* between 1997 and 2003. Colours and stark imagery are used to contrast "before" and "after" narratives, with depression and anxiety framed as biochemical problems. Peppin (2003) points out that the ads decontextualize mental illness, presenting psychiatric diagnoses such as depression and anxiety as conditions of everyday life. Only biological explanations are offered; poverty, abusive relationships, intense life stresses, unemployment, or poor housing are not mentioned. Slogans like "Welcome back" present drug treatment as removing a surface layer of mental illness, leaving the real person underneath. The related message is that there is a known biological cause for depression. For example, a Zoloft (sertraline) ad states: "While the cause is not known, depression may be related to an imbalance in the natural chemicals between nerve cells in the brain." No reliable scientific evidence supports the theory that depression is caused by a serotonin imbalance (Lacasse & Leo, 2005).

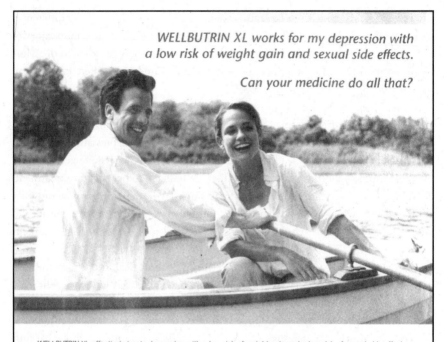

WELLBUTRIN XL works for my depression with a low risk of weight gain and sexual side effects.

Can your medicine do all that?

WELLBUTRIN XL effectively treats depression with a low risk of weight gain and a low risk of sexual side effects. Clinical studies prove it. Ask your doctor about WELLBUTRIN XL. And to find out more, visit www.wellbutrin-xl.com or call 1-800-366-2500.

Experience Life.

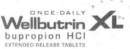

ONCE-DAILY
Wellbutrin XL
bupropion HCl
EXTENDED-RELEASE TABLETS

gsk GlaxoSmithKline

visit www.wellbutrin-xl.com and learn about a $10 savings

Important information: WELLBUTRIN XL is not for everyone. There is a risk of seizure when taking WELLBUTRIN XL, so don't use if you've had a seizure or eating disorder, or if you abruptly stop using alcohol or sedatives. Don't take with MAOIs, or medicines that contain bupropion. When used with a nicotine patch or alone, there is a risk of increased blood pressure, sometimes severe. To reduce risk of serious side effects, tell your doctor if you have liver or kidney problems. Other side effects may include weight loss, dry mouth, nausea, difficulty sleeping, dizziness, or sore throat. WELLBUTRIN XL is approved only for adults 18 years and over. In some children and teens, antidepressants increase suicidal thoughts or actions. Whether or not you are taking antidepressants, you or your family should call the doctor right away if you have worsening depression, thoughts of suicide, or sudden or severe changes in mood or behavior, especially at the beginning of treatment or after a change in dose (see Patient Information: What is important information I should know and share with my family about taking antidepressants?).

Results may vary.   *Please see Medication Guide and Patient Information on following page.*

Figure 2.8: A Wellbutrin advertisement that appeared in *Family Circle*, January 2006

The FDA has found several direct-to-consumer advertisements for antidepressants to be illegal because of a blurring of boundaries between normal sadness and a psychiatric diagnosis of depression. A 2004 radio ad for Effexor (venlafaxine) failed to communicate "important characteristics necessary to distinguish between major depressive disorder and variations of normal daily functioning" (Mintzes, 2006, Table 1). An ad for Paxil (paroxetine) suggested "that anyone experiencing anxiety, fear, or self-consciousness in social or work situations is an appropriate candidate for Paxil CR" (Mintzes, 2006, Table 1).

Does DTCA lead to antidepressant prescribing for people without depression? U.S. researchers used women actresses in their 40s as "standardized patients" making unannounced visits to family doctors (Kravitz et al., 2005). They were randomly assigned to two different scenarios: symptoms of clinical depression or of "adjustment disorder" in response to a stressful life situation. The latter is not a psychiatric condition and does not need drug treatment. If the women asked for a prescription for Paxil, a heavily advertised antidepressant, they were as likely to receive an antidepressant prescription if they had adjustment disorder or depression. The request for an advertised medicine was a stronger predictor of the prescribing decision than whether the "patient" had the condition the drug was intended to treat.

Problems also exist with prescribing for psychiatric conditions that may not exist. The first drug in the U.S. to be approved for premenstrual dysphoric disorder (PMDD) was fluoxetine (Sarafem; the same product as Prozac). Drugs to treat PMDD are not marketed in either Canada or the European Union. The European Medicines Agency (EMEA) raised concerns about the validity of this diagnosis, and possible "widespread inappropriate short- and long-term use of fluoxetine" among women with normal premenstrual mood fluctuations (EMEA, 2003).

Soon after the launch of Sarafem, the U.S. FDA found that the first TV ad "broadens the indication and trivializes the seriousness of PMDD" (Stockbridge, 2000). In this ad, a woman becomes enraged as she tries to pull a shopping cart out of a line of carts. Two other antidepressants have also been approved for PMDD, Zoloft and Paxil, and both have also been advertised to the U.S. public, although the validity of PMDD as a diagnosis continues to be controversial.

Beyond the message in these advertisements, when antidepressants are advertised for PMDD, the focus is entirely on women of reproductive age. More frequent antidepressant use for PMDD is likely to result in more exposures in early pregnancy, particularly if pregnancies are unplanned. These drugs have not been adequately tested for effectiveness or safety in pregnancy, and have been rated category C by the U.S. FDA. Category C medicines are products that have been shown to be harmful in pregnancy in animal studies—in other words, they have led to either birth defects or effects on the viability of the fetus (Code of Federal Regulations, 1997).

Third-trimester exposure to SSRI antidepressants can lead to distress and a withdrawal syndrome in babies, and there is evidence that paroxetine exposure in the first trimester increases the risk of heart defects (Health Canada, 2004; U.S. Food and Drug Administration, 2005).

Conclusion

The fundamental problem with advertising of prescription drugs is that these are serious medical treatments, not consumer products like a pair of jeans or a soft drink. DTCA, like any other form of advertising, aims to sell a product. A simple connection is drawn between the pill and its intended effects. The seductive image is of a magic solution, 100 percent effective. Often ads focus on the idea that a mild symptom may be the sign of a more serious disease, or that a healthy person may be at risk for disease problems. Thus, the overall message is that you should be anxious about your health and that a pill can take away that worry.

Like negative ads in political campaigns, ads for medicines sometimes present the "untreated condition" in a negative light. If this "untreated condition" happens to be a normal part of being a woman, like menstruation or menopause, the underlying message remains negative. There is not necessarily anything consciously misogynistic in this; marketers are just trying to sell a product. Similarly, if normal human sadness is presented as a psychiatric condition—depression—and is abstracted from a person's lived experience, this is unlikely to be a conscious attempt to trivialize human suffering. Manufacturers are just trying to increase sales. The problem is that both these messages can distract people and communities from real solutions. The problem is also that the decision to take any medicine is a balancing act, juggling potential benefit against potential harm. As medicines are used for milder problems or non-problems, the balance is likely to shift so that harm outweighs benefit.

Women are often the focus of these ad campaigns simply because they tend to be at the doctor's office more often. In 1995, the UN Platform for Action on Women's Health called for action to "eliminate harmful, medically unnecessary or coercive medical interventions, as well as inappropriate medicalisation and over-medication" (United Nations, 1995, Section C, Article 106 (h)). Thirteen years later, with spending on U.S. DTCA surpassing U.S. $5 billion, a court case in Canada in which corporate freedom of expression is being pitted against public health, and pressure for legal change in every wealthy industrialized country that prohibits DTCA, the need for appropriate measures to eliminate overmedication of women is as pressing as ever.

Chapter 3

Preventing Disease
Are Pills the Answer?

———— ◆ ————

Sharon Batt
and
Abby Lippman

Introduction

In April 1998, front-page headlines described an apparent breakthrough in preventing breast cancer: "We know for the first time in history that we can prevent cancer through pharmaceuticals," said one of the researchers. Others involved in the study called it a "historic milestone" (Semenak, 1998). The story, which made international headlines, reported the early results of the Breast Cancer Prevention Trial (BCPT), a clinical trial involving 13,388 Canadian and American women. The trial showed that Nolvadex-D (tamoxifen) lowered the risk of breast cancer. But buried beneath the headlines was news that it also raised the risk of endometrial cancer, cataracts, and blood clots.

In the realm of health policy, primary prevention is a strategy to identify and remove the causes of disease before they can do harm. Public health practices are developed to implement primary prevention strategies and it is now well recognized that health gains from these strategies (e.g., the provision of potable water and anti-tobacco regulations) far outstrip those that treat sickness after the fact. In the past two decades, however, the distinction between public health and medicine has been blurred. Medical interventions, usually reserved for the sick, have been introduced for use by those deemed *at risk* of sickness. A strategy of prescribing drugs to healthy people—promoting "pills for prevention"—now threatens to overtake, and even displace, traditional primary prevention goals. And this is especially true for chronic diseases of adult onset.[1]

In this chapter, we argue that government-industry partnerships and the risk management ideology that currently shape federal health protection policy implicitly favour this use of drugs as a form of prevention. The same policy climate discourages traditional primary prevention initiatives such as, for example, the elimination of environmental contaminants. We make the case for a public health approach to disease prevention that is based on the precautionary principle and contend that true primary prevention must remain the gold standard for public health policy in Canada; chemoprevention should be confined to those situations where its use has been shown to be ethical, safe, effective, and the most appropriate intervention to solve the problem.

The Debate over Pills for Prevention

In the BCP trial referred to above, three women in the tamoxifen arm of the trial died from pulmonary embolisms despite screening to eliminate women at high risk of blood clots. Many women's health organizations and some scientists who were not involved in the trial testified at a hearing of the U.S. Food and Drug Administration (FDA) that these results argued against approving the drug for breast cancer prevention. Nonetheless, the trial was stopped early because the benefit in reducing breast cancer risk was deemed to be so great that denying eligible women in the control group the opportunity of taking tamoxifen was considered unethical. Six months after the trial was halted, the FDA approved the use of tamoxifen for women "at high risk" of developing the disease. Tamoxifen has been approved for the same indication in Canada.

Soon after the BCPT was stopped, researchers began recruiting healthy Canadian and American women for a follow-up project that compared tamoxifen to raloxifene. Sold under the brand name Evista, raloxifene was already in use for its approved indication to reduce the risk of osteoporosis. This second prevention trial found that raloxifene, like tamoxifen, reduced breast cancer rates. But also like tamoxifen, raloxifene increased the risk of blood clots in the lungs and legs, although it did not increase endometrial cancer risks (Cummings et al., 1999).

Once again, the findings evoked a mixed reaction. Proponents framed the new study as scientific progress toward an ideal preventive drug. Researchers conducting the trial called the preliminary finding "very exciting" because it "gives women a real choice for reducing their risk … for osteoporosis and breast cancer" (Stein, 2006). By contrast, other scientists, and women's health advocates, sounded cautionary warnings about the absence of long-term data and the lack of clarity about whether cancers were being prevented or simply delayed (Bean, Kimler & Seewaldt, 2006; Stein, 2006). The design of the trial adds to this concern: there was no placebo group, so it was not possible to know whether women on tamoxifen or raloxifene did better or worse in terms of all types of health outcomes than they would have without drug treatment. American physician and women's health activist Adriane Fugh-Berman opposed the Breast Cancer Prevention Trial from the outset, arguing that testing a drug with known toxic effects on healthy women expanded the concept of disease prevention to include disease substitution (Fugh-Berman, 1991).

Breast cancer is not the only disease for which drugs used for treatment have been tested as preventive medications. In April 2000, a trial to test the schizophrenia treatment drug Zyprexa (olanzapine) on people judged to be at high risk for that disease was launched in Toronto, with participating hospitals in Calgary and at Yale University (Shuchman, 2000). In 2003, an article published in the *British Medical Journal* proposed a polypill comprising statins, three drugs to lower blood pressure, Aspirin, and folic acid, which the authors claimed would reduce cardiovascular disease by 88 percent if given to everyone over the age of 55 and everyone with existing heart disease (Wald & Law, 2003). In late 2007, researchers at Mount Sinai Medical Center in New York were studying whether hypertension drugs can prevent Alzheimer's disease (Wang et al., 2007).

The group Citizens for Responsible Care and Research (CIRCARE) called the schizophrenia-prevention trial "highly unethical" because healthy children as young as 12 would be exposed to the risks and serious side effects of a powerful antipsychotic (Alliance for Human Research Protection, 2000). Schizophrenia cannot yet be accurately diagnosed, much less predicted, the group pointed out. Moreover, what would be the impact on children of labelling them as "at risk" for a condition that carries so much stigma? Similar questions can be posed for the polypill or for the use of hypertension drugs as prevention for Alzheimer's disease: What is the potential for generating dangerous side effects in studying clearly hypothetical risks of disease development? Over time, evidence has mounted to support a cautionary approach to the use of new, and even some older, drugs. Why, then, is the practice of testing potent and potentially lethal drugs on healthy populations so prevalent today? We argue that the answer lies in the socio-economic policy environment.

Neomedicalization: A Product of the Socio-economic Policy Environment

Neomedicalization (see box below) fits seamlessly into neo-liberal economic policies that put the emphasis on economic growth and free market forces, and minimize the government's role in social programs. These policies encourage the consumer orientation that dominates contemporary North American society. If the economics of neo-liberalism can be said to embrace corporatism, consumerism, and capitalism, these same forces nourish neomedicalization.

Box 3.1: Medicalization and Neomedicalization

Medicalization is a process that involves seeing and treating natural experiences and socially created problems as biological diseases or illnesses that require medical surveillance or intervention.

Neomedicalization goes significantly further and involves the corporate-driven creation and marketing of diseases to sell drugs, as well as the framing of natural experiences as causes of future diseases. It emphasizes an individual's supposed risk of developing a problem and the use of some drug or device to manage this risk. In its most expansive form, neomedicalization makes being "at risk" a disease state[2] and frames the individual as responsible for ensuring that the risk does not become a reality.

In neomedicalization, the owners and makers of medical knowledge are not only physicians and medical researchers, but also corporate entities, government, the media, and consumers (see Timmermans & Kolker, 2004). Neomedicalization has a broader reach than medicalization, since we all can be found to have some behaviour, some characteristic, some "marker"—genetic or otherwise—that can be called a "pre-disease." As new technologies are devised to identify more and more distant features in a possible disease-causing chain, the likelihood grows that each of us will acquire the label of "pre-diseased." Thus, elevated body mass index (BMI) is now a "pre-disease" for diabetes; low bone mineral density (BMD) is one for hip fracture, etc. The increasing applications of genetic testing will only expand the list (Bureau of Women's Health and Gender Analysis, 2005).

Neomedicalization is both a cause and an effect of the growing use of imaging and measurement technologies that reveal ambiguous "things" of which one is not even aware. Sales and use of the technologies stimulate the economy. The more screening is done, the more things are found. These "things," including DNA patterns and brain images, are not just early stages of a disease. The latter could be useful to detect. More often, however, they are either of unknown or of limited meaning with regard to a person's future health, as with mammography-detected ductal carcinoma in situ (DCIS) as a potential precursor of breast cancer, prostate-specific antigen (PSA) levels as potential warning signs of prostate cancer in healthy men with no previous diagnosis of this condition, and common DNA variations labelled as genetic susceptibilities.[3]

Neomedicalization, like the neo-liberalism that fertilizes it, constructs health as a commodity, a malleable entity that can be a base for economic growth. Thus, we find in at least one government document a reference to "health services as ... a leading edge economic sector for employment, innovation, research and exports" and a description of health care as a "dynamic engine of economic growth" as well as an "export platform with economic spin-offs" (Courchene, 2003). Further, by framing life experiences as causes of disease, neomedicalization generates a whole "Selling Sickness" (Moynihan & Cassels, 2005) industry to create pills for prevention; in the words of the U.K. Health Committee report, there is a "pill for every ill" (Standing Committee on Health, 2004). And by further manufacturing, through their marketing strategies, new diseases for old drugs, grounds are established for the extension of patent protections on existing products and continued profitability of old drugs, a process known as "evergreening" (Commission on the Future of Health Care in Canada, 2002, p. 209). This phenomenon was first described in Lynn Payer's 1992 book, *Disease-Mongers: How Doctors, Drug Companies, and Insurers Are Making You Feel Sick.*

The economic roots of neomedicalization nourish the expansion of drug interventions to manage risks. Given that there are more healthy than sick people in the world, offering a product that is claimed to help manage their risks can capture increasing numbers of those in need of some treatment. Finding the "not yet sick" and the "worried well," who could be offered a drug or device, is the goal, and since likely we are all at risk for something, we are all potential candidates for a clinical prevention trial.

Neomedicalization and Offers of "Choice"
Both neo-liberalism and neomedicalization emphasize increasing women's choices by offering tests, screening exams, etc. However, the concept of "choice" in this context

is manipulated to create markets for both drugs and the tests that will uncover our risks (Lippman, 1999). This conception of choice is problematic, being perhaps more an illusion than authentic. It provides women with a list of options, but not the ability to make choices, since this ability is distributed along the lines of privilege in society that leave many marginalized. And this illusion can be harmful, particularly when it distracts us from looking upstream at the sources of the problems for which response choices are offered.

Pharmaceutical companies and others have borrowed feminist language and converted it to consumer dialect. Most prominent here is the huge expansion of direct-to-consumer advertising (DTCA), whether this is with actual ads for specific drugs or awareness campaigns that encourage us to "ask the doctor" about a particular problem or to fill in a survey in a magazine that will tell us what problem(s) we have so that we can act or take control of our health (see, for example, Mintzes, 2003 and also Chapter 2).

Disease Prevention and Health Protection Policy
To avoid the further growth of neomedicalization, and to create the conditions that allow women authentic autonomy, it helps to recall the goal of health protection: to prevent disease and other causes of disability. The Epp Report, an influential Canadian paper on health promotion, defines disease prevention as "identifying the factors that cause a condition and then reducing or eliminating them" (Epp, 1986, p. 5). This definition reflects the public's intuitive understanding of what is meant by preventing illness and accidents. By contrast, widely used chemoprevention of common chronic diseases threatens to displace these traditional objectives of identifying and removing causes of disease. Indeed, the introduction of pills for prevention poses a new threat to health—iatrogenic illnesses and deaths (i.e., illnesses and deaths caused by medical interventions) in the name of preventing illness.

The single most important public health measure in history remains clean drinking water.[4] Even in recent times, medication has contributed relatively little to the overall gains in health. Of a 30-year increase in lifespan for Americans over the past century, 25 years are attributable to public health initiatives, such as safer workplaces and better nutrition for mothers and babies. Public health interventions tend to carry minimal risks, as is the case with the addition of iodine to salt and of vitamin D to milk (Centers for Disease Control, 1999). There are well-studied examples where the addition of, for example, a dietary supplement is an acceptable way to prevent or delay onset of a serious disease (e.g., folic acid use by pregnant women, calcium supplementation for older women), but even such interventions should not be routinely adopted unless studies have shown that benefits outweigh risks and that other methods with fewer side effects are not equally effective.

Figure 3.1: The Fall in the Standardized Death Rate (per 1,000 Population) for Nine Common Infectious Diseases in Relation to Specific Medical Measures, United States, 1900-1973

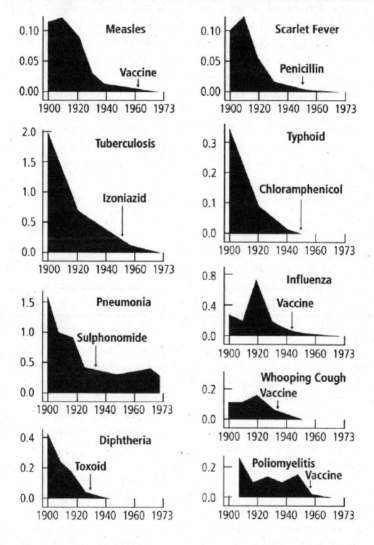

Source: McKinlay, J.B. & McKinlay, S.M. (1977). The questionable contribution of medical measures to the decline of mortality in the United States in the twentieth century. *Milbank Memorial Fund Quarterly, Health and Society*, 55, pp. 422 and 423.

Where then, does one draw the line? In a critique of the Breast Cancer Prevention Trial, bioethicist Charles Weijer proposed four prerequisites to even testing a drug for disease prevention in healthy subjects:

- The drug ought to be relatively safe and should certainly not be life-threatening.
- Subjects should be drawn from a population clearly at risk for the disease, not one defined merely by superficial demographic conditions, such as being a 61-year-old woman (as in the breast cancer-prevention trial) or the sibling of a youth diagnosed with schizophrenia (as in the Zyperexa [olanzapine] prevention study).
- Risk factors for the disease should be fairly well understood, so that the drug will not end up harming too many and benefiting too few.
- The drug must stand on its own merits; that is, if a drug is being tested as a means of preventing heart disease, other potential benefits it may have, such as making people happy or their skin baby-soft, are irrelevant.

"The tamoxifen study fails on all four counts," Weijer concluded (1995, p. 43). These particular criteria may not be the last word, but clearly strong guidelines are needed to limit the testing and use of chemoprevention drugs.

Box 3.2: The Precautionary Principle

Chemoprevention is one of many recent risky health innovations. Alarmed by the hasty introduction of untested technologies and by a perceived slippage in government resolve to eliminate risks to the environment and to health, a number of citizen groups have articulated the precautionary principle as a formal guideline for dealing with situations of scientific uncertainty (e.g., Wingspread in the U.S., Institute for Science in Society in the U.K.). In 2001, the Canadian government incorporated its own version of the precautionary principle into federal policy (Environment Canada, 2001).

The precautionary principle dictates that we frame and enforce our environmental and health regulations to emphasize safety rather than risk when science cannot yet provide clear answers. A formal statement of the precautionary principle reads: "Where an activity raises threats of harm to the environment or human health, precautionary measures should be taken even if some cause and effect relationships are not established scientifically" (Science and Environmental Health Network, 1998). A corollary is that the burden of proof to demonstrate harm should not be borne by the public, but rather that the proponent of an activity or product must demonstrate safety (VanderZwaag, 1994). The precautionary principle argues against intervening with risky medications as a strategy to prevent disease.

Canada's Health Protection Review

Any discussion of health protection must address strategies to prevent disease. The federal government's 1998 discussion document, *Health Protection for the 21st Century: Renewing the Federal Health Protection Legislation*, states that "Health protection helps Canadians to avoid illness or injury" (Health Canada, 1998, p. 1). The document confirms that health risks can arise from prescription drugs, food and water contaminants, air pollution, radiation, and chemical hazards (Health Canada, 1998, p. 6). These statements set the stage for a public health strategy in which the public is protected from these risks by reducing or eliminating exposures to the hazards listed.

However, rather than discussing strategies to remove disease agents or minimize human exposure to prevent the diseases they cause, the document embraces a "modern risk management framework." Canada's guidelines for risk management, the document explains, will be consistent with those adopted by other health agencies around the world (Health Canada, 1998, p. 6).

Risk management was introduced to American health and environment agencies in 1983 after the Reagan administration had slashed budgets and personnel for health and environmental protection. Key to the new approach was the concept that risk is an unavoidable fact of life. No longer would pollution be viewed as a problem to be remedied; rather, toxins in the environment had become negotiable evils. Science historian Robert Proctor observes that with the risk management approach, "risk assessors [scientists] would determine the magnitude of a given risk, while risk managers [policy makers] would determine whether that risk was acceptable" (Proctor, 1995, p. 83). The net effect "was almost invariably to stymie health and environmental regulations" (Proctor, 1995, p. 84).

Canadian government documents describe risk management as "a systematic approach to setting the best course of action under uncertainty by identifying, assessing, understanding, acting on and communicating risk issues" (Robillard, 2001, p. 9). Our thesis in this chapter is that inherent in a risk management framework is the acceptance of whatever it is that is risky, with this then leading to the routine promotion of a chemoprevention model for preventing disease rather than to the development of non-drug-based public health strategies that focus on removing (or reducing) risks at their source. Thus, the risk management approach can be seen as a component of neomedicalization.

Women's Health and Disease Prevention

Policies for disease prevention are women's concerns. The Canadian government subscribes to policy statements that commit Canada to protecting women from overmedicalization and from the overprescribing of drugs. These include Health Canada's Women's Health Strategy (Health Canada, 1999), which states that "Efforts will be continued to educate health care professionals and women themselves to reduce over-medicalization and over-prescribing of drugs" (Objective 3.16) and the Beijing Platform for Action (United Nations, 1995), which gives direction to "Take all appropriate measures to eliminate harmful, medically unnecessary or coercive medical interventions, as well as inappropriate medication and over-medication of women. All women should be fully informed of their options, including likely benefits and potential side-effects, by properly trained personnel" (Strategic Objective C.1, 106 h). Similarly, Health Canada's Women's Health Strategy commits Canada to reducing exposure to toxic substances in the environment, work place, and food supply that threaten women's health (objectives 2.11, 4.7, 4.8, 4.17).

The history of unnecessary surgeries (e.g., many hysterectomies and radical mastectomies) and of poorly tested drugs and medical devices marketed to women (such as thalidomide, Diethylstilbestrol (DES), the Dalkon Shield, and silicone breast implants) has sensitized women's health activists to the issues of overmedicalization and iatrogenic illnesses. Feminist health theorists have also been critical of gendered, guilt-inducing messages that hold women personally responsible for their own health problems as well as those of their families (Sherwin, 1998, pp. 29–33). Similarly, many feminist theorists and activists point out that "lifestyle" explanations and policies tend to promote individual solutions while ignoring political ones. In reality, "lifestyle choices" are not made in a vacuum; they are strongly influenced by social, economic, and political factors (Sherwin, 1998, pp. 31–33).

As noted earlier in the chapter, the term "medicalization" has been developed to encompass how experiences are placed into the medical arena. The BC Advisory Council on Women's Health defines this process more specifically as "the tendency to take a life passage such as childbirth or menopause and turn it into a medical problem requiring drugs or surgery, often ignoring the social and psychological aspects of this passage" (Minister's Advisory Council on Women's Health, 1998). In this light, prescribing drugs to alleviate hot flashes for all women going through menopause, rather than recommending them as a last resort for a few, medicalizes menopause. In the second half of the last century, the medicalization of menopause expanded to a neomedicalization of old age: the medications used to treat menopausal symptoms gradually entered standard practice as preventative therapies for a range of conditions that have their onset as women get older, but for which their use had not been tested (see Box 3.3). As we suggest in the previous section, this practice was facilitated by the neo-liberal socio-political environment that began its ascent in affluent countries in the 1980s.

The Application of Risk Management in Canada
Health Canada documents that review cancer risks from radiological and chemical hazards, as well as risks from endocrine-disrupting chemicals, illustrate how risk management defeats public health objectives.

Box 3.3: Hormone Replacement Therapy: The Social Construction of a Youth Potion

In July 2002, the Women's Health Initiative (WHI) was halted. It was the largest clinical trial ever conducted to evaluate hormone replacement therapy (HRT). Rather than preventing diseases of aging in women as was popularly believed, the study found that Prempro (estrogen + Progestin) actually increases a woman's risk of two common causes of death in post-menopausal women: breast cancer and heart disease (heart attacks, strokes, and blood clots) (Writing Group for the Women's Health Initiative Investigators, 2002). Physicians' organizations quickly revised guidelines that had recommended hormones as health-promoting and women's use of the drugs declined dramatically. By 2004, statistics showed an unprecedented drop in the incidence of hormonally related breast cancers (Kerlikowske, Miglioretti, Buist, Walker & Carney, 2007).

Industry marketing strategies (see ad below) had helped shape the widespread myth that hormone replacement therapy would keep women from aging. In a more covert example, American physician Robert Wilson wrote the bestselling 1966 book *Feminine Forever*, which promoted estrogen therapy as a youth potion for women after menopause. Wilson did not reveal that Ayerst (now Wyeth-Ayerst), the company that manufactures Premarin, underwrote his efforts. Throughout the latter half of the 20th century, the pharmaceutical industry continued to construct scientific knowledge about the effects of hormones on health "not only through the direct funding and control of research, but also by funding the training and continuing education of scientists and physicians alike" (Krieger et al., 2005, p. 744).

The terms "estrogen replacement therapy" (ERT) and "hormone replacement therapy" (HRT) entered everyday language and reinforced the assumption that menopause is a deficiency disease rather than a normal transition in women's lives. The very fact that manipulating women's hormones in the interests of health was deemed plausible and acceptable reflects reductionist, gendered assumptions about women's "nature" (Krieger et al., 2005). Sex hormones have been viewed as more essential to a woman's well-being in old age than her economic security, even though we know poverty is a major determinant of health.

Some analysts argued that stopping the WHI trial was an overreaction because any one woman in the trial had a relatively small increased risk of developing heart disease or breast cancer caused by hormone therapy. But individual risk is the wrong measure to evaluate a population-based intervention. Rather, we need to ask how many extra cases of a disease will result when the drug is prescribed to millions of healthy people. In the U.S. alone, a 34 percent decline in the use of post-menopausal hormone therapy following the WHI study was associated with an estimated 17,500 fewer breast cancer cases annually in women aged 50–69 years of age (Kerlikowske et al., 2007). By the stringent safety standards of public health, the risks of taking hormonal drugs are so high that estrogenic hormones can have no role in disease prevention.

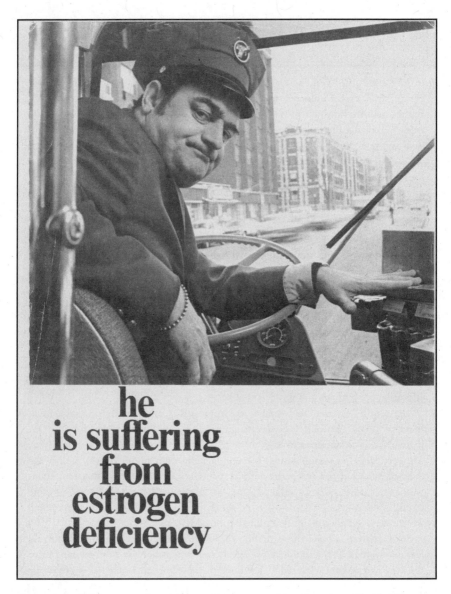

Figure 3.2: A Premarin advertisement that appeared in *Canadian Family Physician*, April 1973

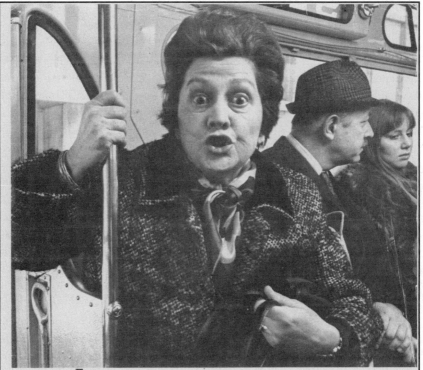

Assessment and Management of Cancer Risks from Radiological and Chemical Hazards (Joint Working Group of the Atomic Energy Control Board, 1998) specifies that strategies for managing the risks of radiation and genotoxic chemicals in Canada endorse the ALARA ("as low as reasonably achievable") principle, according to which "exposures are kept as low as reasonably achievable, social and economic factors being taken into account" (p. 49). A joint working group with members drawn from Health Canada's Health Protection Branch and the Atomic Energy Control Board found that the ALARA principle was not applied in a completely systematic manner either for radiation or chemicals (Joint Working Group of the Atomic Energy Control Board, 1998, p. 9). The joint working group was unable to reach consensus on acceptable levels of risk and, indeed, found that "The *acceptable* levels of risk associated with established guidelines vary up to a million-fold" (Joint Working Group of the Atomic Energy Control Board, 1998, p. 9; italics in original). These large differences reflect the fact that guidelines are based on individual judgments of what is, and is not, acceptable. They highlight a key problem with risk management as it is practised in Canada, which is that judgments about acceptability or unacceptability of a certain level of health risk are often tempered by economic considerations that have nothing to do with public health.

Members of the working group concluded nonetheless that risk management strategies to regulate both radiation and chemicals "provide a high degree of health protection based on the *absence of observable health effects using epidemiological methodology*" (Joint Working Group of the Atomic Energy Control Board, 1998, p. 42; italics added). The absence of observable health effects cannot be taken as demonstrating "a high degree of health protection." The committee failed to consider that while large numbers of studies over time in different populations can demonstrate a *harmful* health effect when it is of sufficient magnitude (as with smoking and lung cancer), epidemiologic tools are not always sufficiently refined to identify harms when they occur at low levels or in complex ways.

A Health Protection Branch document on endocrine-disrupting substances (EDSs) reached a similar conclusion about the limits of epidemiologic methods. A review of the literature failed to find compelling evidence that EDSs had caused widespread adverse health effects in humans, but neither could the current evidence rule out such effects (Wade, 1998). The author finds justification to continue basic laboratory and epidemiological research to determine the true extent of human health impacts, but does not recommend any action to protect public health.

Yet the evidence that EDSs may pose a public health threat points primarily to altered endocrine signals that arise after *in utero* exposures to environmental insults at very specific points in fetal development. Furthermore, the problems researchers have identified are subtle health deficits, not diseases. They include impaired cognitive and sexual development, as indicated by short-term memory and attention disorders, undescended testicles at birth, and lowered sperm counts later in life. "They erode human potential and undermine the quality of human life. They undermine the ways in which humans interact with one another and thereby threaten the social order of modern civilization" (Colborn, Dumanoski & Myers, 1996, pp. 202–203). At what point does such evidence become "compelling," and who decides?

Canada has a tradition of leadership in health protection policy. Key Canadian documents, such as the Lalonde and Epp Reports, strongly advocate disease prevention by means of public health initiatives and are regarded by international observers as models of public health policy (Epp, 1986; Lalonde, 1974). Canada helped to strengthen the protection of women's rights, including rights to health, in the Beijing Platform of Action. Canadian initiative is evident in environmental documents that promote the precautionary principle, such as the 1987 Montreal Protocol on Substances That Deplete the Ozone Layer (Parson, 2003) and the report of the 1992 International Joint Commission on the Great Lakes (Fulton et al., 1992), a bilateral Canada–U.S. proposal to phase out entire classes of chlorinated compounds worldwide. In addition to its international statements, Canadian women's health and human rights documents provide a framework for preventing harm to women and vulnerable subpopulations. In the light of this history, Canada's endorsement of risk management seems paradoxical.

In a discussion paper on the Canadian Environmental Protection Act (CEPA) and the precautionary principle, environmental law professor David VanderZwaag addresses the apparent contradiction between Canadian policy statements and our public record on health protection. He observes that while Canada has signed many international treaties and declarations that articulate a precautionary approach, we have at the same time been slow to acknowledge the precautionary principle at the domestic level (VanderZwaag, 1994, p. 9). Elsewhere, the same author likens the Canadian government's acceptance of the precautionary principle to "hesitant hugs" rather than a "passionate embrace" (VanderZwaag, 1999). When the CEPA was revised in 1999, he notes, although the precautionary principle was cited in the preamble and invoked as an administrative duty, "the revamped CEPA stops short of strong precautionary approaches …" (VanderZwaag, 1999, p. 371). Industry lobbying led to last-minute amendments that weakened the act. One member of Parliament, the Hon. Charles Caccia, expressed his dismay at the result:

> Following the intervention of industry there is no guarantee under the bill
> that virtual elimination would achieve zero or near-zero emissions. There is
> no requirement to push toward that desired result. What comfort is it to
> Canadians if toxic chemicals get catalogued and assessed, but not necessarily
> eliminated? … We had a strong articulation of the precautionary principle.
> It was defeated. (VanderZwaag, 1999, p. 371)

Under Health Canada's current risk management framework, Canadians continue to be subjected to dangerous levels of toxic and radioactive wastes in their environments, especially in poor communities inhabited by racial minorities. Residents of Sydney, Nova Scotia, where a century of steel-making has created one of the most polluted regions in North America, suffer elevated cancer rates of the stomach, cervix, breast, brain, prostate, bladder, lung, and colon/rectum, at levels ranging from 22–134 percent higher than the provincial average. They suffer higher rates of Alzheimer's, multiple sclerosis, asthma, liver disease, cardiovascular and respiratory diseases, and birth defects (Barlow & May, 2000, p. 144). In order to protect the Quebec-based asbestos industry, Canada has blocked international efforts to curb the asbestos trade, despite recognition among scientists that the substance causes a deadly cancer. The bulk of Canadian production is exported to underdeveloped countries, where workers and communities are likely to be poorly protected from exposure to hazardous substances. In 2008, findings from an expert report commissioned by Health Canada were withheld and two scientists who took part in the panel on asbestos's health impacts complained to the minister of health that their views had been misrepresented in the House of Commons (Daubs, 2008). The rationale given for risking lives is that people in poor communities need jobs. Despite growing evidence of health problems linked to pollution, federal and provincial budgets for environmental protection and health have been slashed in the past two decades (Barlow & May, 2000).

In this regard, the increased use of prescription drugs for preventive purposes may have the paradoxical effect of contributing to health problems in a way that has received little attention. Pharmaceuticals enter the environment through human excrement, an ever-increasing source of pollution that holds significant potential to affect human health (see Chapter 9). Virtually nothing is known about the actual effects of these compounds on human health, yet Canadian law allows the application of sewage sludge to croplands. In 1998, Environment Canada reported high levels of estrogens and birth control compounds in the effluent of sewage-treatment plants nationwide (Ternes et al., 1999).

Under a risk management framework, companies are not forced to clean up toxic sites or modify polluting technologies. Such steps become one of several possible approaches to managing risks and an industry can pressure government to implement a different risk management strategy, one with lower short-term costs for companies. A key question, however, is who bears the ultimate cost for these sorts of management strategies? Is it those producing a toxic substance or those exposed to it? In the long term, strategies that reduce and eliminate the causes of disease promote both health and sustainable development. They have finite costs, provide long-term health benefits to entire populations, and usually alleviate a range of illnesses rather than merely one.

The Individualization of Public Health

Chemotherapy for disease prevention focuses on individuals and their risk(s) of disease, in contrast to a public health approach that would apply the precautionary principle. Pharmaceutical companies build on this individualizing by promoting measurement technologies that ground these risks in actual numbers, such as bone mineral density and cholesterol levels, which then become the objects of management by specific pills. Because the environment gets identified as a seemingly non-removable trigger that leads to illness in those who are susceptible, one's biochemistry, hormones, and lifestyle become the focus for management—with a pill to fix each of these conditions. This framing depoliticizes the determinants of health and shifts the emphasis to the individual, who must work to be well by managing her risks. In fact, risk itself becomes medicalized and managing risk becomes a social obligation, albeit an obligation that not all have the resources to carry out.

Using prescription drugs to prevent disease individualizes what could be addressed with public health strategies. Classic public health measures like the chlorination of water, workplace safety measures, taxes on tobacco, and mandating the use of seat belts are designed to prevent disease and disability in everyone exposed to a particular risk. Chemoprevention, by contrast, shifts disease prevention to the individual treatment sphere. The individualized approach to prevention channels more and more of our limited medical treatment resources into testing and monitoring healthy people, leaving fewer resources available for those who are actually sick.

Advocates of breast cancer chemoprevention trials argue that the medication provides women with choice, implying that merely choosing the mode of disease prevention was a positive feature (Ford, 1995). In fact, preventing disease by methods that rely on individuals' decisions is extremely inefficient and contrary to the principles of public health and social solidarity. By characterizing patients as "at high risk" in the broadest possible ways, still more health care resources are channelled toward healthy people and away from the sick.

The prospect of introducing chemopreventives into standard health care holds profound implications for Canada's public health care system. For example, the financial cost of reducing disease by means of drugs would be formidable—and potentially contribute to increasing inequities in women's health, both by diverting resources away from initiatives that could begin to address the structural determinants of health and by further disadvantaging women who are poor and/or marginalized. As well, the use of prescription pharmaceuticals for long-term prevention is a high-maintenance approach to prevention that requires careful evaluation of candidates and close follow-up. Moreover, because people living in the community who take drugs are not monitored as closely as they are in clinical trials, the incidence of side effects is likely to be greater than is found in research reports and dealing with these, too, will have an impact on the public health care system.

Social stigma and insurance and employment discrimination are yet other potential problems for those who have been labelled high risk. Conversely—and ironically—the question could arise whether people who fit a chemoprevention risk profile can successfully sue their physician or provincial health ministry if they are not informed of, or provided with, a drug that might lower their disease risk. When tamoxifen was approved for breast cancer risk reduction in the United States, American physicians became liable for litigation if they didn't discuss the drug with eligible patients. At least one physician who failed to discuss the drug as a preventive option was sued by a woman who later developed breast cancer (McMaster University-based oncologist Mark Levine, personal communication, July 10, 2000). Such discussions add to the time and cost of routine physician consultations.

Treating drugs as ordinary products of consumer choice does nothing to empower women (see Chapter 2 for further discussion of this point). Instead, the process removes the state's responsibility for health protection. Moreover, to say that the Breast Cancer Prevention Trial provided women with a right to choose and that women "understand how to weigh the potential benefits and potential risks" (Ford, 1995, p. 12) is mere flattery if potential volunteers for a trial are denied full access to risk-benefit information, and put at risk in ways that undermine medicine's public health tradition and the ethical foundations of medicine.

Globally, many people do not have access to needed medicines, such as treatments for HIV/AIDS or oxytocin to prevent serious bleeding in childbirth. Consequently, women in poor countries have justifiably demanded greater access to medications. In rich, industrialized countries, however, many of women's demands for expanded health choices have been for options that decrease medicalization and increase possibilities for self-care. These include such things as legalized and publicly funded midwifery, insurance coverage for massage therapy, and non-toxic alternative therapies. With respect to disease prevention, any meaningful discussion of choice must put options in a broad relational perspective and must go beyond the personal to include societal choices, such as the priority set on maintaining clean, safe environments and the many structural constraints that make real choice inaccessible to too many women.

The factors associated with disease, which are usually described as lifestyle factors (in the case of breast cancer, these include exercise, alcohol, and delayed child-bearing), are often presented as governed entirely by individual choices. These behaviours exist in a complex social context, however, and will not likely alter in the absence of social policies that take this context into account. Structural determinants of health, such as gender and impoverishment, greatly influence people's behaviours. Simply exhorting women to exercise more and reduce alcohol intake will not be effective if most women cannot take time off from work or domestic chores for daily physical activities, and if the social reasons for excessive alcohol use are not addressed. Similarly, as long as women who have children in their early 20s have their employment prospects severely limited, many women will continue to postpone child-bearing until they have completed an education.

Conclusion

A pharmaceutical approach to prevention threatens to displace the public health ideal of preventing disease by maintaining clean, safe environments. Canada's health protection system needs to counter the industry-driven enthusiasm for chemoprevention with a regulatory framework that promotes and ensures true primary prevention, and it must be sufficiently funded to do this work. Further, its regulations with regard to the testing, sales, and monitoring of drugs must be enforced.

Decisive action is needed to reduce exposure to known and suspected causes of disease. To continue with the example of breast cancer: one commonly hears that there are no known or proven modifiable environmental causes of this disease, that environmental causes make only a small contribution to rising breast cancer rates (e.g., Sibbald, 1999), or that such factors need "more study." In fact, much of what we know about the environmental causes of cancer is not translated into policy because of political pressures (Davis, 2007; Proctor, 1995). Where evidence is compelling but inconclusive, policies based on the precautionary principle would actively promote an environment as free as possible from known and suspected hazards to human health.

Within the current risk management framework, measurable levels of radiation, genotoxic chemicals, and endocrine-disrupting substances are assumed to be safe because epidemiological studies do not yet show observable health effects. This is what London mathematician Peter Saunders calls "the mathematical fallacy that absence of evidence is the same as evidence of absence" (Saunders, 2000). Rather than looking to drugs to prevent disease, Canada desperately needs a health protection policy built on the sound and proven principles of public health. And rather than assuming individuals should manage the risks to which we are all exposed, Canadian policy needs to follow more closely the precautionary principle and remove these risks. A survey of Canadian investments in cancer research in 2005 found that only 2 percent of the $253,568,130 spent that year went to "prevention research," which the authors defined as lifestyle, drugs, or vaccine interventions "which reduce cancer risk by reducing exposure to cancer risks and increasing protective factors" (Canadian Cancer Research Alliance, 2007, p. 7). The report's authors point out that some projects that they classified under "cancer etiology" (i.e., origins and causes of cancer, including environmental exposures) qualify as prevention research, as do some coded as "surveillance," but even including these two categories would raise the proportion spent on prevention research to only 7–10 percent of the total (Canadian Cancer Research Alliance, 2007, p. 16).

The public health principles of disease prevention provide the best framework for protecting Canadians against disease. The health risks, ethical dilemmas, and financial burden of medicating large numbers of people are too formidable to justify allowing a chemoprevention strategy to displace public health objectives. The lure of apparent economic benefits and the "quick-fix" appeal of drugs, as well as major pressures on governments to adopt industry-friendly policies, have tilted government momentum away from public health principles. However, chemoprevention is less a detour than a wrong turn. Policy changes are needed at the highest level to affirm the precautionary principle as the basis for health protection and to confine chemoprevention to situations where its use is safe, economical, and ethical. Even in these instances, chemopreventive applications should not distract from the search for long-range public health solutions.

Notes

1. Childhood vaccines are generally an exception here; they are aimed at acute conditions and are provided in Canada almost always within public health program contexts.
2. For a recent example, see Moynihan and Cassels (2005), and also Pollack in the *New York Times* (May 9, 2005), "marketing a disease, and also a drug to treat it."
3. This also raises concerns about iatrogenic harm if the intervention on these "early" findings itself has adverse effects and/or leads to unnecessary treatment.
4. Some argue that improvements to the food supply through advances in agriculture have saved more lives over the past 300 years than any one public health measure, including improved water quality. Benefits from the provision of adequate food, like those deriving from clean water, clearly outweigh the relatively modest gains obtained by advances in medicine.

Chapter 4

Who Pays the Piper?
Industry Funding
of Patients' Groups[1]

———

Sharon Batt

Introduction: Hijacked by Pharma?

In November 2007, the *Lancet* published an online letter titled "WHO's Web-Based Public Hearings: Hijacked by Pharma?" In it, five correspondents from public health ministries in Thailand, the Maldives, India, and Sri Lanka expressed their collective dismay that public consultations carried out under the auspices of the World Health Organization (WHO) appeared to have been undermined by pharmaceutical industry funding to groups that ostensibly represented the interests of patients. The consultations were intended to gather public input on a draft global strategy and action plan to promote research and development into neglected diseases and access to medicines in developing countries. Many of the submissions supported · strong intellectual property (IP) protections. Predictably, 11 out of 12 responding organizations that were directly affiliated with the pharmaceutical industry wanted strong IP protections. The authors of the letter were surprised, however, that 14 patient advocacy groups adopted the same stance, often using "near identical phrases or concepts in their submissions." Their suspicion that the process had been hijacked was based on their discovery that 11 of the 14 groups received financial support from the pharmaceutical industry. "For example," they wrote, "a Canadian patient advocacy group whose submission was in favour of IP received financial support from Actelion Pharmaceuticals, Amgen Canada, Bayer, Gilead Sciences Canada, INO Therapeutics, Merck Frosst Canada, Novartis Pharmaceuticals Canada, Ortho Biotech, Amicus Therapeutics, Apopharma, BioMarin Pharmaceutical, Hoffmann-La Roche and Sigma-Tau Pharmaceuticals" (Wibulpolprasert, Moosa, Satyanarayana, Samarage & Tangcharoensathien, 2007).

This example is far from an isolated case. Partnerships between patients' groups and pharmaceutical companies ("pharma") are now commonplace, raising important questions of ethics and policy. Within Canada's community of consumer health, patient, and disease-specific organizations, the issue has been a topic of intense debate for at least a decade (e.g., Ford, 1998; Mintzes, 1998) with media reports bringing the issues to public attention (Johnson, 2000; Nebenzahl, 2003; Picard, 2001; Weeks, 2007). This chapter examines the phenomenon and its implications from the perspective of a women's health organization that does not accept pharmaceutical company funds and whose members have argued against pharma funding to patients' groups (e.g., Mintzes, 2007).

Background

Advocacy by disease and consumer groups is not a new phenomenon. Organizations like the American and Canadian Cancer Societies and the March of Dimes (established to defeat polio) date to the first half of the 20th century. In the 1980s, however, AIDS activism raised patient group advocacy to a new level of visibility and political sophistication (Epstein, 1996, 2008). Since then, patient and health activist causes have proliferated, attracting the interest of social analysts (Landzelius, 2006). Governments are eager to engage the public in health policy decision making and once-passive patients have organized to have their voices heard (Bucchi & Neresini, 2008; Epstein, 2008).

To advocate effectively, organizations need money. In Canada, however, federal government policies, which once supported community-based advocacy, have eliminated or restricted most funding to advocacy groups (Jensen & Phillips, 1996). Instead, governments fund projects that support government goals and encourage charitable groups to diversify their sources of revenue. A strict interpretation of the "10 percent rule" that limits the proportion of donated funds a registered charity can spend on advocacy further limits the ability of these groups to speak out; meanwhile, groups in the voluntary sector have seen their advisory role expanded (Harvie, 2002; Laforest, 2004).

Partnerships between non-profit groups and the private sector are one funding strategy that emerged from the 1990s climate of deficit-reduction and privatization (Cossman & Fudge, 2002). Although some provinces (e.g., British Columbia and Quebec) still have core funding programs for non-profit organizations, fundraising and grant writing have become overwhelming requirements for community groups and many in the non-profit health and disease sector welcome the advent of pharmaceutical industry partnerships as an alternative source of funding (Picard, 2001).

Companies whose sales are directly affected by government policies donate funds from their marketing budgets to groups positioned to influence these policies. Disease-specific organizations receive tens or hundreds of thousands of dollars annually from pharma for conferences, publications, websites, and advocacy training. Exact figures are difficult to compile systematically because groups are not required to disclose this information and seldom do. Amounts quoted in newspaper articles, however, include 70 percent of the Colorectal Cancer Society of Canada's $500,000 budget in 2000, $1.8 million of the Arthritis Society of Canada's $30 million budget in 2000, and $100,000 of the Canadian Breast Cancer Network's budget in 2000. Surveys based on annual reports, websites, and interviews confirm the prevalence of pharmaceutical company donors as well as concerns about disclosure, not only in Canada but in the U.S., Europe, Australia, and New Zealand (Ball, Tisoki & Herxheimer, 2006; Herxheimer, 2003; Kent, 2007; Lofgren, 2004; Mintzes, 2007; O'Donovan, 2007; Patient View, 2004).

For the past decade, red flags have been raised in many countries over the ethics of pharma funding of medical researchers (Bekelman, Mphil & Gross, 2003; Krimsky, 2003), contributors to medical journals (Goozner, 2004), physicians (Oldani, 2004), bioethicists (Elliott, C., 2001, 2004), universities (Schafer, 2004), and drug regulatory agencies (Abraham, J., 2004). As in these other sectors, neo-liberal policies in Canada and elsewhere support partnership arrangements between patient groups and pharma by encouraging collaborations with industry while systematically weakening state funding programs. If public consultation processes are indeed being "hijacked by pharma," these processes, as well as the practices of individual groups, may need to change to ensure that the public interest is properly represented.

Women's Health Advocacy and Health Protection

When the modern era of pharmaceuticals began in the 1940s, many drugs and medical devices were marketed solely or primarily to women, sometimes with disastrous effects. By the time the women's health movement took shape in the late 1960s and early 1970s, thalidomide and diethylstilbestrol (DES) had alerted women to the dark side of prescription drugs, legally sold with false promises and no safety warnings. Even the birth control pill, although generally welcomed by women, was rushed to market without adequate testing for dosage and harmful effects; when deaths from blood clots began to mount, drug companies suppressed the information (Seaman, 1995). Women's health organizations, such as DES Action Canada, the Toronto Women's Health Network, *A Friend Indeed*, and the breast implant group Je Sais/I Know, to name only four, advocated for strong health protection legislation and raised awareness of potential harms of drugs and medical devices marketed to women. These groups, as part of the women's health movement, helped create a new model for thinking critically about pharmaceuticals and women's health. Small grassroots organizations, drawing from their members' own experiences and from feminist understandings of socially constructed knowledge, re-examined prevailing medical practices, particularly as they affected women.

Women's health issues have since moved into the mainstream. Sheryl Burt Ruzek and Julie Becker (1999) analyzed the institutionalization of women's health in the United States and concluded that in the late 1980s and the 1990s newer, "professionalized" women's health groups emerged. These differed from the grassroots groups. The professionalized groups often advocated providing women with greater access to drugs and other treatments rather than protecting them from unsafe or unnecessary medical interventions. They also strove to make educated women aware of scientific information, while grassroots groups tried to educate women to improve their own health. Some women's groups, in both Canada and the U.S., still monitor the overmedicalization of women's health, adopting a watchdog role toward both industry and government; for other groups, however, the overarching goal is to expand women's access to health services and treatments. This evolution has obscured rather than highlighted problems of drug safety and overprescribing to women because competing messages blunt the feminist critique of unsafe or overpromoted pharmaceuticals and medical devices. Consistent with their contrasting perspectives on biomedical intervention, grassroots advocacy groups are likely to express concern about corporate sponsorship, while women's health organizations with a focus on access often rely heavily on corporate funding (Cossman & Fudge, 2002; Ruzek & Becker, 1999).

As noted in the introductory example, the discourses within "professionalized" advocacy groups often echo those of the pharmaceutical industry: patients need rapid access to new medications; pharmaceutical innovation will cease if pharmaceutical companies are reined in; expensive drugs reduce costs in other parts of the system, etc. However, drugs harmful to women's health continue to make headlines (e.g., HRT, Diane-35). A major contribution of the women's health movement has been its willingness to challenge the medical establishment. The marginalization and disappearance of independent groups that act as watchdogs for women in the realm of unsafe or unnecessary medical interventions erode the critical understanding of health politics that women's health activists developed over decades.

Health Advocacy Groups and Canada's Health Policy Environment

In 2000, the Health Products and Food Branch (HPFB) of Health Canada established the Office of Consumer and Public Involvement (OCAPI) to encourage public involvement in the branch's priority-setting, programs, and policy decisions. The *Policy Toolkit for Public Involvement in Decision Making*, published by Health Canada, defines the public as "individuals, consumers, citizens and special interest groups and/or stakeholders," where a stakeholder is "an individual, group or organizations having a 'stake' in an issue and its outcome (e.g., specific matters relating to health, environment, consumers, volunteers, industry, science)" (Health Canada, 2000, p. 26). Canadian consumer, health, and patient groups testify regularly at public hearings on pharmaceutical issues; sit on policy committees where drug policy decisions are made; attend workshops and consultations; and meet with health department decision makers to discuss changes to drug policy. Canadian groups that take an active interest in pharmaceutical policy issues include Best Medicines Coalition, a national umbrella lobby for patients' groups, and its members (many of which are disease-specific patients' organizations), the Consumer Advocare Network, the Canadian Health Coalition, PharmaWatch, the Consumers' Association of Canada, the Canadian Women's Health Network, *la Fédération du Québec pour le planning des naissances*, *le Réseau québécois d'action pour la santé des femmes*, and Women and Health Protection.

Concerns about conflicts of interest on the part of industry-funded groups purporting to represent the public interest at HPFB led Women and Health Protection and several other organizations to urge the HPFB and OCAPI to address the issue. In response, OCAPI developed the Voluntary Statement of Information, a policy to encourage groups participating in policy consultations to voluntarily declare their industry funding sources and other organizational information (Health Canada,

2005). This policy was a step toward greater transparency; however, experience in other sectors demonstrates that voluntary statements without enforcement do not ensure disclosure. Top scientists at the National Institutes of Health in the U.S., for example, failed to disclose lucrative industry contracts to their bosses as required (Weiss, 2004); similarly, Goozner (2004) found that authors do not always comply with conflict-of-interest disclosure policies of leading academic journals. A more serious concern is that disclosure of conflicted loyalties does nothing to remove the conflict.

Current government policy actively promotes partnerships with industry, in the voluntary sector as well as within government itself. Non-profit groups that reject this model as inappropriate for their mandate risk marginalization, both because they are perceived as "not playing by the rules" and because their access to funds is severely limited. As an example, OCAPI formed a partnership with Best Medicines Coalition (BMC), a group that describes the pharmaceutical industry as "a major supporter" (Best Medicines Coalition, 2007). At a meeting between OCAPI staff and coalition members, participants recommended that OCAPI "use BMC as an umbrella group in its patient consultation strategy" (Office of Consumer and Public Involvement & Best Medicines Coalition, 2003, p. 6). While the report noted that OCAPI would also consult with groups representing the healthy population, BMC was characterized as "more appropriate to represent the Canadian *patient* population" (Office of Consumer and Public Involvement & Best Medicines Coalition, 2003, p. 7; italics in original). Some patient advocates and patient groups, however, have found that an organization that accepts funding from the pharmaceutical industry cannot meet patients' needs for unbiased information about medications and their disease (see Box 4.1). If the official voice of patients in drug policy consultations is a pharma-funded coalition, how can independent patients and patient groups believe their perspective will be fairly heard?

Conflicts of Interest and Pharma's Culture of Gift-Giving

A conflict of interest (sometimes called a "competing interest") is said to occur when a person or organization has a primary moral obligation to act on behalf of another and, at the same time, has a relationship (financial or otherwise) with a third party that could interfere with proper judgment in the first relationship. An organization that presents itself as a voice for a specific constituency, such as people with diabetes or breast cancer, women, Canadian consumers, or the public, has a primary moral duty to represent the interests of this sector. Pharmaceutical companies are problematic funding sources for these groups because they often have a direct interest in the outcome of the group's advocacy, which in turn can cloud the judgment of decision makers within the organization. Alliances with pharmaceutical companies may also involve non-monetary exchanges, such as the provision of expertise, published materials, and networking opportunities.

Box 4.1: The Alzheimer Society

---

by Linda Furlini, PhD

Both my parents were simultaneously affected by Alzheimer's disease when they were 60 years of age. I was 23 years old at the time, had no medical background, and knew little about the illness. My father's illness lasted approximately 10 years and my mother's about twice as long. When she died, I returned to academe and completed a doctoral thesis focused on the experiences of caregivers of people with dementia-type diseases.

When my parents initially became ill, like most caregivers in my situation, I had to learn about the disease through trial and error. In desperation, I approached the Alzheimer Society for assistance. Eventually, I joined as a volunteer. My purpose was to acquire knowledge, contribute to greater awareness about the consequences of Alzheimer's disease, and support the development of appropriate and desperately needed resources. My work at the local, provincial, and national levels culminated, in 1996, in a mandate as president of the Federation of Quebec Alzheimer Societies (FQAS) and as an Executive Committee member of the Alzheimer Society of Canada (ASC). My involvement with these groups turned out to be one of my greatest educational experiences. However, it also involved some illuminating and heartbreaking revelations, insights into the realities of the way the pharmaceutical industry does business.

In the late 1990s, a new drug was approved by Health Canada for the treatment of mild to moderate Alzheimer's disease. Shortly after its approval, the drug's manufacturer began lobbying the Quebec Ministry of Health to have the drug added to the Quebec Provincial Drug Formulary (so that its cost would be covered by the Quebec government). The drug manufacturer exerted great pressure on the federation to concentrate its lobby efforts on this drug. The pressure was very intense and, in the end, lobbying efforts in support of this drug ended up supplanting other FQAS objectives set out in the organization's strategic plan. In addition to the FQAS lobby efforts, a separate drug lobbying group was created, formed, and funded by the drug manufacturer. It was headed by two doctors and comprised of caregivers whose loved ones were early in the disease process. This group gained quick and easy access to the media and the Ministry of Health and shortly thereafter the new Alzheimer's drug was approved for partial payment on the Quebec Drug Formulary.

This may be a typical story of how a new drug gets approved, but we must be cognizant of the extreme vulnerability of the patient and the patient's advocates and relatives, especially in light of the pressure and incentives that drug companies can and do exert. There is an understandable tendency for caregivers, early in the disease process, to be overwhelmed and vulnerable. Initially, they know very little about the disease's insidious, variable, and unpredictable symptoms. They may attribute any improvement in behaviour, memory, or cognition to a drug rather than to the erratic nature of the disease. We all expect some positive effects when we take medication.

Caregivers, facing a new and confusing situation, with few resources and no effective treatments in sight, are even more susceptible to attribute all changes to a "new miracle drug."

Some drugs clearly lead to greatly increased life expectancy and quality of life. However, as business enterprises, the mandate of drug manufacturers is to maximize profit. Drug approvals usually involve a delicate balancing act among many interests. I often wonder how much further advanced we would be today if the public funds spent on this drug had been allocated toward research into Alzheimer's disease, the development of resources for those affected by it, and on assistance to their caregivers.

[More detail about Ms. Furlini's experience can be found in a letter written by her to the British Medical Journal (BMJ). The letter was published by the journal on September 26, 2007, where it formed part of an exchange about disease charities, industry funding, and the challenges of evaluating the cost-effectiveness of drugs. The original letter and "rapid-response" letters are available on the BMJ website. See "Further Readings" at the end of this book.]

Richard Smith, former editor of the *British Medical Journal*, proposed adopting "competing interest" as a more neutral descriptive term than "conflict of interest" in the hope that authors who received industry funds for their research would be more likely to comply with the journal's disclosure policy (Smith, 1998). He argued that a conflict of interest is a common condition that does not imply wrongdoing, whereas "authors think an admission of conflict of interest implies wickedness." Subsequent research, however, has shown that Smith's analysis does not fully grasp the complexity of industry funding. Bero, Glantz, and Hong (2005) used documents from the Legacy Tobacco Documents Library at the University of California to study the adequacy of competing interest declarations by two authors with an extensive history of research on tobacco and its effects on health. Although the authors had fully complied with the *BMJ*'s disclosure requirements in a 2003 article, the researchers found that:

> Even an extensive financial disclosure statement that meets the journal's requirements can still provide an incomplete understanding of the tobacco industry's relationship with a project. The documents show how the tobacco industry funds research for multiple reasons, including gaining credibility or developing relationships with scientists that might be useful to the industry in the future. (Bero, Glantz & Hong, 2005, p. 123)

The declaration of competing interests did not show, for example, how the authors' ongoing relationship with the tobacco industry enabled the industry to influence the researchers' protocols and collegial networks. Based on the available evidence, the present author believes that the pharmaceutical industry likewise systematically develops relationships with patient groups (and other players in the medical system) for multiple reasons that are not evident from a mere statement of competing interests. The more political term "conflict of interest" is therefore used to emphasize the likelihood that companies cultivate partnerships for strategic gain.

Ethicist Carl Elliott worries that the term "conflict of interest" individualizes what is in fact a systemic undermining of institutions meant to serve the public good. He points to particular practices, such as pharma-funded ghostwritten articles in peer-review journals and the suppression of negative clinical trial results, which go beyond mere conflict of interest to corruption (Elliott, C., 2004). In the case of advocacy groups, the pharmaceutical industry's use of voluntary groups to "hijack," or covertly manipulate policy debates, arguably falls into the latter category. More generally, the very pervasiveness of pharmaceutical money within medical structures creates a for-profit environment that inhibits healthy and balanced debate of pharmaceutical policy issues. The pharmaceutical funding of advocacy groups is best understood as one component of a broad marketing strategy in which advocacy groups are only one player. In the words of Arthur Schafer, director of the Centre for Professional and Applied Ethics at the University of Manitoba, "all of modern medicine is floating on a sea of drug company money and the result has been utterly corrosive" (Taylor, 2008).

While the terms "corruption" and "corrosive" seem apt when discussing these systemic effects, it is important to keep in mind that the nature of systemic influences is to constrain individuals and groups acting within the system, including employees of pharmaceutical companies. Furthermore, many of these structural factors are invisible or resistant to change. The intent of this analysis, therefore, is not to demonize the actors but to bring to light underlying conditions that could be modified through improved understanding and policies.

Another question debated vigorously in the medical literature is how large a gift must be to constitute a potential conflict. The Canadian Medical Association's guidelines place limits on what gifts a physician may accept, but allow "modest meals or social events that are held as part of a conference or meeting" and "patient teaching aids appropriate to [a physician's] area of practice provided these aids carry at most the logo of the donor company and do not refer to specific therapeutic agents, services or other products" (Canadian Medical Association, 2007, pp. 4–5). No Free Lunch, a physicians' organization concerned about conflicts of interest in medicine, takes a tougher, "zero-tolerance" position on pharmaceutical company gift-giving. The group makes its point humorously with a "pen amnesty" program to encourage physicians to turn in pens bearing drug company logos in exchange for pens with the "No Free Lunch" logo.

Another initiative in this regard is the Brownlee List, managed by two American medical journalists. It is a listing of resource people and experts who have indicated that they do not receive or have not received drug company funding within the last five years. The list is available for use by national and international media and others seeking independent medical information.

One rationale for the zero-tolerance stance is the culturally widespread expectation of reciprocity in gift-giving. Anthropological studies show that gifts play a key role in many cultures and even small gifts create social obligations of loyalty and friendship (Mauss, 1967). Anthropologist Michael Oldani, a former pharmaceutical company sales representative, describes gift exchange as the core of the relationship between the prescribing physician and the pharma sales rep. The resulting gift economy creates a "feel-good" culture that glosses over the fact that all drugs come with the risk of drug-induced side effects, including death (Oldani, 2004).

Psychology experiments show that the ways in which conflicts of interest bias decision making are very subtle and unconscious. Even when researchers educated volunteers in a decision-making experiment about the way bias operates, the participants assumed they would not be biased by a reward, but their opponent would be, or they vastly underestimated how strong their own bias would be. The same experiments found that people were unable to avoid bias even when it was in their best interest to do so. Finally, bias was indirect: self-interest changes the way people seek out and weigh information (Katz, Merz & Caplan, 2003).

Studies of actual physician behaviour suggest that these findings translate to the medical environment. House staff who attended grand rounds given by a pharmaceutical company speaker were more likely than their colleagues to prescribe that company's drug as treatment, even though they did not remember which company sponsored the grand rounds. A study of medical residents found that 61 percent believed promotions did not influence their own practice, although only 16 percent believed that other physicians were impervious to influence from promotional gifts (Steinman, Shlipak & McPhee, 2001). Another study found that 19 out of 20 physicians who attended medical education seminars sponsored by two drug companies denied the seminars would influence their behaviour before attending; in fact, use of the companies' drugs did increase after the seminars (Orlowski & Wateska, 1992). Research with physicians has found that bias is strong, even with small stakes (Katz et al., 2003; Krimsky, 2003). Based on a review of the psychological and physician practice literature, two researchers concluded that attempts to control bias by mandatory disclosure, limiting gift size, or educational initiatives are likely to fail because they rest on a faulty model of human behaviour (Dana & Loewenstein, 2003). They conclude that industry gifts to physicians should be prohibited.

Conflicts of Interest and Government Funding

Some health policy groups, including Women and Health Protection, receive funding from the federal government. Because governments have a budgetary and political interest in what policies are enacted, government funding of such organizations must be characterized as conflicted. Unlike the private sector, however, governments have a responsibility to develop policies in the public interest. Ultimately, government funds come from tax revenues paid by citizens. Unlike industry, which has a fiduciary responsibility only to a small segment of the population, in a democratic society governments have a responsibility to represent the interests of the whole population. Therefore, a fundamental difference exists between public and private interests.

Paul Pross, an analyst of pressure groups in Canada, acknowledges that public funding of interest groups "brings with it problems of uncertainty, dependence, and a tendency to distort the goals of their organization" (1992, p. 22). Despite these problems, Pross argues that government support of groups is necessary if all points of view are to be included in public debate. A decision not to fund anyone would automatically favour the views of well-resourced sectors and weaken the quality of the discourse. The real issue, he concludes, is finding ways "to structure the processes of group-state relations so that the dangers of intimidation, favouritism, and manipulation are minimized" (Pross, 1992, p. 17).

Advocates for Better Care: Myth or Reality?

Groups that have chosen to work in partnership with the pharmaceutical industry often reject suggestions that these partnerships lead to co-optation. In a *Globe and Mail* article (Picard, 2001), representatives of several Canadian charities vigorously defended their decisions to accept funding from the drug industry. They saw such partnerships as a way to meet the medical and information needs of an increasingly sophisticated, demanding consumer. As Barry Stein, of the Colorectal Cancer Society of Canada, put it, "People want better patient care, [and] that includes better drugs." Denis Morrice asserted the Arthritis Society of Canada's independence, stating, "People with arthritis have to benefit or there won't be a partnership, no matter how much money is offered."

Leaders from each charity spoke of the steps they had taken to maintain independence and uphold ethical standards. These included being "upfront" about industry financial assistance (Stein), taking money from multiple companies, including those in direct competition with one another (Morrice), and selecting "truly benevolent" companies as partners (Durhane Wong-Reiger of the Consumer Advocare Network). Murray Elston, a spokesman for the pharma lobby group Rx&D Canada, described the charities as part of an empowered vanguard, "starting to use that power to demand changes, and to ask some tough questions" (Picard, 2001).

If these groups represent an empowered public, how is that power being exercised? What "tough questions" are being asked? The article in the *Globe and Mail* notes that groups like the Arthritis Society have become "far more militant and outspoken about issues like the slow approval of new drugs and reluctance to place new drugs on formularies." Denis Morrice, the former Arthritis Society's president and CEO, considered it coincidental that these same issues also "happen to be foremost on the minds of corporations" (Picard, 2001). In 1999, a story in the *Toronto Star* quoted Morrice as saying that the launch of the arthritis drug Celebrex was "truly a breakthrough" and that, "Basically it means that Canadians suffering from arthritis no longer have to fear the serious side effects of their medications" (Boyle, 1999). It was later found that the drug did not to lead to any reduction in potentially life-threatening gastrointestinal problems, including perforated ulcers, obstruction, or serious bleeding, as originally claimed.

The claims of pharma-funded patient advocacy groups need to be closely examined since their collective mission is to represent the health interests of millions of Canadian patients. Recurring themes are: the assumption that the "newest" medications are the "best" treatments and that unlimited access to new medications promotes better health; that slow approval of new drugs is a pressing policy problem and a threat to health; that advertisements provide information that empowers patients; that sick people have a right to new medications on the market, with full insurance coverage; and that groups can ensure independence from corporate sponsors with internal policies such as openness or having multiple pharma partners. These questions are examined below.

Are New Medications the Best Treatments?

New drugs are not necessarily better than older drugs; in fact, they are often neither as effective nor as safe. Despite the many cases where older, less expensive drugs are equal to or better than their newer counterparts (Prescrire International, 2007), the conviction that a newer drug must be better than an old one is pervasive.

The myth that new drugs are always better than old ones persists partly because new treatments are rarely tested against competing older drugs; rather, they are tested against a placebo. The fact that a drug is approved by a national drug regulator (in Canada, the Health Products and Food Branch or HPFB) may simply mean it was found, in a small, limited-term experiment, to be better than nothing. Most "new" drugs are not actually therapeutic advances either. A substantial number are minor molecular modifications of drugs already on the market, known as "me too" drugs. Drug companies, however, make most of their profits on new drugs and promote the belief that new means "improved."

Table 4.1: Therapeutic Value of New Drugs and New Indications for Older Drugs Introduced in France

Drug Category	Number	Percent
Major therapeutic innovation in an area where previously no treatment was available	2	0.2
Important therapeutic innovation but has limitations	38	3.9
Decision postponed until better data and more thorough evaluation	67	6.8
Without evident benefit but with potential or real disadvantage	77	7.8
Some value but does not fundamentally change the present therapeutic practice	106	10.8
Minimal additional value and should not change prescribing habits except in rare circumstances	251	25.5
May be new molecule but is superfluous because does not add to clinical possibilities offered by previously available products	442	45.0
Total	983	100

Source: Adapted from Prescrire International. (2007). A look back at pharmaceuticals in 2006: Aggressive advertising cannot hide the absence of therapeutic advances. *Prescrire International, 16*(88), p. 84.

Are Slow Drug Approvals a Problem?

Before drugs can be sold on the Canadian market, the HPFB reviews and assesses the safety and efficacy data that pharmaceutical companies are required to provide. For many years, the industry complained that bureaucratic approval processes caused a "drug lag," thereby denying life-saving new treatments to sick patients (Hilts, 2003). Best Medicines Coalition[2] promoted essentially the same position. Independent researchers questioned these arguments, however.

In the early 1990s, the HPFB, then called the Health Protection Branch, and the Food and Drug Administration (FDA) in the U.S. instituted user fees payable by industry, and at the same time took steps to speed drug approvals. Health Canada has committed to completing drug application reviews in a maximum of 300 days for non-priority drugs and 180 days for priority drugs. It has devoted substantial resources to achieving this goal. While this policy shift benefits the industry by bringing new, expensive drugs to market sooner, a number of studies suggest that lower standards of drug safety are a result (Abraham & Davis, 2002; Lurie & Wolfe, 1998; Office of Inspector General, 2003). Estimates suggest that in the United States, during the period 1990–1995, for every one-month reduction in a drug's review time, there was a 1 percent increase in expected reports of hospitalizations due to adverse drug reactions (ADRs) and a 2 percent increase in expected reports of ADR deaths (Olson, 2002).

The FDA has a statutory requirement to approve 90 percent of new drug applications within specific periods of time. If it fails to meet that obligation, renewal of the Prescription Drug User Fee Act (PDUFA) may be endangered and user fee revenue would be lost. Carpenter and colleagues (Carpenter, Zucker & Avorn, 2008) have concluded that when drugs are approved in the immediate pre-deadline period, there is a substantially higher rate of withdrawals and/or safety labelling changes compared to drugs approved at other times during the review cycle. In other words, it appears that if the deadline is imminent, the FDA does a less thorough job of reviewing drugs in order to avoid missing the deadline.

Similarly, revenue to Health Canada's Therapeutic Products Directorate (TPD) will suffer if service standards—that is, approval of new drugs within the targeted time—are not met. If the review time in a given fiscal year is more than 110 percent of the target for that fee category, fees are then reduced for the next reporting year by a percentage equivalent to the review time beyond the target, up to a maximum of 50 percent (Health Products and Food Branch, 2007). Faced with the prospect of penalties, it is possible that the TPD might follow the pattern set by the FDA and rush their reviews of new drugs to avoid incurring a financial loss in the following year.

Speedy access to experimental drugs is a hollow victory for patients if those drugs cause more health problems than they remedy. A number of independent health groups—including Women and Health Protection, PharmaWatch, the Consumers' Association of Canada, and the Canadian Health Coalition—argue that the push to speedy drug approvals draws attention and resources away from the careful drug review and post-market surveillance needed to assure drug safety.

Does the Ban on DTCA Deny Information to Patients?

Prescribing physicians have traditionally been the intermediaries between the commercially motivated manufacturers and vulnerable patients. All Western countries except the U.S. and New Zealand ban the advertising of prescription drugs to consumers. Pharmaceutical companies have contested these restrictions and lobbied for the right to advertise their products directly to consumers. Their greatest success was in the U.S., where the FDA relaxed restrictions on direct-to-consumer advertising (DTCA) in 1997.

Some patient groups have lobbied strenuously to have DTCA legalized in Canada, while others have opposed DTCA. A brief to Health Canada by the Consumer Advocare Network,[3] a national advocacy organization supported by the pharmaceutical industry, argues that the Canadian ban on DTCA denies patients their "fundamental right to information about prescription drugs, which includes direct-to-consumer advertising, or promotion, of drugs" (Wong-Reiger, 2003). Opponents of DTCA respond that advertising does not provide patients with the unbiased information they need to make informed health decisions (see Chapter 2).

Do People Have a "Right" to New Medications, with Full Insurance Coverage?

Each province has a formulary that restricts drug coverage to a subset of all available drugs. After Health Canada approves a drug, each provincial or territorial government assigns that drug to one of three categories: (1) covered; (2) not covered; or (3) limited use (i.e., the government will pay for the drug only under certain conditions or, in some cases, prescriptions for that drug will be filled by a comparable, lower-priced drug). The high cost of many new drugs creates a dilemma for provincial governments, working within strained health budgets. A drug that has been approved will not necessarily be added to all (or any) provincial formularies if a government decides its cost exceeds the health benefit or if the drug is simply unaffordable.

Advocacy groups differ in their responses if a province decides not to add the drug to its formulary. A common response has been for groups of patients who feel they are being denied a drug to demand that it be added to the formulary. Lobbies for drug access may include a media appeal by a suffering patient, demands for formulary inclusion by the spokesperson from a relevant disease group, and statements dismissing concerns about the cost. These campaigns may be developed in close collaboration with a company or companies that support the organization financially (see Box 4.1).

The idea that drugs should be added to provincial formularies as soon as they are approved rests on the contention that patients have a "right" to a new treatment that might help them, regardless of costs. A *Globe and Mail* article about disparities between provincial drug formularies cited Kathy Kovacs Burns, then president of Best Medicines Coalition, saying that cost containment should not be part of any national drug plan (Abraham, C., 2004). Kovacs Burns also stated that the "best drugs" are not likely to be the "cheapest or oldest" drugs available. Other industry-funded advocacy groups have suggested that patients have the right to sue provincial governments that don't add drugs for their condition to formularies (Somerville, 2000). In November 2004, the Supreme Court of Canada ruled unanimously that Charter protection against discrimination does not require a province to add an expensive treatment to its formulary.

Clinical practice guidelines are another means by which pharmaceutical companies collaborate with patient groups to influence prescribing practices. The Canadian Diabetes Association (CDA) recommended the insulin analogue glargine (brand name Lantus) in its industry-sponsored practice guidelines (Canadian Diabetes

Association, 2003) more than a year and a half before the drug was on the Canadian market. Based on the guidelines, physicians prescribed Lantus to patients, who had to get the drug in the U.S. When Lantus was available in Canada, the CDA organized patients to demand that it be funded through provincial drug plans (Lazaruk, 2005). The Ministry of Health guidelines in British Columbia are now based on the CDA's industry-sponsored clinical practice guidelines and included Lantus before the drug was placed on the provincial formulary with a "special authority" status ("Special authority coverage of insulin glargine," 2007).

Groups that have remained independent of industry are more likely to ask whether exaggerated claims have been made for the new drug, whether it is significantly more effective and/or safer than less costly treatments, and whether the pricing is excessive. A brief by Richard Elliott for the Canadian HIV/AIDS Legal Network specifically addresses the question of drug pricing and recommends amendments to the Patent Medicines Prices Review Board guidelines and the Patent Act. The brief recommends distinguishing between the pricing of "breakthrough" drugs and those that offer little or no therapeutic advantage over existing drugs. Another recommendation from the same brief is to allow a "reasonable" profit margin over and above the costs of development and manufacture (Elliott, R., 2003).

No health care system, whether publicly or privately insured, can give every sick person everything he or she wants. A public health care system implies sharing resources, spreading available funds across many services and prioritizing on the basis of need and evidence.

Do Industry-Funded Groups Empower Patients?

Patient empowerment is prominent in the discourse of industry-funded groups. The power supposedly comes from providing patients with information about new drug treatments for their disease, and from the muscle to lobby regulators and politicians for access to these products. The close correspondence of advocacy group views with those of their industry sponsors suggests this empowerment is more illusory than real. True empowerment comes from having independent information about diseases and their treatments, and tools to critically analyze a problem. Is it coincidence that pharma-funded groups focus their criticism of government on issues like "drug lag," formulary access to new drugs, and the ban on DTCA, while groups independent of the industry critique government partnerships with industry that have weakened the government's monitoring of drug safety and misleading claims? Based on the analysis presented in this chapter, the answer is no.

This critique is not meant to imply that patient advocacy groups that form partnerships with pharmaceutical companies intentionally align their goals with their industry sponsors. Drug companies look for individuals and organizations who share their perspective. In addition, many groups would prefer not to accept funding from the pharmaceutical industry, but they see few alternatives. The dilemma for many is that any funding is better than no funding, and industry funding allows them to mount programs to serve their communities that they could otherwise not afford. Having accepted industry money, however, organizations may become blind to its co-opting effects. The most obvious bias is that, in order to avoid biting the hand that feeds them, they may restrict their lobbying to governments, not to industry. As discussed above, studies in the medical community and psychology experiments on decision making show that conflicts of interest create very subtle biases. They are unintentional, unconscious, and indirect, but the good intentions of patient advocacy groups and their partners don't diminish their potential for harm.

Perspectives on Partnerships

How Organizations See Partnerships
Groups within the health consumer and patient communities have varied reactions to the explosion of pharma partnerships within the sector. Some are reluctant or cautious partners, accepting funds on a case-by-case basis; others welcome funding from drug companies. Still others have explicit written policies not to accept support from drug companies.

The most cynical partnership model is the front group, an organization created to covertly promote a product or political perspective. Such groups are often dubbed "Astroturf" groups because of their fake claim to grassroots status. The fact that a group receives funding from the pharmaceutical industry is not sufficient to warrant the "Astroturf" label, however (O'Donovan, 2007). Some groups begin as legitimate grassroots organizations, but undergo a process of "mission drift," which makes them hard to distinguish from Astroturf groups. American health journalist Alicia Mundy (2003) described such an evolution in an article about the Society for Women's Health Research, a group founded to promote research on women's health. The group accomplished many of its goals and its founders moved on; the new executive director began to collaborate in seminars and other events with pharmaceutical companies and formed a corporate advisory board that included Eli Lilly, Johnson & Johnson, Merck, Pfizer, and Wyeth, all manufacturers of popular drugs for women.

Canadian policy researcher Barbara Mintzes points out that drug companies can use patient groups to exploit policy loopholes. Because information and educational materials produced by patient groups are not subject to advertising regulations, a company that produces or co-produces information with a patient group can circumvent regulations that require information about a drug to be accurate and balanced. Patient groups are not obliged to acknowledge drug company sponsorships of their public events or educational materials (Mintzes, 2007).

One example of this strategy is a series of public seminars on migraines organized across Canada. Ostensibly sponsored by a patient group, the Canadian Migraine Foundation, the seminars were actually organized by Glaxo Canada in the pre-launch stage of the company's new migraine treatment, Imitrex (sumatriptan) (Mintzes, 1998). The Migraine Foundation of Canada had been dormant for some time, but the company gave it grants to hold the meetings. Participants were charged $5 for the popular seminars, a marketing strategy to increase the illusion that the events were independent of industry. When the foundation in time objected to the company's heavy-handed involvement, Glaxo transferred its support to another group, the Canadian Association of Neuroscience Nurses (Mintzes, 1998).

Groups that accept pharmaceutical company funds sometimes develop strategies that they hope will maintain their independence and credibility. Project Inform, a San Francisco-based AIDS service organization, suggests three guiding principles for AIDS groups seeking to develop ethical partnerships with the pharmaceutical industry: (1) disclosure of financial support; (2) a structured communications policy of who should talk to whom; and—most critical—(3) independence and ownership: community agencies should control their own agenda and create their own programs (Delaney, 2005).

Pat Kelly, of the Campaign to Control Cancer (C2CC), argues that corporate sponsorship can be a source of "principled, positive experiences" that enables "delivery of much-needed advocacy programs and services." In a review of sponsorship guidelines used by Canadian disease groups to set the parameters for their corporate partnerships, she found best practices guidelines include: maintaining autonomy of the group's mission, educational materials, and agenda; relying on the expertise of scientific advisers when advocating for regulatory and drug plan listings; accepting funds from corporations that have a "logical fit" with the organization's mission; disclosing corporate support on an annual basis and responding openly to inquiries about said support, while disclosing exact amounts received from a partner company only with the permission of that company; allowing use of the organization's logo only with permission; and not endorsing specific products or services (Kelly, 2002).

Other patient organizations have concluded that accepting funds from the pharmaceutical industry is inconsistent with their mission. In August 1998, the San Francisco group Breast Cancer Action (BCA) rejected a policy that allowed the group to accept donations from any company or person in favour of one that excludes pharmaceutical companies, chemical manufacturers, oil companies, tobacco companies, health insurance organizations, and cancer-treatment facilities. BCA's rationale was that the funding of any advocacy organization can appear to affect its political legitimacy. The list of off-limits corporations was compiled to exclude organizations whose interest in cancer diagnosis and treatment could bias, or be perceived as biasing, the information BCA provides about cancer treatments. Breast

Cancer Action Montreal has a similar policy on corporate funding, as do the Canadian Women's Health Network, *La Fédération du Québec pour le planning des naissances*, and *le Réseau québecois d'action pour la santé des femmes*.

Inter Pares, a Canadian social justice organization that builds relationships of common cause with activist groups around the world, critically examines the neo-liberal underpinnings of partnerships in a paper called "Rethinking Development":

> A devalued ideology of partnership has become pervasive, in which the conditions and terms of partnering relationships are determined and dictated by the partner with the money, whether donor governments, international financial institutions, corporations, or international NGOs. The symbolism of partnership usually masks the bitter realities of fundamentally unequal relationships that often represent a repudiation of sovereignty and self-determination. (Inter Pares, 2004, p. 12)

Inter Pares uses the term "counterparts" to capture an ideal of co-protagonists and colleagues who collaborate, co-operate, and conspire to change the structures and relations that perpetuate injustice and inequalities. The typical collaboration between pharmaceutical companies and patient advocacy groups is a far cry from this ideal.

How Drug Companies See Partnerships

Murray Elston, then executive director of Canada's pharmaceutical industry association Rx&D, acknowledged to the *Globe and Mail* that "at the end of the day, our focus is to have patients use our products," and described the approach as long-term: "Ultimately informed patients will be allies because they will demand the latest and most effective treatments and press politicians and bureaucrats to get them" (Picard, 2001, p. A8).

Drug companies target their support to patient groups in three areas: (1) education; (2) "disease awareness"; and (3) advocacy. Understanding the industry's goals and the infrastructure used to achieve these goals helps bring the ethical issues into clearer focus.

A survey of corporations and non-profit organizations in Canada, conducted by the public relations firm Cohn & Wolfe, found that, whereas companies used to sort through and select from requests for funding, they now use a targeted model, actively seeking partners that can provide a measurable return on investment. This model, characterized as "layered" or "multifaceted," involves a team whose members are drawn from various departments within the company, and formal relationships with groups that share the company's vision and goals. Voluntary organizations no longer see themselves as supplicants seeking handouts. They are aware that they can provide the company with tangible benefits, including credibility and the ear of regulatory agencies. In partnerships between patient advocacy groups and pharma, survey respondents described a multilayered "synergistic" arrangement in which the drug company might provide targeted educational programs about its products to patients within the organization's membership, as well as seed money to allow the organization to grow by raising additional funds in the local community. In return, the patient group could help the company develop materials that will "pique physicians' interest." Companies may set up a partnership advisory board with members from different departments, including communications, product management, and corporate and government affairs (Cohn & Wolfe, 2003, p. 32).

Two consultants from the firm PriceWaterhouseCoopers studied the factors that facilitate or inhibit pharma alliances with non-profit disease organizations in the U.S. and Canada (Chapman & Rule, 1999). They found that pharma companies and disease non-profits entered into the partnerships for very different reasons. The chief motivations for companies were to "impact corporate image" (100 percent), "share resources" (75 percent), and to "offer community support" (63 percent); additional incentives for 50 percent of corporate respondents were: "add value to a product/service," "impact marketing strategy," and "gain access to data collection." For non-profit disease organizations, the overwhelming driver was "access to financial resources" (100 percent). Other factors were the opportunity to "share resources" (60 percent), "partner request" (i.e., the group responded to a corporate overture) (60 percent), and "associate with a winning organization" (50 percent) (Chapman & Rule, 1999, p. 26). The report concluded that these alliances could be effective and meet the goals of both organizations. The following guidelines were suggested: (1) communicate overriding objectives upfront; (2) ensure accountability and gain senior management support; (3) establish trust; (4) meet regularly to compare progress and intended milestones; and (5) discuss strategies to resolve differences of opinions.

Pharmaceutical companies and groups have begun to develop "best practices," such as contracts that spell out the expectations of both sides to avoid misunderstandings. If a contract is considered too rigid to accommodate a multilayered relationship, the partners may opt for a document that specifies "principles of partnership" to which both sides agree (Cohn & Wolfe, 2003, pp. 33–34). In 2005, the Consumer's Health Forum (CHF) of Australia and Medicines Australia developed a guide and a manual called *Working Together* to assist Australian consumer health organizations and Australian drug companies with developing and maintaining mutually satisfactory working relationships. The manual includes a sample agreement (Consumers Health Forum and Medicines Australia, 2005, p. 8). A striking feature of these partnership guidelines is that they are fashioned to support harmonious collaborations between the two partners. The public, which arguably has a vested interest in the terms of these alliances, has scant opportunity to influence the relationships, the terms of which are typically confidential.

Public Relations Firms, Invisible Intermediaries

Public relations (PR) firms frequently act as intermediaries between the drug company and the patient group. In a radio documentary on the pharmaceutical industry's promotional practices, Victoria researcher Alan Cassels interviewed people who work in educational and public relations firms arranging partnerships for drug companies. The vice-president of strategic development for one such agency told Cassels that the main value of the group's support is to lend credibility to promotional material that a physician will perceive as unbiased. Credibility might actually be enhanced if the company's product brand is not mentioned, or was mentioned along with the names of competing brands:

> The manufacturer recognizes the value of having advocacy group support … mostly, truly, as an endorsement of the credibility of its content. And when you look at surveys of physicians, their top request, of course, is for unbranded, "unproduct-specific" information to be provided to them to give to their patients. (Cassels, 2003, p. 4)

The managing director of a PR firm explained how her company helped manufacturers of osteoporosis drugs raise awareness of the disease among women who were usually too young to exhibit symptoms. The goal of the campaign was to convince women in their 40s, 50s, and 60s to begin thinking of themselves as at risk for osteoporosis so that they would have bone density tests and ask their doctors about bone-strengthening drugs. The company formed a coalition made up of women's groups, health groups, and companies that employed a lot of women. The groups then promoted "osteoporosis education" among their respective memberships and eventually became a lobbying force for funding and education.

> And I think what we've succeeded in doing certainly was really putting osteoporosis higher on the agenda, certainly for public funding.… If the [bone mass measurement] test wasn't paid for, there were a lot of women who, even if their awareness was heightened, weren't going to seek that test and find out whether or not they, in fact had the early signs of that disease. (Cassels, 2003, p. 7)

Marketing professor Reinhard Angelmar and colleagues argue that a condition or disease can actually be marketed, in the same way as its drug treatment is marketed, a process they call "condition branding" (Angelmar, Angelmar & Kane, 2007). They argue that condition branding "is becoming a necessity in the increasingly fierce 'war of conditions'" in which conditions battle for limited health care resources (Angelmar, Angelmar & Kane, 2007, p. 343). The authors note that patient advocacy organizations are among the stakeholders strongly motivated to "improve the management of their respective conditions" (Angelmar, Angelmar & Káne, 2007, p. 348).

The goal of promoting drug safety is notably absent from these industry initiatives, as is information about how diet, exercise, or other non-pharmaceutical approaches contribute to health. In addition, since the campaigns are framed using the language of education, it is not clear that the organizations are aware that they are actually part of a drug marketing strategy.

In sum, industry partnerships with patient groups lack transparency in both process and spending. Even with the best intentions of groups, the partnerships can shape the public's understanding of health and illness in a way that promotes excessive drug use and compromises safety measures. The partnerships also have the potential to undermine public trust in voluntary groups. Finally, the prevalence of the partnership model marginalizes women's health advocacy groups and other health advocacy organizations whose primary concern is drug safety and accurate information.

Conclusion: Conflicts of Interest or Corruption?

Contradictory policies within Health Canada promote public participation in drug policy development, but ignore the unequal terms under which pharma-funded and independent groups participate. The lack of transparency in funding agreements between industry and health advocacy groups could eventually undermine public trust in all voluntary groups in the health sector. Because neither groups nor pharmaceutical companies are required to declare the existence of these partnerships or make public the terms of agreement, drug companies are able to use their relationships with patient organizations to avoid regulatory controls on drug promotion.

These problems are embedded in the ideology and political structures of neo-liberalism; merely requiring greater transparency in these funding arrangements would be a woefully inadequate response. We need to ask why one industry has been allowed to so thoroughly dominate the many structures that make up our health system. If there is any truth to the saying that "He who pays the piper calls the tune," the few remaining voices that contest the marketing messages of the pharmaceutical industry will soon be lost. Public funding of advocacy groups that challenge powerful interests is a legitimate public policy that should be revived.

Notes

1. In addition to funding from Women and Health Protection through the Bureau of Women's Health and Gender Analysis, Sharon Batt received financial support through Dalhousie University from the CIHR Training Program in Ethics of Health Research and Policy, from Dr. Janice Graham's CIHR grant MOP 74473—Risk and Regulation of Novel and Therapeutic Products, and from a Norah Stephen Oncology Summer Studentship.

2. In testimony to the Parliamentary Standing Committee on Health, on March 6, 2008, the vice-president of Best Medicines Coalition acknowledged that the organization receives at least half of its funding from major pharmaceutical companies.

3. On its website (www.consumeradvocare.org), Advocare describes itself as a national network of health care consumer organizations and individuals in Canada, but there is no information about who these organizations and individuals are. They also do not provide an annual report.

Part II

The Canadian
Drug Regulatory Process

There is no question that medicinal drugs must be regulated and that government must assume this responsibility. Understanding how drugs are regulated in Canada, and how effective the regulation is in protecting women's health, is therefore critically examined in this section, again with an emphasis on how these issues relate specifically to women. This examination covers the life cycle of a drug, from its development through to its potential "afterlife."

In Chapter 5, Abby Lippman examines aspects of the clinical trial process used to test the safety and efficacy of new drugs and to provide the data on which approval decisions are based. She expands her critique to question the whole system and context in which drug approvals occur.

Chapter 6, by Ann Silversides, focuses specifically on the extent to which the Canadian drug approval system is transparent to the general public. The chapter points out some of the problems caused by a lack of transparency. Ann is a journalist and author who is currently working part-time for the *Canadian Medical Association Journal*.

Taking a complementary approach in Chapter 7, Colleen Fuller discusses what happens after new drugs have been approved and are in use in the real world (as opposed to the restricted world of clinical trials). Issues related to harms caused by approved drugs and how these are reported, monitored, and followed up are discussed. Colleen is a freelance writer and activist and a co-founder of Pharma Watch.

In Chapter 8, Anne Rochon Ford provides a detailed critique of the Canadian government's plans to "update" the legislation related to drug regulation. She shows how over the past decade the government has consistently shifted from an emphasis on the precautionary principle to one of risk management. Anne is the coordinator of Women and Health Protection and the author of numerous writings on women and pharmaceuticals.

The final chapter in this section adds another dimension to the evidence that we need to rethink our relationship to pharmaceutical drugs. Sharon Batt summarizes the growing body of data on the contamination of our waterways and examines the Canadian government's approach to addressing this issue.

Chapter 5

Trials on Trial
Women and
the Testing of Drugs[1]

———•◆•———

Abby Lippman

Introduction

Prescription drug sales in Canada topped $22 billion in 2007, and well over half the medicines sold were used by women. But have these women—and the thousands taking drugs in previous years—been taking substances that had been tested only in males and might, therefore, not work, or work differently, for them? This concern has led regulatory agencies to develop guidelines and recommendations about the inclusion of women in clinical trials of drugs. However, while including women in clinical trials may begin to provide data that address average biological differences between males and females with regard to drug metabolism and kinetics, the dictum "to include" glosses too quickly over gender differences that may play a substantial role in how women use and respond to drugs. It also glosses over the multiple differences among women that mediate their responses to medicines.

In fact, wider questions about whether drugs are the best way to deal with a problem, as well as about what problems to address, are left unexamined by a singular focus on the "inclusion of women" in trials. This chapter, therefore, addresses both the narrow and the broader issues evoked in considering the inclusion of women in clinical trials, highlighting especially where gender, even more than sex, is pertinent. It goes beyond a critique of randomized clinical trials themselves to examine this research method in context so as to shed light on its meaning for women, women's health, and women's drug use.

Women and Clinical Trials: From Exclusion to Inclusion

Women have different relationships with drugs than do men, with the differences based in gender at least as much as in biology. For example, women are more likely than men to be poor and following a prescribed medication regimen may, for cost reasons alone, be quite difficult and lead to pill splitting or skipping (Lippman, 2005). Women are also more likely than men to live longer and, in consequence, experience more chronic diseases needing treatment with a range of medications, opening the door to an increased risk of harmful drug interactions. As well, the marketing of drugs is often geared primarily to women and girls, so they may be preferentially exposed to misleading information (Mintzes, 2004) (see Chapter 2).

Nevertheless, most of the discussion about including or excluding women from clinical trials has stemmed from awareness that biological variables may, on average, differ between males and females, and these differences may affect how a drug functions within the body. As Wizemann and Pardue (2001) have noted, "It has become increasingly apparent that many normal physiological functions—and, in many cases, pathological functions—are influenced either directly or indirectly by sex-based differences in biology" (p. 13). These biological differences, found among women as well as between women and men, have implications for the development of drugs and other health interventions and thus for clinical trials.

In 1994, Health Canada published guidelines about the inclusion of women in clinical trials of medications. These guidelines advocated the inclusion of women of child-bearing potential and of post-menopausal women at all stages of research to develop drugs, and urged their inclusion in sufficient numbers to enable the "*detection of clinically significant sex-related differences in drug response*" (Health Canada, 1997, p. 2; italics added). In other words, investigators were not only to bring women into studies, but to analyze the results by sex so that if there were any male/female differences, these could be identified. How did this come about? And where are we now?

Women and Pharmaceutical Research: A Brief Overview

Following the thalidomide and diethylstilbestrol (DES) disasters of the 1950s and 1960s, when it was recognized that major damage could be done to offspring of women exposed to drugs during pregnancy, it became common practice (for research purposes) to assume that all women from the time of first menstruation until menopause were "potentially pregnant." Thus, in the late 1970s, the U.S. Food and Drug Administration (FDA) adopted a policy of exclusion that basically prohibited all women—irrespective of their status with regard to sexual activity, gender identity, sexual orientation, etc.—from pharmaceutical research for fear of causing fetal harm. While this was supposed to refer only to phase 1 trials (done either on healthy people or those at the terminal stages of a disease to determine toxic levels of a drug—see Table 5.1), it was not long before the rule was applied to *all* pharmaceutical research (Stevens & Pletsch, 2002).

In the 1990s, various women's health advocates, recognizing that women were taking medications that had been tested for efficacy and safety only on men, began to lobby for inclusion of women in clinical trials. As well, health care professionals, who wanted more options for their female patients, pushed for including women in clinical trials and for trials of drugs to treat conditions that affected primarily women—and not only in their reproductive capacities. A consensus developed fairly rapidly that women had to be included in trials so they could share in any resulting benefits.

In response, the U.S. National Institutes of Health (NIH) began to formulate guidelines and then policies for the inclusion of women in clinical trials. The NIH Revitalization Act, adopted in 1993, specifically required that research funded by the NIH include women as subjects in all clinical studies.[2] It also required that NIH-funded clinical trials be adequate in size to allow analyses to determine if women were differentially affected by whatever was being studied. The U.S. FDA developed a parallel policy, but unlike the NIH approach, including women was not made mandatory.

Canadians, too, were attentive to the possible harms and injustices to women if they were excluded from clinical trials. In 1997, then Minister of Health Allan Rock announced a guideline on "Inclusion of Women in Clinical Trials" (Health Canada, 1997). Unlike the NIH policy in the U.S., this guideline only sought to "*encourage*" (my emphasis) the inclusion of women; it did not make it a requirement. It also proposed that "patients of both sexes ... be included in the same trials in numbers adequate to allow detection of clinically significant sex-related differences in drug response" (p. 2), but again, this was not made mandatory. The guideline did acknowledge, however, the importance of including, and then examining for differences, women using oral contraceptives or estrogen replacement therapy.

In both Canada and the U.S., "inclusion" referred almost exclusively to being research subjects; there was no serious mention of the need for inclusion of women in the community of researchers or in the decision-making groups that set research agendas.[3] It is also worth noting that the calls for inclusion were not always attentive to the particular role in drug research that had been played by women with disabilities and racialized and other marginalized women over the years. In fact, women in these groups actually had all too often been included in research studies, specifically of methods of contraception and, equally all too often, included without having given proper informed consent.

Internationally, the issue of including women in clinical trials of drugs has also been discussed, in particular by the International Conference on Harmonization (ICH). The ICH has specific guidelines on the conduct of clinical trials in geriatric and pediatric populations, reasoning that because of age effects (both groups) and the effects of "concomitant medications" (geriatric populations), these two populations warranted special attention in drug development. However, following a review of existing policies from the U.S., the E.U., and Japan, as well as of its own "good practice guidelines," the ICH concluded that no guidelines specifically addressing gender issues were necessary, despite requiring that a study population represent the target patient population (Guideline E8, European Medicines Agency, 2004).

At first glance, the various policy announcements on the inclusion of women appear straightforward—and uncontroversial. But, as Epstein (2004) has pointed out, they actually raise some important questions about just what "differences" between men and women require the inclusion of women in clinical trials. In other words, what is being claimed? That sex and gender are used as shorthand for biological differences? As social concepts? A combination? Why, and for what reasons, has taking account of difference "come to seem like a good thing" (Epstein, 2004, p. 189)?

At first, most of the clinical trial policy recommendations from 1993 on addressing the inclusion of women seemed to be based on the notion of distributive justice.

Women needed to participate in the trials of interventions that might be applied to them to ensure they could properly benefit from any advances. With time, and the growing numbers of women in trials, some shifts in emphasis occurred to underline how effects needed to be assessed separately in women to account for ways in which they might differ biologically—or otherwise—from men.

Table 5.1: Characteristics of Clinical Trial Phases

Phase	Purpose	Number of Patients (on average)	Type of Patients	Risks
I	Determine pharmacological actions of the drug and side effects (toxicity) associated with increasing doses	20–50	Healthy (often paid) subjects or patients in the terminal phases of an illness	Drug has never been administered to humans before; safety information is based on assumed (chemical and other) properties of drug and animal testing
II	Preliminary evaluation of efficacy of the drug; determine side effects and risks	100–300	Medical condition to be treated, diagnosed, or prevented	Wider group of patients exposed; disease in question may alter the drug's action leading to unexpected side effects
III	Gather additional information about efficacy and safety needed for further risk/benefit assessment of the drug	Several hundred to several thousand, often at multiple sites	Medical condition to be treated, diagnosed, or prevented	Wider group of patients exposed; drug administered for longer periods of time; disease in question may alter the drug's action, leading to unexpected side effects

Source: Adapted from Lexchin, J. (2008). Clinical trials in Canada: Whose interests are paramount? *International Journal of Health Services, 38*(3), 525–542.

Inclusion of Women in Clinical Trials[4]: Current Status

Over the past several years, various investigators have attempted to capture what is happening to fulfill these guidelines and regulations on inclusion. The most vigorous has been what is now called the Government Accountability Office (formerly the General Accounting Office) in the U.S. It is perhaps thanks to its reports that policies have become increasingly explicit and binding so that today, investigators in the U.S. may not obtain NIH funding if their plans for including and separately analyzing data on women are not spelled out in protocols submitted for support (National Institutes of Health, 2001).

Non-governmental groups and individuals have also assessed the inclusion of women in trials. Some focus on specific health problems, while others have looked at trials in general. Until recently, they have generally found a continuing underrepresentation of women, which is especially apparent when ethnic and minority status intersect with gender. This is underlined in a recent report from the Eliminating Disparities in Clinical Trials (EDICT) initiative, which makes it clear that reducing disparities of sex (and of age and race) in clinical trials remains an elusive goal (EDICT, 2008). It is also reported by the Australian Gender Equity in Health Research Group (Ballantyne & Rogers, 2008) who note, too, the difficulty in actually obtaining the data needed to assess the "myth or reality" of the exclusion of women.

Yet, even when more women are enrolled in trials, there has been little, if any, in-depth reporting of sex-disaggregated data, and perhaps even less clarification of how gender categories are used or conceptualized when they are presented. In fact, the current situation remains generally what it was in 2003 when Caron examined "initiatives and evaluations" carried out to "promote or support research taking into account gender and sex differences" (Caron, 2003, p. 5). His focus was on the degree to which existing guidelines and regulations were being monitored. Two of his findings remain relevant:

- While there have been major efforts in the U.S. to increase the numbers of women in clinical trials, there are no data to show "beyond doubt" that these efforts have "resulted in the desired quantitative objective" (p. 66).
- There is still insufficient disaggregation by sex of research findings, although in some areas (e.g., cardiovascular disease) this may be changing, albeit not necessarily in ways that provide solid, valid conclusions (Aulakh & Anand, 2007).

In Canada, despite the 1999 promise of the Women's Health Strategy of Health Canada to monitor the clinical trials policy on the inclusion of women, there are, even now, only general guidelines from Health Canada encouraging the inclusion of women in clinical trials. There is, as well, a federal government commitment to the application of gender-based analysis to policy and program development, but there is nothing systematic in place to evaluate what is being done in this regard. The Tri-Council policy on the ethical conduct of research involving humans states (Section 5.B, Article 5.2) that "Women shall not automatically be excluded from research solely on the basis of sex or reproductive capacity" (Canadian Institutes of Health Research, National Sciences and Engineering Research Council of Canada & Social Sciences and Humanities Research Council of Canada, 2005, p. 5.3), but there is nothing specifically about the inclusion of women in the section addressing clinical trials and there is still no *mandate* in Canada to include women in clinical trials. Moreover, most researchers still make only a statistical adjustment for sex differences rather than performing separate analyses by sex. This makes it impossible to know if a difference in sex leads to a difference in response to the drug being tested. And finally, while much has been written about where and how women and men differ biologically in ways that could underlie sex differences in drug availability and action, there continues to be almost no attention to gender matters, to questioning the binary use of gender, or even to intersectional analyses—other than to reduce these to questions of biological sex. And in a recent report (Simon et al., 2005), apparently there is minimal attention even to studying sex differences in NIH-supported research.

Clearly, there is much to criticize in the current implementation and monitoring of when and how women are included in clinical trials. When drugs are the appropriate option for the treatment of a diagnosed medical problem, women want to know that the substance(s) they will take is of proven effectiveness and safety. Have the drugs prescribed for women been tested on sufficiently large—and representative—groups to provide the information needed to assess the potential benefits and harms of their use and allow a woman to make an informed decision? All too often, these concerns remain unaddressed.

(Why) Do We Need to Include Women in Clinical Trials?

In epidemiological terms, demands for including women in clinical trials often reflect concerns about the external validity or generalizability of the research on drugs: If those who would eventually take the drug had not been studied in its development, how could we know the drug would work and be safe for them? And the past few years have demonstrated clearly the importance of studying drug effects in women separately from in men. For example, a recent analysis (Yerman, Gan & Sin, 2007) indicates that Aspirin may be less effective in decreasing non-fatal myocardial infarctions (heart attacks) in women compared to men, a difference that is hidden when all participants in a trial of this drug are lumped together.

Calls for inclusion have both justice and "scientific" rationales, and these don't always fully overlap. While inclusion is "right" to ensure that the benefits of research are shared by all and that the risks, too, are distributed fairly, including a group because they are identified as women needs to be justified on other grounds: Are sex/biology or gender questions to be addressed? Further, if expectations of biological differences are the basis for inclusion, are there reasons to anticipate that differences between sexes will be more important than those within a sex? In other words, while the biological impact of sex differences must be considered, we must also be cautious and not assume that all women are alike and/or that there is something fundamental ("essential") about being a woman that pertains to all females.[5] As well, we need to guard against making false assumptions that all male/female differences are necessarily biologically determined—or even that gender identity is a simple binary. Most important to avoid are assumptions that arbitrary biological traits are markers of innate differences between males and females.

Efficacy versus Effectiveness

Randomized clinical trials generally address questions about efficacy (how a drug works in an ideal situation among highly selected individuals), not about effectiveness (how it works—does it do what it's supposed to do—in the "real world" among the general population), and the transition from efficacy to effectiveness is neither necessarily smooth nor linear. This means that applying average results obtained in ideal circumstances to individual patients requires caution, and warns against reifying traditional clinical trials as necessarily the "best" research approach when it is, at most, "a means to an end, not an end in itself" (Oakley, 1990, p. 193).

Without question, the inclusion of a range (in age, in pre-existing conditions, etc.) of women in appropriate, well-designed, ethical clinical studies *is* important prior to a drug receiving approval. Important, too, is the development of independent, thoughtful, specific processes for post-marketing investigations and surveillance of approved drugs. However, it is important to recognize that randomized controlled trials (RCTs), even if followed by rigorous monitoring of marketed drugs, are not the only way to get useful, valid information of the kinds needed to promote and protect women's health.

A further question, therefore, is whether there is information to show that a drug is, in fact, the best option for dealing with a condition of concern. A focus restricted only to issues of inclusion of women in trials and to sex-disaggregated analyses of the data they provide may actually distract us from obtaining the possibly more important kinds of information many women actually need, including information about non-drug or holistic ways of addressing their problems, as well as about the factors that influence a woman's ability to follow a recommended drug regimen when medication is clearly needed.

Power relations in society provide women with differing resources associated with their ability, class, gender identity, etc., and as women age, these will play out in how they experience the multiple chronic conditions with which they may live for many years. Clinical trials generally involve short-term exposure to a single drug to treat or prevent a specific condition, and often exclude potential participants if they are taking other medications, have other disorders, or are deemed to be unable to comply with a

---

Box 5.1: Trials and Drugs for the Elderly

Drug trials almost always have an upper age limit for participants, and researchers continue to exclude older people. This leads to what McMurdo, Witham, and Gillespie (2005) call a "yawning chasm between patients in the real world and patients who participate in clinical studies" (p. 1037). Paula Rochon and others have noted how this practice is particularly prejudicial to women who, on average, develop some diseases later in life than men, take more medications as they get older, and also live longer than men (Rochon, Clark, Binns, Patel & Gurwitz, 1998). An arbitrary limit of age 75 for trial participation, for example, means that drugs could be prescribed for an ever-growing population of women for whom their safety and effectiveness is unknown.

This problem is compounded by there being very few, if any, trials of drugs for the elderly that have compared a new active medication with one being used in current practice. These "head-to-head" trials are not required for Health Canada approval and there is little incentive for pharmaceutical companies to mount them, in part because such comparisons might reveal the new entity to be no better, or even worse, than the existing one. In addition, such trials are more expensive to run: it is easier to show a difference between an experimental drug and a placebo than between an experimental drug and an active control. But without these comparison trials, the health and well-being of the elderly may be put at especial risk, exposing aging women to drugs that, though they have shown efficacy in placebo-controlled trials, may not be safe. This is particularly the case when there is more than one drug in a class and it is assumed, with no scientific basis, that they are interchangeable.[6]

This issue has specific relevance with regard to the development of drugs to treat or prevent cardiovascular disease (CVD). Because women tend to develop CVD at later ages, on average, than men (Avorn & Shrank, 2008), and because the probability of having other chronic diseases that may require medication also increases with age, it is not unlikely that women with CVD will be taking drugs to address other conditions (for example, hypertension, osteoporosis, multiple sclerosis). Yet, clinical trials are still set up to examine one product at a time, with those taking other medications often excluded from trials. This raises the fundamental question of whether this kind of trial has any real relevance to older women. As well, with adverse drug reactions very common among older patients, and insufficient attention to how these may be mistakenly thought to be some new disease and not a drug effect, the urgency of studying drug effects in older women becomes clear.

regimen (often a classist assumption). Thus, even when drug treatments for women's medical problems are studied in clinical trials, the very set-up of the trials—especially those that compare an active drug with a placebo rather than with a medication already in use—seriously limits the answers they can provide to questions women have about how to manage their individual situations (Petryna, 2007). Trials, by their design, primarily study medicines, not treatments, which are context-dependent.

Research Climate and the Commercialization of Research

An October 2008 listing showed 25,015 trials in the process of recruiting subjects (Ghersi & Pang, 2008). In the U.S. alone, "total grant spending for clinical trials involving human subjects [in 2002] was approximately $5.6 billion" (Getz & Zisson, 2003). Of this, more than 70 percent came from the biopharmaceutical industry (American Medical Association, Council on Scientific Affairs, 2004). This kind of monetary investment (e.g., a probable U.S. $55.2 billion research and development budget for the entire biopharmaceutical industry in 2006 [Pharmaceutical Research and Manufacturers of America, 2007]) gives this industry great power in setting research agendas, influencing the questions that will be asked, the ways in which answers will be sought, and the extent and nature of the results that are disseminated. (For more on this topic, see Chapter 4.)

The growth in contract research organizations (CROs) that design and carry out studies, offer in-house ethical review of protocols, and even provide writers for research publications is one sign of the extent to which clinical trials are becoming an industry (Association of Clinical Research Associations, n.d.). Another is the frequency of ads in community newspapers and on the radio seeking participants for clinical trials run by these private groups.

This kind of heavy industry investment leads to the development of clinical trials that are designed more with patents and profits than with women's health in mind. Compounding this is the extent to which academics are pressured into research partnerships with industry, so that even work supported with public funds—as from the Canadian Institutes of Health Research (CIHR) or provincial agencies—is privileged if it will bring benefits back to the university.[7] For example, the GlaxoSmithKline (GSK) CIHR Research Chair Award Competition notice mentions, as a specific objective, establishing chairs in disciplines where GSK has a "clear scientific interest" and fields that are "important to specific elements of development and commercialization …" (Canadian Institutes of Health Research, 2007, para. 9).

If we consider only drugs being developed to treat what probably all would agree are "real" diseases (such as breast cancer, for example), we find a pro-trial bias is also being created at the individual patient level. With trials and consent forms written in ways that may lead to what has been called a "therapeutic misconception," overstating the possible advantages of being in a study, one can raise questions about whether consent is truly informed. Pro-trial attitudes are also fostered because women are generally expected to "want to help"[8] and may feel they must conform to this expectation.

By contrast, when a woman *does* express resistance to participation in a trial despite all the lures dangled before her, and makes an informed decision not to take part, she may find herself treated as a second-class patient, if not overtly criticized.

It is essential that trials not be viewed as a default option by women who might otherwise not have access to proper care, and this is especially true in countries without publicly funded health insurance and in resource-poor countries (see p. 111 on "Outsourcing"). At the same time, it is important to recall that this "default" can be inequitably distributed: women with disabilities may be seen as ineligible for trial participation and relegated once again to what is perceived as "lesser" care, as well as deprived from knowing just which drugs are effective and safe for them to take.

Prevention Trials

The situation described above pertains primarily to those with serious medical problems who are "invited" into clinical trials that can be termed *therapeutic* trials: these trials test a product for its ability to cure, delay, or interfere with the progress of a disease. However, research today probably focuses as much on treating *risk factors* as on treating disease, so that one may also find a pro-trial bias among women when researchers and the media hype the benefits of the miraculous panaceas needed to ward off diseases such as breast cancer and chronic conditions such as osteoporosis (see Chapter 3). The constant messages of rescue and of hope, in the face of all the "risks" with which we live, may lead individuals to assume there are more benefits than harm to participating in these *preventive* clinical trials.

Primary prevention trials raise special concerns with regard to potential harms and safety since they involve giving potent drugs to healthy individuals. Prevention trials, it can be argued, must be larger than therapeutic trials because here, especially, adverse effects must be identified before marketing is approved. But, paradoxically, their very size and the need to recruit healthy participants—often by public advertising—can turn prevention trials into marketing activities, a way to make a brand name known, and a product seem desirable, even before the drug has been approved for sale!

Alternatives to "Pills for Prevention"

Although it is important and necessary to enrol women in ethical and scientifically valid clinical trials and to analyze trial data in ways that take potential sex/gender differences in responses into account, this is not sufficient if the goal is to recognize and meet women's health needs. Safe, effective medicines are important, but pharmaceutical products are not always the best—or the primary—response to women's health problems. For example, many consider prescriptions for physical exercise, rather than antidepressant medication, to be the most appropriate intervention for those with mild forms of depression, but these types of interventions are rarely studied in randomized clinical trials.

Box 5.2: Women and Statins

by Danielle Allard and Harriet Rosenberg

Cholesterol-lowering drugs, called statins (e.g., Lipitor, Crestor) are the most widely prescribed pharmaceuticals in Canada and the world. Within Canada, women account for half of those who take a statin daily.

The commonly held rationale for prescribing these drugs is based on the cholesterol hypothesis, an assumption that lowered cholesterol protects the heart and prolongs life. But even though half of those using statins are women, no gold-standard trial has tested statins' benefits or safety for this population. In fact, women are significantly underrepresented in the 14 major statin trials that do exist. U.S. cholesterol guidelines suggesting that women should be treated the same as men are based on studies that include few or even no women.

People with pre-existing heart disease are considered to be most at risk. They are called a secondary-prevention population. "Primary prevention" is the term used for treating healthy people who have some risk factors, but no overt heart problems.

The Framingham study of the 1950s was the first significant study to point to a relationship between cholesterol levels and heart disease (Kannel, 1976) and is often cited to support the mass prescription of statins. This study, however, focused only on young and middle-aged men. The authors noted that their findings were not applicable to either seniors or women.

Independent researchers who have assessed the major statin trials that did include women have concluded that there is some benefit in taking cholesterol-lowering drugs for women with pre-existing heart disease (secondary prevention). Statin use in this population of women reduced non-fatal heart attacks and strokes, and death from coronary heart disease (CHD), but did not reduce the overall death rate (Walsh & Pignone, 2004). A 2008 trial indicates that 175 women would need to be treated with Lipitor for close to five years to prevent one cardiac death in this secondary population (Wenger, Lewis, Welty, Herrington & Bittner, 2008).

However, about 75 percent of women who take statins do not have pre-existing heart disease (primary prevention). The available trial information for this category reveals that the use of cholesterol-lowering drugs does not reduce coronary or overall deaths. There is insufficient evidence to know whether CHD events (e.g., heart attacks, strokes) are reduced (Therapeutics Initiative, 2003; Walsh & Pignone, 2004).

On the basis on this research, many women's and consumer health advocacy analysts urge women to be cautious in considering drug therapy. They note that other risks like smoking, lack of exercise, air pollution, poverty, and stress are generally more important in influencing women's heart health than statin use. Furthermore, they point out that heart disease is the leading cause of death for women only after the age of 80 (Statistics Canada, 2006, p. 57).

Beyond the question of whether statins are actually effective in reducing heart disease in women are questions about the safety of this class of drugs for women. Statins have commonly been described as so safe they should be in the drinking water. There are, however, reasons to be concerned.

- Many safety assessments based on the data that are publicly available do not disaggregate their findings for women.
- Health Canada has issued an advisory that cautions women who are pregnant, intending to become pregnant, breastfeeding, or intending to breastfeed to consult their physicians before taking a statin, but has not published the sources it used to come to this conclusion.
- Statins are prescribed to women in age categories in which they have not been tested, including women of child-bearing age. Research indicates that statin exposure in younger women is associated with higher risks of miscarriage and of children born with rare and profound birth defects (Edison & Muenke, 2004).
- There is no significant research on the health implications for women taking statins and birth control drugs concurrently.
- There is inadequate research on the troubling association between statin exposure and breast cancer. In addition to a history of association between cholesterol-lowering drugs and cancer, two statin trials saw a statistically significant increase in breast cancer (Lewis et al., 1998; Shepherd et al., 2002). A 2008 trial indicates an excess in cancer mortality for women taking high-dose Lipitor (Wenger et al., 2008). Further research, beyond the relatively short duration of trials, is required to assess the long-term impact of statin use and its relation to breast and other cancers.
- Of special concern is the dual exposure of menopausal women to statins and hormone therapy. The small amount of research that currently exists on this topic found an elevated risk of breast cancer with concomitant use.

When women are asked to take a drug for life, the research underlying such guidelines should be of the highest quality; it should demonstrate clear benefit to all categories of users in comparison to non-drug alternatives. Research on potential serious adverse reactions should be extensive and publicly available for analysis. These criteria have not yet been met with regard to statin therapy and suggest that women should proceed with caution.

Perhaps if women's health advocates were among those setting research agendas, structural determinants of health might get more attention. Women's health advocates would likely ask different questions, such as: What improvements in neighbourhood facilities will promote increased time in physical activity? What policies help to reconcile paid/home work demands? Where are the clinical trials of—and other research on—these kinds of interventions? And these advocates would likely also push for the kinds of qualitative (and participatory) research needed to give us these understandings. Similarly, if "social values and consequences" were included in the "range of arguments that may be taken under consideration during deliberations on regulations," as Fox (2008, p. 3) has called for in a somewhat different context, attention would be given to the social consequences of a drug and not merely its safety and efficacy, the only grounds for approval at present.

Policy Environment and Clinical Trials[9]

As noted in a report from the James Lind Alliance, there are four major drivers of the biomedical research agenda: (1) industry, (2) government, (3) patients, and (4) the general research community. These are not, if ever, easily reconcilable (James Lind Alliance & the Association of Medical Research Charities, 2007). Nevertheless, understanding their often-competing needs and goals emphasizes that the policy environment is no less likely to influence the nature of clinical trials than is the research environment. In this light, the ongoing overall restructuring of Health Canada—and other branches of government—under the umbrella of streamlining regulations becomes relevant (see Chapter 8). Space limits preclude discussion of this major policy shift here, but some have suggested that this move to join economic growth with the development of "safe" drugs and devices is not a plan for health-protecting regulations and can only set the stage for what bioethicist Sue Sherwin has called "incoherence" in policy values with respect to drug regulation: Can government commitment to health and well-being be compatible with its support of industry and the economic development of the biotech/pharmaceutical sector?

The answer is probably obvious when we learn that the use of cost-recovery mechanisms and decreases in the time for drug approvals, components of "streamlined regulations," lead not only to reduced vigilance in testing the safety of drugs and devices, but to a host of policies and mechanisms that favour industry over the individual (Council of Canadians, n.d.; Lexchin, 2005). Thus, the new clinical trials regulatory framework that became active in 2001 had, as an explicit goal, a decrease in the time taken to review new drug applications. This approach is apparent as well in some of the features of Bill C-51, introduced to Parliament in April 2008.

This climate provides at least a partial explanation for the lack of adequate surveillance and monitoring of drugs in the marketplace, a lack especially relevant to women, since of 10 drugs recalled recently in the U.S. because of dangers they posed, eight were substances that caused greater risks for women than for men (Simon et al., 2005). It is true that, even if there had been women in all the pre-marketing trials of these drugs, harm might not have been seen until after the substance was in wide use in the population. But regulations designed to accelerate drug approvals tend to lead to therapeutic trials of very limited size and of short duration, as well as the use of homogeneous populations and surrogate end points. (A trial has a surrogate end point when the outcome measure, for example, cholesterol level, is used as a substitute for a clinically meaningful end point that measures directly how a patient feels, functions, or survives.) In this scenario, uncommon harms—and if there will really be any meaningful effectiveness—are often not revealed before a drug is put onto the market. Clearly, this underscores the importance of vigilance after, as well as before, a drug is marketed.

As for prevention trials, these must have the most stringent regulatory overview and post-market monitoring, with advertising completely prohibited until there are solid data about the long-term safety and specific effectiveness of the drug.

The regulatory system is woefully remiss in ensuring that phase 4, or post-marketing, trials are carried out after a drug is for sale and being taken by those who have probably not been represented in earlier study populations. And this is particularly problematic given that commitments to such trials, often a condition of regulatory approval, are frequently not fulfilled (Schuchman, 2008). Thus, the Canadian government's plan to initiate a "Drug Safety and Effectiveness Network" is a positive step, but one that may be insufficient given it will have only $1 million in funding to get it started (Health Canada, 2008).

Key Clinical Trials Issues

Concerns about clinical trials—and about all aspects of the pharmaceutical industry and its regulation—are multiplying daily. Parliamentary committees (in Canada and the U.K.), journalists, and academic scholars are examining and critiquing current and past practice, each taking on different drugs (e.g., SSRIs and Vioxx [rofecoxib]). How clinical trials are funded, the length of the trial, what is used for comparison with a study drug, and what outcomes (end points) are considered relevant are among many issues of concern. However, even those who have voiced these concerns tend to do so as if they were gender-neutral.

With the exception of rare calls for public financing of drug trials (Lewis, Reichman & So, 2007), solutions for some of the problems that have been identified have generally emphasized the full reporting of trial data, as well as an open/public registry of the protocols of all drug trials on an easily accessible website.[10] These are clearly necessary steps, but they are not sufficient, even if there were not already signs of non-compliance and of limited transparency (Zarin, Tse & Ide, 2005). To begin to address specifically gender-related concerns about clinical trials of drugs, the following issues are among those needing particular attention.

Beyond Numbers

Most studies related to inclusion have focused on the numbers of women in trials. This focus is far from sufficient. Not only must women be included in studies of all drugs that they may use, but all resulting data must, at a minimum, conform to existing guidelines and be sex-disaggregated when they are presented, so that lessons for women can be obtained.[11] There must be sufficient numbers in any subgroup to be analyzed for the data to be robust and useful, and these analyses must be planned in advance to avoid the false inferences that can come from data dredging (the inappropriate search for statistically significant relationships in large quantities of data): underpowered analyses may do more harm than good if the results are seen as definitive. Moreover, other relevant features (ethnicity, class, age, etc.) need to be accounted for in study protocols and described in published studies in meaningful ways. Above all, when differences are found between male and female participants, between individuals of different ethnicities, etc., it should not be assumed automatically that they have only or necessarily a biological basis. As well, study designs and analyses must take into account the diversity among women and carefully conceptualize how gender, sex, and other markers of "difference" are to be understood.

Further, if women are underrepresented in a trial, we must be told why: Were they not asked to take part? Were they asked, but declined? Were they appropriately ineligible? Did they lack the resources that would allow participation? Without knowing *why* there is underrepresentation (overall or only some groups of women), appropriate remediation is impossible, as is the ability to make valid inferences from the data presented. And assessing the nature and the full implications of underrepresentation will require an integrated and intersectional gender-based analysis. This will mean that current guidelines about the inclusion of women in trials and for sex-disaggregated analyses become not only mandatory requirements for regulatory approval and funding decisions, but that full justification for how the concepts are used be provided. It will also require that research ethics boards reviewing study protocols be provided with training and resources that will equip them to consider these issues appropriately (cf. Ballantyne & Rogers, 2008).

Safety and Effectiveness as Gender Issues

Numbers alone cannot cover the absence from trials of women (older, impoverished, stigmatized, with co-morbidities, etc.) for whom the intervention being studied may be most relevant. Often, only when it is in "real world" use can the true nature of a drug's benefits be assessed and potential lost opportunity costs and social consequences emerge. And it is in the real world that gender differences—and differences among women—with regard to a drug's safety may be most relevant. Clinical drug trials have inherent limits. This means that independent, broadly conceived post-marketing studies of new therapeutic drugs must be made mandatory. Monitoring adherence to phase 4 trial commitments and applying sanctions for non-compliance are also important. Moreover, any drug that has been given accelerated approval must be labelled specifically with this information noted on mandatory patient leaflets to warn potential users of the minimum testing the drug has received in advance. As well, this information should include the numbers, sex, and ages of those in clinical trials of the product.

- *Consent Forms and Literacy*
It is essential to ensure that informed choices about participation in trials are more than pro forma. This requires attention to informed consent material and to the informed consent process. Given the limited health literacy levels of many Canadians, with particularly low levels among immigrant and older women (Rootman & Gordon-El-bihbety, 2008), there are serious doubts that many women can give truly authentic consent to trial participation. Even for women who are print literate, other factors related to expectations of medical care, understanding of random assignment, placebos, and probability, can compromise the ability to give truly informed consent (Stead, Eadie, Gordon & Angus, 2005).

As the number of those who use languages other than English and French increases in Canada, the common requirement for women to be able to read and/or write in one of the official languages may be an inclusion criterion that keeps many out of a study. This may lead to underrepresentation of immigrants and other minorities. In addition, given gender- and class-based differences in doctor-patient relationships, one needs to be attentive to the possibility of gender-based differences in how the informed consent process itself is carried out.

Tracking Inclusion of Diverse Groups
"Women" are a diverse lot; it is important to pay attention to subgroups and to socially relevant features that may be operative in women's health studies. Policies about trial registration (for example, by the CIHR and by peer-reviewed professional journals) that mandate the public posting, prior to the start of any research, of basic information about a trial (e.g., purpose, funding source, patient population, etc.) on an easily accessible website, and the requirement for the prior submission of complete protocols that clearly indicate the end points to be analyzed in a study are a first—and necessary—step in promoting improved clinical trials. However, it is not clear that these practices will facilitate the kinds of tracking needed to monitor the status of women in clinical trials, to address gender-based concerns, or even to ensure unbiased and complete reporting of results from all registered trials. Registering trials in a global register, provided there are sufficient data, including results from completed and aborted trials, will provide a "snapshot," but an active process for tracking the research and the ways in which inclusion is considered is needed.

Pregnancy and Pregnant Women

In the past, concerns about pregnancy and fetal exposures were the basis for the exclusion of women from drug research. This gendered inequality is most obvious in phase 1 and phase 2 trials. Paradoxically, however, it may be safer to expose women in phase 1 and 2 trials (as opposed to phase 3 trials) since these are often very short in duration, making it unlikely that a woman would conceive during such a trial. Further, without the basic physiologic and other data these early stage trials provide, the medication dose to which women in phase 3 trials are exposed may be inappropriate and even harmful.

With the focus on possible effects on the fetus of drugs a woman might take (and these are far from trivial), research attention has been diverted from the potential harms to women if they are *excluded* from trial participation. These include the harms that might occur if safe drugs for treating a pregnant woman for an established medical condition are not developed.[12] And sometimes treatments are widely used during pregnancy, although they have not been tested in clinical trials that included pregnant women. For example, a population-based study in British Columbia found that 5 percent of pregnant women took antidepressants in 2001, over twice as many as did in 1998 (Oberlander, Warburton, Misri, Aghajanian & Hertzman, 2006).

As maternal age at first pregnancy increases, it is becoming more likely that a woman will have some problem needing medication to maintain her health when she is pregnant. Thus, it is essential to get information about the safety of these drugs. For this reason, as well as to avoid treating heterosexuality as the norm (heteronormativity), and to ensure that women are not treated with a lack of trust with regard to being able to make decisions about their sexual activities and contraceptive use (Downie, Munden & Butler, 2003), trial criteria for in/exclusion must be based on individual realities, not false assumptions about women's sex lives, sexual orientation, and capacity for responsibility. Standard consent procedures must allow a woman to decide for herself how to balance the possible risks to her, her pregnancy, or her fetus, with the possible advantages of participating in a clinical trial. Moreover, pregnancy exclusions should apply equitably to men and women given the evidence that damage to a fetus can be transmitted via sperm.

Clearly, there are obvious safety reasons to avoid enrolling pregnant women in trials unless the drug is one that is likely to be prescribed for them and there is a strong likelihood of benefit and little expectation of harm. However, widespread untested use of antidepressants, for example, may put many more women at more risk than if clinical trials had been carried out under controlled conditions on specific volunteers. In discussing births to women who took the antidepressant paroxetine (Paxil), Einarson et al. argue that drug exposure is less dangerous than untreated depression, and that "For obvious reasons, it is impossible to conduct a randomized controlled study of women taking drugs during pregnancy" (Einarson et al., 2008, p. 751).

It is inappropriate to assume that any product used during pregnancy is either safe or harmful. In the case of depression, such an assumption takes for granted—as Einerson et al. did in the absence of supportive data—that antidepressants offer greater therapeutic benefit than non-drug approaches.

Trials as a Way to Better Care and Outsourcing

Against a background of media reports in Canada about growing waiting lists, a shortage of physicians and nurses, and increasing privatization of health services, it is essential that clinical trials do not become a default option for women who might otherwise not obtain access to proper care. Thus, any hospital that participates in clinical trial research must ensure that no woman's care is jeopardized in any way by *not* taking part in research.

Conversely, there has been an increasing outsourcing of research[13] to lower wage markets, and a growing enrolment in trials in Canada by women seeking paid employment. Drug companies may move trials (to test interventions that will be used by privileged women) to emerging markets under the cover of good business (i.e., to allow for cheaper drug development). This will, however, shift harms and burdens onto poor and otherwise vulnerable women, women from whom, experience has shown, informed consent is not always obtained and who are less likely to have access to the drug if it eventually reaches the market (Schipper & Weyzig, 2008). These trials, too, have occasioned concern about their research ethics: Was truly informed and freely given consent obtained? Was this compromised by direct or indirect financial inducements? Is there appropriate oversight of trials done elsewhere? Women in Canada should not gain at the expense of others.

What Does and Does Not Get Studied

It is not clear that the frequency of drug trials corresponds with the conditions most prevalent among women and for which there is most need for safe, effective pharmaceutical intervention (Perell, Miranda, Ortiz & Casas, 2008). This is not to presume that all that ails women needs drug treatment, but to acknowledge that there remain serious medical conditions for which appropriate pharmaceutical interventions are unavailable or of unproven safety or about which substantial uncertainties regarding their effects remain—and this is painfully true for those living in resource-poor countries.

To promote the development of these innovative and potentially beneficial treatments, the added value of new products should be considered in drug approval decisions, as should be the degree to which they meet unmet and real needs. As noted above, regulators need to have authority to make decisions on matters such as social value and the impact on health inequities of a product and not merely on its safety and efficacy. Moreover, especially rigorous standards must be applied in judging the safety and effectiveness of "me too" formulations. Both therapeutic importance and cost effectiveness need to be considered and this often requires head-to-head comparisons of interventions. Perhaps a policy to withhold public funds from drug trials unless they address important health questions and are unbiased by commercial interests in their design, implementation, analysis, and reporting should be developed.

Conclusion

Randomized clinical trials can provide useful, albeit limited, information related to pharmaceutical treatment and the prevention of health problems among women. However, merely involving (more) women in clinical trials will not guarantee that the information will be truly reliable and useful, and it certainly must not be the sole concern in examining the relationship(s) between women and clinical trials. Fundamental is first asking *why* a drug trial is being proposed; whether—and *how*—gender and sex have been taken into account in the development of a drug; and whether a drug is the most appropriate means for addressing a problem. This latter concern is particularly relevant in prevention trials. Only when a drug trial seems appropriate as the answer to a specific problem—and ideally, a question that women themselves want addressed—do technical questions about the trial protocol (recruitment of participants, analyses, etc.) become relevant. Even the best of trials may be wrong if they are not suited to an actual problem women face. And they will certainly risk being irrelevant if they do not study outcomes that women themselves find interesting and desirable. Obtaining these critical insights may require qualitative research prior to the designing of a clinical trial.

Consequently, clinical trials must not only accommodate gender differences, they must also become a site for the transformation of gender relations in the biomedical/ health care world, including the strengthening of women's roles in health research. Some of the issues requiring attention are: the training of those carrying out trials to privilege the involvement of women; promotion of user/patient input into choosing questions, designing studies, and performing analyses; challenging all inferences from men to women; studying end points that are gender-sensitive; and ensuring that interventions recognize the social positions of women participating in trials.

In this regard, gender concerns should be addressed in choosing study questions as well as in study design so that women do not face either improper inducements encouraging participation, or structural barriers preventing participation. Furthermore, specific—and authentic—attention must be given to issues of diversity, so that the drugs studied meet the needs of a full range of women, including women with disabilities, racialized women, and bisexual, lesbian, and transgendered women. Using the terms "appropriate" or "adequate" representation of women in guidelines and policy statements is insufficient; specifics about the women (e.g., details about who and how many they are), not generalities, are required.

Moreover, choosing the outcome to be used as a measure of success of a drug tested in a therapeutic trial must take into account its relevance to the women who will be given the drug if it works (e.g., with regard to an increase in survival, an improvement in quality of life, an easier management regime, etc.). With the increasing support of industry for clinical trials, there is a concomitant increase in the use of surrogate laboratory-based markers to define effectiveness, but too often such things as a decrease in tumour size or in some biochemical measurement does not indicate longer survival or a better quality of life. If a surrogate marker of success is used, it must at the least be shown to be relevant to the women to be studied.

Last, but perhaps most important, women (including women's health advocates) must be included when decisions are made about what research to do and how to do it. It is not sufficient to include women as research subjects; they must also be included further upstream, helping inform research and funding decisions, and, of course, priorities. Involvement of patients and patients' groups is increasingly accepted; however, there is need for vigilance to ensure that these individuals and groups are truly community-based and not speaking for industrial funders (see Chapter 4). Who is being represented and to whom one is accountable are critical questions to ask, with recent concerns about pharmaceutical funding of the European Patients' Forum (Health Action International Europe, 2005) underscoring the need for involving community-based individuals.[14]

Clinical trials answer specific—and very narrow—questions. These *do* need to be asked if we are to have safe and efficacious medicines to treat real diseases, and we must answer these questions with the best study designs and analyses. However, we need to recognize that RCTs are *one* way, but not the only way, to get the information we need about how to respond to women's health problems. We also need to recognize and apply as study outcomes human risks and benefits that cannot be commodified (Hankivsky, 2007). In this regard, we need to validate and credit observational and other forms of expertise, and develop health promotion and disease treatment options outside a reductive medical model and separate from commercial influences.

Notes

1. While several students helped me locate references—and were perhaps exhausted by my seemingly endless quest for more—two warrant particular thanks: Elizabeth (Liz) Turner, for all she did—and her patience in doing it—in the earliest stages of the research from which this chapter derives, and Emilia Ordolis, for her contributions to bringing things to closure here.

2. Several authors (e.g., Baird, 1999; Mastroianni, Faden & Federman, 1994, 1999; Merkatz, 1998; Prout & Fish, 2001) have detailed the historical events leading up to this decision and will not be repeated here.

3. Something beyond mere inclusion that women wanted was good research on the problems that were most prevalent among us, as well as studies to learn if medications already marketed were safe and effective. These wants remain mostly unaddressed.

4. This report uses the term "clinical trials" to refer primarily to phase 3 trials.

5. For example, studying males and females separately may be of less importance in a drug study than separating subgroups on the basis of weight or some other feature related to how a drug may work.

6. In October 2008, the World Medical Association Declaration of Helsinki was revised, and the changes to these guidelines that govern much medical research include a tightening of the limits on using placebos and a statement that "a new intervention must be tested against ... the best current proven intervention" (World Medical Association, 2008, para. 32).

7. Sheldon Krimsky (2003) has referred to the pharmaceutical business as a "vertically integrated industry" in which drug development, guideline development, physician education, drug promotion, etc., are all under the same aegis.

8. A particularly problematic paper suggesting that "scientific research is a moral duty" by John Harris in the March 2005 issue of the *Journal of Medical Ethics* is further cause for concern.

9. For a more detailed discussion of the issues raised in this section, see Downie (2006).

10. For example, www.Clinicaltrials.gov operated by the NIH in the U.S., with such registration recently becoming a requirement for consideration of later publishing of results by peer-reviewed medical journals (DeAngelis, Drazen, Frizelle, Haug, Hoey et al., 2004).

11. Because there can be basic biological differences between males and females at all levels, from cells to the whole organism, the possibility of sex differences needs to be considered even when cell or non-human animal models are employed in the development and testing of drugs in the laboratory.

12. In September 2007, the American College of Obstetricians and Gynecologists (ACOG) published ACOG Committee Opinion #377, "Research Involving Women," in which the critical importance of including women in research trials was emphasized (American College of Obstetricians and Gynecologists, 2007).

13. Outsourcing takes several forms, including the running of trials by for-profit commercial research organizations (CROs), ghostwriting of medical papers, and the hiring of paid spokespeople to promote company products (Healy, 2005).

14. In this regard, it is of interest that as of January 1, 2006, the Association of the British Pharmaceutical Industry has changed its code of practice so that all drug companies must "make public their involvement with patients' advocacy groups" (Day, 2006).

Chapter 6

Lifting the Curtain on the Drug Approval Process

———◆◆◆———

Ann Silversides

Introduction

In the fall of 2004, Canada's federal minister of health took the unusual step of criticizing Health Canada's policy of keeping secret the results of clinical trials submitted by drug companies when they apply to have new prescription drugs approved for marketing. The Hon. Ujjal Dosanjh told a gathering of health researchers:

> Questions have been raised as to whether Canadians are well served when the results of all clinical trials are not publicly disclosed. As an advocate for public health, it is difficult to me to defend such secrecy.... I want to make it clear tonight that I have a bias on this issue in favour of disclosure, and except for legitimate and compelling reasons of privacy or commercial confidentiality, this is the direction in which our Department of Health shall move. I encourage industry and other parties to work with Health Canada toward that goal because there is no turning back. (Dosanjh, 2004, para. 62)

The former health minister's comments came in the wake of well-publicized revelations of serious harm associated with heavily marketed and widely used prescription drugs, such as Vioxx (rofecoxib) and the SSRI class of antidepressants. The revelations threw a spotlight on concerns that vital information about drugs is routinely withheld from the public not only by the drug industry, but also by government regulators, who are presumably mandated to make known vital information that is in the public's interest.

This chapter provides a brief history of the controversy about Canada's drug approval system, an outline of how the system works, and an examination of the usefulness of the Access to Information process as a way to obtain drug approval information. The chapter examines the extent to which transparency does or does not exist—what is made public and what is not—and argues that, currently, far more is kept secret than can be legally justified and, further, that this lack of transparency is not serving the public interest. The approval procedures for two other key jurisdictions, the United States and the European Union, are outlined briefly, and the implications of industry funding of the drug approval process are considered.

Drug Approval Secrecy: Some History about the Controversy

Two key events drew attention to the importance of public access to all clinical data about drugs authorized for marketing: the September 2004 worldwide recall of the widely prescribed arthritis medication Vioxx and, that same year, revelations about the dangers associated with the use of the selective serotonin reuptake inhibitors (SSRIs) class of antidepressants. Pharmaceutical giant Merck withdrew its drug Vioxx after a clinical trial proved that it increased the risks of heart attacks and strokes. But for several years before that, serious problems with the drug had been documented and were on file with regulators, including Health Canada, and internal company documents showed that Merck's scientists were concerned about risks (Berenson, 2005). (Three years after the withdrawal, Merck agreed to spend $4.85 billion to settle 27,000 lawsuits launched by or on behalf of individuals who said they suffered harm from taking the drug [Berenson, 2007].) Meanwhile, the dangers associated with the SSRI antidepressants were discovered in clinical trials that had never been published, but were also known to health regulators (Whittington, Kendall, Fonagy, Cottrell, Cotgrove et al., 2004). The clinical trials revealed the drugs were of negligible benefit and sometimes harmful for young people and adolescents.

Why is important information being withheld? The definition and treatment of "confidential third-party information" appears to be the key factor cited by Health Canada in keeping clinical trial information from the public. However, drug agencies and inspectorates "often maintain secrecy to a much greater extent than law or logic actually demand," according to the International Working Group on Transparency and Accountability in Drug Regulation, a group convened in Uppsala, Sweden, in 1996 by Health Action International and the Dag Hammarskjoeld Foundation (Health Action International, 1996). The fact that the U.S. drug approval process is significantly more transparent than Canada's underscores this point (see Table 6.1).

Health Canada repeatedly assures Canadians that its drug-approval process is rigorous and of the highest standard (see Box 6.1), but external expert groups complain that too little information is provided to the medical community, researchers, and consumers. It is not just clinical trial results, but also related information, such as full reports of expert advisory groups and names of drugs refused authorization for marketing, that are withheld. Notwithstanding Health Canada's assurances, it is difficult, perhaps impossible, to evaluate the integrity of a process when you can't get basic information about it. Health Canada makes public far less information than does its U.S. counterpart, the Food and Drug Administration (FDA), and even Health Canada officials have referred to the "black box" nature of their own agency's operation.[1]

Drug approval decisions are most important to Canadians in terms of benefit and harm, as the Vioxx and SSRI stories reveal, but costs also factor into the equation. Drugs are the second largest category of health care spending in Canada, after hospitals, and spending on prescription drugs was expected to reach $22.5 billion in 2007, an increase of $1.6 billion over the previous year (Canadian Institute for Health Information, 2008, p.v). Meanwhile, total spending on prescription drugs in Canada rose an average of 11.2 percent a year from 1997–2004—faster than spending in any other health care category, except capital costs (which represent a much smaller dollar amount). Put another way, per person expenditures on prescription drugs in Canada almost doubled from 1998–2004.

Box 6.1: Health Canada Repeatedly Assures Canadians That Its Drug-Approval Process Is Rigorous and of the Highest Standards

- Canada has one of the most rigorous drug-approval systems in the world and one of the best safety records (Medical News Today, 2004, para. 2)
- HPFB strives to ensure that the potential benefits of all health products outweigh their risks. Our highest priority is public safety. Before any health product or veterinary drug is authorized for sale in Canada, the manufacturer must provide HPFB with substantive scientific evidence of its safety, efficacy, and quality. Highly skilled HPFB scientists review this evidence carefully to determine whether the potential risks from the health product are acceptable when balanced against its positive effects (Health Products and Food Branch, 2007).

Unfortunately, it is difficult, if not impossible, to evaluate the integrity of the process if you cannot get basic information because such information is not public.

Another aspect of the controversy is that the pharmaceutical industry now co-funds Health Canada's drug approval system and critics charge that this arrangement has led to a situation where the regulator is inclined to view industry, not the public, as its client.

The level of secrecy maintained around Health Canada's drug approval process has long been criticized by medical and scientific bodies, at least one parliamentary standing committee, consumer groups, and the media. Health Canada, meanwhile, has publicly endorsed the concept of greater transparency in the drug approval process, especially in the past few years, but action on this front has been slow in coming.

During Canada-wide public consultations about replacing the *Food and Drugs Act*, one of the "consistent strong messages was that the lack of public confidence in Health Canada cannot be fully addressed until the activities of the department are made more transparent" (Health Canada, 2003, Section 2.2.1). Another strong message during the 1998 consultations was that "the right of Canadians to be informed should prevail over the right of industry to have confidential commercial information protected, when disclosure of this information is necessary for the protection of public health" (Health Canada, 2003, Section 2.2.2).

A report from Health Canada's own Scientific Advisory Board, released in early 2000, found that the current drug review process is "unnecessarily opaque." Canada can "at least emulate the standards of our nearest and largest trading partner," concluded the report: "No observer can fail to be struck by the fact that the same companies that insist on secrecy when it comes to their applications in Canada are perfectly prepared to send senior scientific and management representatives to public hearings in Washington, there to present details of their research and answer detailed questions on the science supporting their applications to the FDA" (Scientific Advisory Board to Health Canada, 2000, Appendix D, 4.2.2). The report dismisses arguments that domestic law and international treaties require that Health Canada maintain a high level of confidentiality: "Canada would not be subject to any action under these treaties if we adopted procedures which were no more transparent than those of our largest trading partner, the United States" (Scientific Advisory Board to Health Canada, 2000, Appendix F, p. 1). The Science Advisory Board report argued that "safety and well-being of the person must take precedence over considerations of commercial advantage or bureaucratic process" (Scientific Advisory Board to Health Canada, 2000, p. 12).

Four years later, in January 2004, an open letter composed by the Canadian Health Coalition and signed by hundreds of Canadians was sent to then Prime Minister Paul Martin expressing alarm about Health Canada's proposal to replace Canada's *Food and Drugs Act*. A key rationale for proposing changes, according to Health Canada, was the act's "too narrow focus on safety." As one of six key demands, the letter urged the prime minister to "allow full public access to the information upon which federal regulators base approval of a product or technology" (Douglas et al., 2004, p. 2).

A couple of months later, in April 2004, the House of Commons Standing Committee on Health's report on prescription drugs observed that individual Canadians "may be harmed by the lack of scrutiny and by a dearth of independently assessed information." The committee "does not support a clinical trial system that discourages openness in order to protect commercial interests" (Standing Committee on Health, 2004, p. 4). The committee recommended that Health Canada introduce measures to ensure public confidence, starting with a public database that provides information on clinical trials in progress, trials abandoned, and trials completed.

In May 2004, the Canadian Association of Journalists awarded Health Canada its annual Code of Silence Award. In bestowing the award for Health Canada's "efforts to shroud open government," the journalists' association press release took particular aim at the drug approval process, quoting from the all-party Standing Committee on Health report, which found "the manner in which drugs are tested and approved is too secretive, in large part due to excessive concerns about the commercial interests of the drug companies" (Canadian Association of Journalists, 2004).

The Prescription Drug Approval System

Canada's drug approval process falls under the responsibility of the Health Products and Food Branch (HPFB), formerly known as the Health Protection Branch. A number of directorates and offices fall under the aegis of the HPFB. The prescription

---

Box 6.2: The Purposeful Creation of Ignorance

---

by Diane Saibil

The lack of transparency in the drug approval process affects everyone, but it is of particular significance to women. As pointed out in previous chapters, women are often the targets of drug advertisements, women consume more drugs than men (in part because they live longer), and women are often the purveyors of health information and the drug purchasers for the family unit.

It is instructive to view the culture of secrecy within the Canadian drug approval process through the lens of Nancy Tuana's writings about the construction of ignorance (Tuana, 2006). Tuana lists and describes several types of socially constructed ignorance, ignorance that is more than a simple gap in knowledge, but rather a gap that is purposefully created. She includes a category called "They do not want us to know" and goes on to say, "One of the aims of the women's health movement was to provide women with access to medical knowledge that had been made inaccessible through professionalization and which had constructed women as objects of knowledge not as authorized knowers" (p. 9).

When it comes to the regulation of prescription drugs in Canada, a great deal is known by drug manufacturers and government regulators, while most people— including both health care practitioners and consumers—are kept in the dark. This appears to be a clear example of Tuana's "They do not want us to know" category. This deliberately imposed ignorance compromises the ability of health care consumers to make informed health care decisions on behalf of themselves and their families.

SSRI antidepressants are a case in point. This class of drugs, prescribed much more frequently for women than for men (Currie, 2005), is also prescribed for children. If a more transparent system had provided timely information about the risks and lack of efficacy of SSRI antidepressants, how many more women would have balked at filling prescriptions for themselves and for their children?

Another example has been documented by Barbara Seaman in her important work on estrogen (Seaman, 2003). Seaman argues that manufacturers of estrogen-based birth control pills were aware of the dangerous health effects of their products quite early on, yet they deliberately kept this information out of the public arena, thereby constructing and maintaining consumer ignorance.

---

drug-approval process is handled by the HPFB's Therapeutic Products Directorate. Biologics—blood products, vaccines, and drugs derived from biotechnology—are approved by another directorate, the Biologics and Genetic Therapies Directorate. Previously, the Therapeutic Products Programme (TPP) was responsible for both prescription drugs and biological and genetic therapies. The TPP was also responsible for monitoring the safety of marketed health products.

To have a drug approved for sale in Canada, the pharmaceutical manufacturer has to test it on cells and tissues, on animals, and, finally, on people in order to ensure that the drug is acceptably safe and effective. The manufacturer must submit to the regulator basic chemistry, laboratory data, animal studies, and manufacturing information, as well as the results of clinical trials. The results of all clinical trials must be submitted, regardless of their outcome.

The information provided to Health Canada by drug companies is considered, by Health Canada, to be proprietary to those companies and thus secret. Researchers and media who seek information about the approval process for a given drug must submit Access to Information (ATI) requests. The amount of information released under ATI can be extremely limited, and the process is usually slow.

Box 6.3: Members of the Public Do Not Have Access—or Have Very Limited Access—to the Following Information from Health Canada

- the names of the drugs in the regulatory approval system
- results of clinical trials
- full comments of Health Canada reviewers about information submitted
- information about indications applied for, but refused authorization, in the case of drugs that are approved for another use
- names of drugs that are refused authorization to market (i.e., drugs that receive a Notice of Non-compliance)
- how long companies have to meet the conditions placed on drugs that receive a Notice of Compliance with Conditions (NOC/c) (see the section on NOC/c later in this chapter) and the company's progress toward meeting those conditions
- the full reports of expert advisory committees, including rules concerning selection of members

---

What We Don't Know

Names of Drugs in the Regulatory Approval Process

In Canada it is not possible, pre-approval, to find out the names of drugs that have been submitted to Health Canada for approval—at least not from Health Canada. Drug companies themselves, on the other hand, are free to make this information available and sometimes do.

Results of Clinical Trials

In order to gain approval for a new drug, pharmaceutical companies must submit to the regulator the results of clinical trials. In Canada, this information is considered proprietary to the drug company. Independent and public interest researchers and the public are unable to scrutinize the basis on which a drug receives approval in Canada. Even provincial drug evaluators, whose job is to recommend whether a drug should be listed in a provincial formulary so that eligible patients can have drug costs at least partially covered, don't have access to all of the clinical trial information.

Meanwhile, evidence about the way some clinical trials are conducted and reported has set alarm bells ringing. At issue are the ways that clinical trials, most of which are effectively controlled by the pharmaceutical companies, can be (and are) manipulated to produce biased results. The results of failed trials for drugs that have been approved (trials that show harm, or no benefit, from a drug) can go unreported or unpublished (Baird, 2003), while positive results from the trials for the same drugs are sometimes published many times in different journals, creating a misleading impression about the drug (Melander, Ahlqvist-Rastad, Meijer & Beermann, 2003).

The International Working Group on Transparency and Accountability in Drug Regulation, in a 1996 statement, observed that, among other consequences, secrecy impedes development of knowledge (particularly dangerous where suspicion arises of a hitherto unknown risk), can serve to hide malpractice (such as "falsification or suppression of unfavourable data by certain companies, or submission of inconsistent files on the same drug to different agencies" [Health Action International, 1996, Section 5]), and may facilitate use of substandard drugs and irrational drug use. Issues that surfaced regarding the clinical trials for SSRIs illustrate these points. In June 2004, Health Canada issued a warning about the class of antidepressants known as SSRIs because of their potential for harm (Health Canada, 2004). This risk of harm applied to everyone, but was of particular concern because of the number of young people taking the drugs. Unknown to the doctors prescribing drugs to this age group, clinical trials that had been conducted in under-19-year-olds showed evidence of harm, no benefit, or extremely modest benefit from the drugs when compared to a placebo (Garland, 2004).

These trials were submitted to Health Canada as part of the drug approval process, but, as is the current policy of the regulatory agency, were not available to anyone outside the agency. Pharmaceutical manufacturers, meanwhile, had simply chosen not to publish those trial results that did not cast a positive light on their product (only six of the 15 trials conducted on children and adolescents have been published). SSRIs are being prescribed to thousands of Canadian teenagers. By 2002, according to IMS Canada, a private health information company, treatment with medication was recommended to fully 80 percent of those 18 and under who were seeking help for depression (Bongers, 2004).

Health Canada's June 2004 advisory notes that SSRIs are not authorized for use in patients under 18 years of age and states that doctors prescribe them for this "off-label" use "at their discretion." The advisory does not provide any more details about the efficacy (or lack thereof) of these drugs.

But in prescribing these drugs to teenagers, doctors had access to "an incomplete and inaccurate representation of the totality of evidence.... When we are guided by meta-analyses carried out of biased datasets, we are operating under the illusion of practising evidence-based medicine," concludes a study of antidepressant medications in children and adolescents from the University of British Columbia's Therapeutics Initiative (Therapeutics Initiative, 2004).[2] (The Initiative is an independent organization set up to provide doctors and pharmacists with timely, evidence-based, practical information on drug therapy.)

An article in the *Canadian Medical Association Journal* put the case more bluntly: "The secrecy that surrounds the drug approvals process means that physicians and their patients may be unaware that they are using a medication in a manner for which the evidence of effectiveness and safety is inadequate. Such policies value commercial interest above that of patients" (Herxheimer & Mintzes, 2004, p. 487).[3]

If Health Canada did not make the results of the SSRI clinical trials on teenagers and children public, how were the results of the unpublished trials scrutinized? They were posted on the U.S. FDA website following the enactment, in 2002, of the Best Pharmaceuticals for Children Act. That law provides incentives, in the form of extra patent protection, to drug companies that conduct clinical trials on children (a practice that Health Canada is currently considering).

Because of concerns about unpublished trials, leading peer-reviewed medical journals gave notice in 2005 that they would no longer accept articles about clinical trials of drugs unless the trials were publicly registered when they began. Registration creates a trail, making it more difficult to suppress unfavourable results, but registration alone will not provide access to the full results of clinical trials that are submitted as part of the drug approval process.

In May 2007, the World Health Organization (WHO) launched the International Clinical Trials Registry Platform Search Portal. As this book was being published, Health Canada "is currently exploring the development of a regulatory requirement for the registration of clinical trials and disclosure of results" (Health Canada, 2007b).

Full Comments of Health Canada Reviewers

The reports of Health Canada reviewers are not made available, except sometimes through Access to Information requests, although they reveal much about the drug approval process and may include the reasoning of those in favour of, and those opposed to, approving a particular drug.

Because provinces pay for drugs provided in public plans, provincial governments have their own drug reviewers who gather information to ascertain a new drug's effectiveness and, if relevant, its effectiveness compared to similar drugs already on the market. Until recently, Health Canada reviewer reports were denied even to these provincial drug evaluators. In early 2004, the reports became available to those evaluators involved with the Common Drug Review (CDR) initiative (personal communication from Dr. Ken Bassett, November 9, 2007). (The CDR is a federal initiative, launched in late 2003, to review drugs and recommend to publicly funded drug plans in all Canadian jurisdictions, except Quebec, whether or not the drugs should be added to provincial formularies.)

Indications Applied for, But Refused Authorization

Information about indications that were applied for, but not approved by Health Canada, is also vital since so many drugs are prescribed "off-label"—that is, for uses that have never been authorized. Sometimes, the companies never sought approval for these uses, but sometimes approval was refused because companies did not submit data that were convincing enough. If a drug company applied for and was denied approval for a particular use, the public needs to know why, especially if that unapproved use is being widely suggested by the drug company and the drug is being prescribed for that unapproved use.

Physicians can prescribe drugs off-label "at their discretion," as Health Canada notes. This is legal even though the regulator has not ruled on a drug's safety or efficacy for the off-label use, and even though there may be no evidence about safety or efficacy. Federal legislation applies only in that it prohibits promotion of a drug for unapproved uses.

Although comparable Canadian figures are not available, a U.S. newspaper investigation found that 21 percent of the prescriptions written for top-selling drugs are prescribed for off-label uses (Knight Ridder Newspapers, 2003). The investigation looked at the three top-selling drugs in 15 classes of medications. It also revealed that off-label prescribing nearly doubled in the five years from 1998–2002. The off-label prescribing of drugs is, increasingly, actively sought after by pharmaceutical firms, since it is an effective way of enlarging the market for a drug without having to undertake expensive clinical trials.

As the International Working Group on Transparency and Accountability in Drug Regulation noted in 1996, if a drug is subject to negative findings, and the drug regulatory agency does not make this public, that omission "can leave the way clear for the sometimes very different and emphatic account given from the manufacturer" (Health Action International, 1996, Section 5).

An example that affects Canadian women is Diane-35, (cyproterone acetate and ethinyl estradiol), a drug approved by Health Canada only as a treatment for "severe acne unresponsive to oral antibiotic and other available treatments, with associated symptoms of androgenization, including seborrhea and mild hirsutism" (Compendium of Pharmaceuticals and Specialties, 2007), but subsequently marketed as an oral contraceptive (see Box 6.4).

Box 6.4: Diane-35: Ferreting out the Secrets

by Barbara Mintzes

Diane-35 is a hormonal drug currently sold in Canada by Bayer HealthCare Pharmaceuticals. Although Diane-35 and its predecessor, Diane (a higher dose form), have been sold in Europe since 1978, it was not approved in Canada until 1998. Diane-35 is approved only to treat severe acne in women who have failed to respond to previous acne treatments, and have signs of high levels of male hormone (androgen).

Soon after its approval in Canada, Diane-35 became one of the first prescription medicines to be advertised to the Canadian public. The ads used images suggesting use for mild acne and birth control, although Health Canada had never approved it for the latter indication. In 2003, because of safety concerns about Diane-35—and the ad campaigns—CBC TV produced a documentary on Diane-35: "CBC Disclosures, Two-for-one." CBC researchers filed numerous Access to Information requests and were successful in obtaining a significant amount of previously unreleased pre-market information from Health Canada.

Secret 1

Before it was approved in Canada, Health Canada rejected Diane-35 twice because of safety concerns. Berlex, which was bought by Bayer in 2006, first applied for approval in Canada in 1993. In 1994, a long-term user in Germany died of liver cancer, prompting a safety review by Germany's regulatory agency. One of Diane-35's ingredients, cyproterone, binds to liver cell DNA. This type of effect on DNA is called "genotoxicity" and is a sign a chemical may cause cancer. Use for birth control and mild acne was prohibited in the U.K., Malaysia, Germany, and most of Europe ("Germany's cyproterone warning," 1995). Health Canada did not approve Diane-35, stating that further long-term animal studies were needed to clarify whether or not Diane-35 caused cancer (Chaudhuri, 1993). Berlex applied again in 1996. Again, Health Canada reviewers raised concerns that cyproterone was genotoxic and likely to pose greater risks for cancer than other forms of progesterone (Chaudhuri & Leroux, 1996). The company carried out a case-control study of risks of liver cancer, concluding that Diane-35 did not lead to increased risks. The published version of this study (Heinemann et al., 1997) has serious limitations. Inadequate attention was paid to the often lengthy latency periods between exposure to a cancer-causing chemical and cancer diagnosis. Additionally, most results for cyproterone were only reported in combination with medroxyprogesterone (Depo-Provera), for which there is not the same evidence of genotoxicity. It is not clear if Health Canada also had other more detailed study results.

How Did This Become Public?
CBC obtained otherwise confidential pre-market correspondence between Health
Canada and the manufacturer and posted these documents on the Internet. If CBC
had not intervened, this correspondence would have remained secret.

Secret 2
Diane-35's effectiveness was never tested in women with severe, unresponsive acne.
Berlex originally applied for approval for Diane-35 for all forms of acne in women.
The drug was approved for a more restricted use—second-line use for severe acne if
other treatments fail—because of safety concerns. However, Health Canada did not
require any additional testing in women with severe, unresponsive acne. There are
no published studies or unpublished placebo-controlled studies specifically in this
population group in Berlex' submission to Health Canada, and none of the materials
obtained and released by the CBC include analyses of effectiveness in women with
severe, unresponsive acne. Thus, a huge question mark exists about whether Diane-
35 is effective for its approved use.

How Did This Become Public?
CBC obtained otherwise confidential pre-market materials and posted them on the
Internet.

Secret 3
Health Canada judged the TV, billboard, and magazine ads for Diane-35 to be
illegal.

How Did This Become Public?
Health Canada's repeated judgments that the ads were illegal became public only
in 2006, in expert testimony provided by Ann Sztuke-Fournier, Health Canada's
advertising coordinator, during the CanWest Charter Challenge on the ban of
direct-to-consumer advertising of prescription drugs (Sztuke-Fournier, 2006). The
public seeing the ads was never informed. Even those making complaints about
Diane-35 ads, including Women and Health Protection, never got a clear answer
from Health Canada about the legality of the ads. Health Canada has never fined the
company, nor levied any other sanctions, despite repeated illegal ad campaigns from
1999–2005 and Health Canada's recognition of the safety concerns associated with
these ad campaigns (Sztuke-Fournier, 2006).

And a Secret We Still Don't Know the Answer to
Health Canada may have also delayed approval of Diane-35 because of concerns
about risks of potentially fatal blood clots (venous thromboembolism).

In 1995 and 1996, while Diane-35 was still being considered for approval in
Canada, several studies comparing risks of venous thromboembolism with different
types of birth control pills found that Diane-35 was riskier (Farley, Meirik, Chang,

Marmot & Poulter, 1995; Pini et al., 1996). At the time, Diane-35 was approved for birth control in a number of countries. These studies were not designed to specifically evaluate the risks of Diane-35, but they did include some users of this medication. While no definitive conclusions about Diane-35 can be drawn, the studies do provide a signal of possible harm. No mention is made of this evidence in the pre-market reports and memos provided to the CBC.

More recent studies provide stronger evidence that Diane-35 is associated with a greater risk of venous thromboembolism than commonly used birth control pills. For example, a case-control study by Vasilakis-Scaramozza and Jick (2001) found a fourfold increase in the risk of venous thromboembolism with Diane-35, as compared with levonorgestrel-containing birth control pills, and Seaman, de Vries, and Farmer (2003) found a doubling of risk compared with all conventional pills. Health Canada has warned doctors not to prescribe Diane-35 for birth control or mild acne.

None of the publicly released pre-market information mentions these risks. Berlex was legally required to provide Health Canada with the 1995 and 1996 studies. Did the company do so? If not, did the company face any consequences?

Notice of Compliance with Conditions

A Notice of Compliance with Conditions (NOC/c) from Health Canada means a company can market a drug on the condition that it undertakes additional studies to verify its clinical benefit. According to a fact sheet from the Therapeutic Products Directorate (TPD), posted on the HPFB website, to receive a NOC/c, a drug "must be of high quality and possess an acceptable benefit/risk profile ... [although] the clinical benefit of these drugs has not yet been verified" (Therapeutics Products Directorate, 2002). When the conditions are met, the conditional tag will be removed, the website states. The NOC/c category was created in May 1998 and first used in July of that year for the AIDS antiretroviral drug Rescriptor (delavirdine mesylate).

The rationale for having the NOC/c is to fast-track drugs for life-threatening conditions such as AIDS and cancer. It was, therefore, a surprise when Relenza (zanamivir), a new drug for "uncomplicated" influenza, received an NOC/c designation in 1999. In the U.S., a Federal Advisory Committee had recommended against approving the drug, since the largest trial in North America showed it reduced the length of time someone suffered from influenza by half a day. (The FDA overruled its advisory committee and approved the drug anyway.) Meanwhile, researchers with the Therapeutics Initiative were unable to find out exactly what conditions were placed on the drug's notice of compliance (personal communication, Dr. Ken Bassett, summer 2004). That was because, for the first eight years that conditional approvals were granted, Health Canada did not make information about them public, leaving prescribing doctors and patients in the dark about what risks might be involved in taking the drugs that were granted conditional approval.

In material prepared for patients, Glaxo Wellcome (Relenza's manufacturer) did not mention the conditional nature of the marketing approval. "The subject of conditional approval is complex and is very unlikely to be meaningful to a patient in the absence of an appropriate explanation from a health care professional," Michael Levy, the chief medical officer of Glaxo Wellcome in Mississauga, Ontario, explained in a letter published in the *Canadian Medical Association Journal* (Levy, 2000). When a complaint was brought to the Pharmaceutical Advertising Advisory Board (PAAB) because brochures did not state that conditions were placed on Relenza's notice of compliance, the PAAB agreed with the complainant and "referred the case to Health Canada for an opinion on the necessity of including the fact that a product was issued a NOC/c, in patient information brochures" (Pharmaceutical Advertising Advisory Board, 2000, p. 4). Three years later, in 2003, Health Canada published a revised policy on NOC/c and accepted the PAAB recommendation.

In 2006, the regulator acted on a February 2003 policy decision to improve transparency by publishing the NOC/c Qualifying Notice (QN) "which provides in general terms (i.e., non-proprietary) the commitments required of sponsors in order to proceed with authorization under the NOC/c policy" (Health Canada, 2007a, 6.A.ii). While more information is now provided about why drugs are granted this kind of approval, and the conditions placed on the approval, the length of time that companies have to meet conditions (such as a requirement for more trials) and their progress toward meeting the deadlines are not made public.

Expert Advisory Committees

Health Canada sometimes convenes expert advisory committees to provide advice about the approval of particular drugs. The regulator now posts on the Internet brief summaries of the deliberations of these committees, which meet in private, but the summaries provide only a glimpse into what was discussed. And the criteria for these committees—for example, the appointment process—are not available to the public.

For example, the report of a March 2000 meeting of Health Canada's TPD expert advisory committee on HIV therapies, posted on the Internet, notes that members were asked to reveal conflict-of-interest information with respect to the drug to be discussed (abacavir sulfate). However, what those conflicts were, and how they were managed, was not made public. Instead the report notes that "actions were taken at the meeting to manage all disclosed conflicts of interest in a preventive manner" (Therapeutic Products Directorate, 2000, p. 1).

More recently, until the publication of a newspaper report that noted that secret meetings had taken place, Health Canada refused to reveal the names and recommendations of a nine-member advisory panel that met in 2005 to consider licensing applications for silicone gel breast implants. Following the press reports, then Health Minister Ujjal Dosanjh directed the department to name the participants and their advice. When a second advisory panel was convened in September of the same year, panel member names and their declared statements of conflict of interest were posted on a public website. Some did declare financial conflicts in the form of payments for work they had done for the manufacturers of the products under review. Health Canada's decision to make these declarations public was laudable, but the regulator's good intentions were weakened by their subsequent decision to dismiss the relevance of these conflicts. An additional, more serious, concern is that it was revealed on the day of the public hearing that four of the panel members had previously been hired as expert witnesses by Health Canada in a related legal case.

Getting Information

Confidentiality and the Access to Information Route

The definition and treatment of "confidential third-party information" is at the heart of the issue when it comes to Health Canada's track record of keeping information from the public. This is not the only problem, but it is central. There are valid reasons to protect manufacturing secrets and the identities of patients in clinical trials. However, Health Canada "protects" far more information than this. Important information from clinical trials and expert reviewers about the safety and effectiveness of drugs is virtually impossible to obtain.

In Canada, at the present time, you must file a request under the Access to Information (ATI) Act if you want to obtain information about the approval process for any given drug. Filing ATI requests can be a "difficult, long, formal process," Serge Durand, the manager of the proprietary and scientific information assessment section of the TPD, acknowledged in a July 2004 interview with this author. Documents that are released are often heavily edited. Section 20 (1) of the ATI Act states that the head of a government institution "shall refuse to disclose any record requested" that contains: a) trade secrets, b) "financial commercial scientific or technical information that is confidential information supplied to a government institution by a third party and is treated consistently in a confidential manner by the third party, c) information the disclosure of which could reasonably be expected to result in material financial loss or gain to, or could reasonably be expected to prejudice the competitive position of a third party, or d) information the disclosure of which could reasonably be expected to interfere with contractual or other negotiations of a third party."

The Information Commissioner of Canada, in a special report to Parliament, called for the abolition of 20 (1) (b) and questioned whether 20 (1) (a) was necessary if 20 (1) (c) was in place. The commissioner comments:

> With government downsizing and privatization, more and more matters affecting the public interest are dealt with by the private sector. Government

officials and private firms should not be able to agree among themselves to keep information secret. Yet paragraph 20 (1) (b) comes perilously close to giving authority to just such a cozy arrangement. (Reid, 2002, p. 67)

The Science Advisory Board report in 2000 found that the procedures of the Therapeutic Products Programme (TPP), now the Therapeutic Products Directorate, are at odds with a 1998 judgment with respect to the ATI Act, which found that the onus rested with a company to show why information should not be disclosed. The TPP procedures "seem to enjoin secrecy unless there is a requirement that information be disclosed.... Significant improvement in transparency can be achieved simply by interpreting the Act as it is meant to be interpreted: with a presumption of disclosure unless an exemption is clearly warranted" (Science Advisory Board to Health Canada, 2000, Appendix F, pp. 2, 3). In any event, the act can be amended to clarify its limited application to the drug review process, the report concluded.

The access-to-information route has not been effective or satisfying, judging from the experience of four public interest applicants. In the late 1990s, Dr. Joel Lexchin sought to discover why Canada had approved several pediatric anti-diarrheal drugs when the World Health Organization had decided the drugs had no place in managing acute diarrhea in children. He waited more than 21 months for a reply to his ATI request and eventually received a document with almost everything blacked out. More recently, in 2004, Lexchin filed multiple ATI requests, some of which were not answered for more than a year (personal communication, Dr. Joel Lexchin, October 2007). As a doctoral student, Barbara Mintzes filed an ATI request to find out more about a contraceptive product in the late 1990s. She waited one year for information. When she applied to obtain the same information from the FDA under the U.S. Freedom of Information Act, she received the information within two weeks. More recently, it took CBC reporters, using ATI requests, more than five years to get access to Health Canada's Adverse Drug Reaction database—a database containing information of direct relevance to the public—in a searchable form. When it finally received the information and analyzed it, the CBC found that, since 1997, there was a threefold increase in adverse reactions, including deaths, among children. Health Canada had not noted this alarming trend because it had not analyzed its own information (Canadian Broadcasting Corporation, 2005).

Before releasing any information under ATI, Health Canada officials must inform the sponsor (the drug company) of intent to disclose the information (Section 27/28 of the act). If a sponsor disagrees with the officials about the extent of disclosure, it can take Health Canada to court, and there are multiple court cases outstanding as a result of such appeals. Meanwhile, Durand, who is responsible for ATI, observed that legislation "may not have intended" the company's use of the appeal process to block disclosure (personal communication, Serge Durand, July 2004).

Applicants can also appeal when they are refused information, as public interest researcher Ken Rubin did after Health Canada refused to release the full text of a report titled "Special Review on the Safety of Calcium Channel Blockers." Controversy surrounded the safety of some drugs in this class and Rubin appealed Health Canada's decision to release only a highly edited version of the review, arguing there was a public interest in having the safety concerns revealed. His appeal failed. The federal court trial decision rested on the point that, while a government official may disclose in the public interest, he or she does not have "the obligation to do so" (Office of the Information Commissioner of Canada, 2002, Chapter IV, p. 2).

Requests from pharmaceutical companies or their agents account for fully 90 percent of the requests about drug product files. These requests, in turn, account for more than half the ATI requests filed with all of Health Canada. The high percentage of corporate ATI requests (presumably for information about competitors) probably goes some way to explaining the delays experienced by others who have filed ATI requests with Health Canada. Ironically, while the government is obliged to keep "third-party information" confidential, the sponsor company is free to make public whatever it wants. Health Canada has found itself in the unusual situation of refusing to release information that is already posted on a company's website, according to Serge Durand of the TPB.

Other Jurisdictions

The United States
Much more information about the drug approval process is publicly available in the U.S. than in Canada. Indeed, Canadians who seek information about a drug approved in both countries can log on to the U.S. FDA website and find their way to a wide range of information that is unavailable in Canada, such as the clinical trials that companies submitted with their application for licensing approval and reviewer notes. Much of the information on the FDA website may be rather too technical for non-professionals, but consumer and public interest groups in the U.S. routinely analyze such information and produce reports.

Unlike the situation in Canada, information is available in the U.S. about some not-yet-approved drugs. For about one-third of new drug submissions, the FDA looks to outside help for their evaluation and convenes a federal advisory committee. Everything the committee examines and discusses is public, although documents are often posted on the Internet only in the 24 hours prior to the committee meeting. Other new drug applications (NDAs) are not made public by the FDA, but drug manufacturers often make them known to investors; information about NDAs can be found in U.S. Securities and Exchange Commission documents and, often, in the U.S. financial press.

In the U.S., unlike the situation in Canada, expert advisory panel meetings are held in public. When a drug is approved by the FDA, the agency posts on the Internet the transcripts of meetings with the pharmaceutical company representatives and the FDA scientists who approved the drug. As well, clinical trial and other information for new chemical entities is posted on the FDA website within a set period after a drug has been approved. Before posting the information, FDA officials edit it to remove any manufacturing secrets and information that would identify patients. They are not required to defer to or consult with the drug company sponsor before posting the information.

While there is greater disclosure of information in the U.S., it is not acceptable for Canadians to have to rely on obtaining information about the drug approval process from the FDA website. For one thing, companies may seek approval in Canada before they seek approval in the U.S. As well, they may seek approval for drugs that have been rejected by the FDA, in which case no information would have been released south of the border. Companies may also use different sets of data to seek approval here, and they may seek approval for different indications. As well, the opinions of Canadian reviewers may differ from those of their American colleagues.

Europe

In Europe, the European Medicines Agency (EMEA), which is the equivalent of Canada's Therapeutic Products Directorate (TPD), issues European public assessment reports (EPARs) that are "supposed to reflect the assessment file submitted by the manufacturers, its analysis by the EMEA's scientific advisory body and the reasons underlying that body's opinion" (Lexchin, 2007). However, the EPARs are written under the supervision of the company concerned, and, in the past, when reports were analyzed by the International Society of Drug Bulletins (ISDB), it found the documents to be uneven and not reliable. The society stated that the documents do not always have epidemiological data or describe the mechanism of action of the drug, and they are not updated regularly (International Society of Drug Bulletins, 1998).[4]

Meanwhile, new European community legislation regarding access to EMEA documents appears to have important parallels to Canada's ATI Act, and to mirror the latter's shortcomings. For example, although there is a "presumption of access," the legislation builds in a requirement to consult with companies before disclosing information. An EMEA spokesman told a June 10–11, 2004 Health Canada consultation that full clinical trial results submitted to the regulator would remain confidential (consultation notes, A. Silversides). An analysis of the operations of the EMEA, published in the *British Medical Journal* in 2007, challenged this policy: "Although disclosure of documentation concerning production and drug technology could help competitors, there is no reason to hide data on toxicology and clinical evaluation" (Garattini & Bertele, 2007).

The EMEA does, however, provide information about the reasons why drugs are not approved and information explaining the withdrawal of drugs from the market. For drugs that are not approved, a press release is issued along with a Q & A document explaining the grounds for the negative opinion. The regulator also publishes a refusal in a European public assessment report (EPAR). When the European Commission

Table 6.1: Information That Is Made Available on Marketed Drugs: A Comparison of Three Jurisdictions

Country	Canada (Health Canada)	U.S. (Food and Drug Administration)	European Union (European Medicines Agency)
Register of ongoing and completed clinical trials	No	Yes (clinicaltrials. gov)	No
List of new marketing authorizations	Yes	Yes	Yes
List of refused marketing authorizations	No	No (limited)	Yes (on the Enterprise Directorate of the European Commission website)
List of cancelled marketing authorizations	Yes (drug product database, but list incomplete)	Yes (not very regularly updated)	Yes
Reports submitted by drug companies for marketing authorization	No	Partially (reports submitted before advisory meetings)	No
Reviews and reports compiled by the regulator and based on information submitted by a manufacturer in support of a new drug application	Yes (summary basis of decision)	Yes (approval packages)	Yes (European Public Assessment Report)

Source: Adapted from a more extensive country comparison in Vitry, A., Lexchin, J., Sasich, L., Dupin-Spriet, T., Reed, T., Bertele, V. et al. (2008). *Provision of information on regulatory authorities' websites. Internal Medicine Journal, 38*(7), 559–567.

issues a decision to withdraw a drug from the market, the background information about the product, the scientific conclusions reached, and any conditions are published in an EMEA document (personal communication, Valvanera Valero, press office of the European Medicines Agency, November 6, 2007).

Health Canada: Small Steps to Transparency
Health Canada maintains a database of Notices of Compliance (NOC), also known as market authorizations, about drugs that have received approval for marketing (Health Canada, 2008b). The information in these NOCs is limited, and includes the brand name of the drug, the manufacturer's name, the active ingredients, the date, and the therapeutic class of the drug. Health Canada has recently undertaken the following steps to provide more information to the public.

Summary Basis of Decision Documents
In 2004, as part of a five-year initiative called the Therapeutics Access Strategy (TAS), Health Canada began to publish Summary Basis of Decision (SBD) documents to provide information about the scientific and benefit/risk considerations that went into the decision to authorize a new drug for the market. The title of the document implies that the decision to refuse to approve a new drug, or a particular application of a drug, will also be summarized. However, this is not the case and information about the refusal to authorize a drug for market—made public in Europe—is not released in Canada.

In its first phase, SBDs are produced for drugs that received market authorization after January 1, 2005 and are new active substances (drugs with a different molecular structure from prescription drugs already on the market). When the SBDs were launched, a Health Canada press release stated they were "intended for Canadians interested in the basis for Health Canada's product-specific decisions for drugs and medical devices." However, although the SBDs are accompanied by readers' guides and background documentation, it is fair to say that their technical jargon makes them inaccessible to most Canadians.

The U.S. FDA published Summary Basis of Approval (SBA) documents until 1994, when this approach was abandoned. Instead, the FDA chose to make public edited versions of drug approval reviews, a less time-consuming task than creating SBAs. While the edited reviews provide far more information than SBAs did, the reviews are also not easily read by non-experts.

An analysis by Lexchin and Mintzes (2004) of the information in the sample Canadian SBDs concluded that the lack of detailed information meant the documents would not be useful in uncovering safety concerns since they will not provide enough information to reveal bias in trials or ascertain the risk-benefit ratio of the medication. In fact, a number of consumer groups told a multi-stakeholder consultation that

SBD documents would be useful only if they served as a user-friendly portal to the simultaneous provision of far more information, such as the details of clinical trials submitted to support new drug submissions and reviewers' notes (consultation notes, June 10–11, 2004, A. Silversides).

Clinical Trial Information Disclosure
Health Canada is undertaking a Registration and Disclosure of Clinical Trial Information initiative. The process started in June 2005 at a multi-stakeholder meeting and, in December 2006, an external working group issued a final report recommending that all trials be registered and that reporting content requirements and time frames for disclosure should be established for all completed trials. Further, the report recommended that trials that were prematurely stopped for clinical reasons (unexpected efficacy, hazards, futility) should be disclosed in an expedited time frame (see Health Canada, 2007b). As this book went to press, Health Canada was "continuing to explore the development of regulatory requirements" with respect to the registration of clinical trials and disclosure of results. No timeline was announced for a final decision.

Posting of Product Monographs
In early 2008, Health Canada began posting product monographs—the approved product information that accompanies a drug approval—on its website. Until that date, product monographs were considered the property of the manufacturer and were not publicly available. A product monograph describes "the properties, claims, indications and conditions of use of the drug and contains any other information that may be required for optimal, safe and effective use of the drug," according to Health Canada. Most, but not all, prescription drugs will have a product monograph available; some drugs with "lengthy market histories and an established safety profile will generally not have an associated Product Monograph" (see Health Canada, 2008a).

The Complications of Industry Funding
While public access to information about the regulatory process remains strictly limited, drug regulators in Health Canada have arguably stronger ties to the pharmaceutical industry as a result of significant changes made to drug regulatory operations in the past decade. A key change has been the way in which the drug regulatory function is funded. In 1992, the Prescription Drug User Fee Act enabled the U.S. FDA to collect fees from drug companies in order to speed up reviews of new drug applications (Office of the Inspector General, Department of Health and Human Services, 2003). Two years later, Health Canada followed suit, although in Canada drug company fees replaced government money, while in the U.S. the money was supplemental to government appropriations.

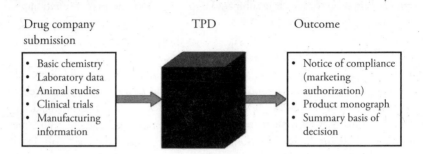

Figure 6.1: The Current State of Transparency in Drug Regulation in Canada

Drug company submission   TPD   Outcome

- Basic chemistry
- Laboratory data
- Animal studies
- Clinical trials
- Manufacturing information

- Notice of compliance (marketing authorization)
- Product monograph
- Summary basis of decision

Source: Lexchin, J. (2007, May). Pharmaceutical secrecy endangers our health. *The Monitor*. Retrieved November 10, 2008, from the Canadian Centre for Policy Alternatives: www.policyalternatives.ca/MonitorIssues/2007/05/MonitorIssue1638

Cost recovery was launched in Canada in 1994–1995, when just over 20 percent of the Therapeutic Products Programme budget came from industry fees, with the balance from government appropriations. By 1998–1999, cost recovery accounted for just under 75 percent of the total budget. In April 2004, 51 percent of revenue came from cost recovery with the balance from government appropriations. The lower proportion of funding from cost recovery was largely because of an injection of more government money. A new initiative, the Good Clinical Practise Fee Proposal, seeks to stabilize the funding arrangement.

A danger inherent in a "user pay" scheme is a tendency to see the "user" as the client and for this attitude to become pervasive. Indeed, by 1997, the director general of the TPP was advising staff in an internal bulletin that "the client is the direct recipient of your services. In many cases this is the person or company who pays for the service." The public, in this bulletin, is not the government's client, but rather its "beneficiary" or a "stakeholder." When companies come to be seen as the customers, the regulators "want to be able to help them, because they realize the enormous research and the resources that have gone into the clinical trials. So they want to be able to deliver a positive message for them" (Mary Wiktorowicz, quoted in Eggerston, 2005).

Instead of directly funding the operations of drug regulators, drug company payments could be added to general government revenues (with regulators being apportioned a budget from there), hence breaking the direct link between companies and regulators. But if any kind of "user pay" system of drug approval is to remain in place, the best way to counter a bias, or perception of bias, is an open, transparent, and rigorous drug-approval process with external scrutiny.

Future Directions

Bill C-51, a broad amendment to Canada's *Food and Drugs Act*, was introduced on April 8, 2008. The bill died on the order paper because of the Fall 2008 federal election call, but as this book went to press, the draft legislation is expected to be reintroduced. Given the recent drug safety scandals involving unpublished clinical trial results that were kept secret from the public, one might expect that the proposed new legislation would finally enshrine the public's right to access the full body of scientific evidence on drug safety and effectiveness submitted to Health Canada. Bill C-51 took the opposite approach, however. Instead, the proposal enshrined the right of companies to keep information secret from the public and introduced a definition of confidential business information into the *Food and Drugs Act* for the first time (see box below). To paraphrase the definition, companies could maintain secrecy if the information is secret, if they want to keep it secret, and if making it public could affect their bottom line. This proposal may not become law; as of this writing, it is still under discussion. However, after the Vioxx and SSRI scandals, the drafting of a proposed law in this way is of grave concern.

Box 6.5: Definition of Confidential Information in Bill C-51

Confidential business information, in respect of a person to whose business or affairs the information relates, means, subject to the regulations, business information

1. that is not publicly available
2. in respect of which the person has taken measures that are reasonable in the circumstances to ensure that it remains not publicly available
3. that has actual or potential economic value to the person or their competitors because it is not publicly available and its disclosure would result in a material financial loss to the person or a material financial gain to their competitors (Bill C-51, 2008)

Conclusion

Drug regulatory agencies are servants of the public, entrusted with the responsibility of maximizing the safety and efficacy of drugs. They must be accountable to the public, and the public and the scientific community must be able to ensure, through access to relevant information, that the agencies are acting in the public interest. The fact that Health Canada's drug approval process is shrouded in secrecy is directly contrary to the public interest.

Recent revelations of the many ways that drug companies have skewed clinical trial protocols and the presentation of clinical trial results in order to promote their products makes it abundantly clear that greater public scrutiny of the whole drug-approval process is essential.

While Health Canada takes small steps toward greater transparency, observers are growing impatient. For women, the question of safety is paramount as they are typically the guardians of not just their own, but their extended families', health. Secrecy can allow unsafe practices to exist, as it did in the case of SSRIs. According to the International Working Group on Transparency and Accountability in Drug Regulation, the risks of excessive secrecy include that "malpractice can be hidden from view," substandard drug use can be facilitated, irrational drug use may be unchecked, and the development of knowledge may be impeded (Health Action International, 1996, pp. 2, 3). This is not in anyone's interest.

To re-establish the perception that Health Canada is an effective, independent institution that acts in the public, and not commercial, interest, much more information about the drug approval system must be made public and posted on the Health Canada website. This information includes: all clinical trials reviewed by Health Canada to approve a drug, whether published or unpublished; all reviewer reports; the reports of expert advisory committees; the progress of companies toward fulfilling the conditions associated with having a drug approved with a Notice of Compliance with conditions; all clinical trial data about drugs denied approval; and drugs that are withdrawn from the market by companies. Further, there should be protection for anyone involved in the drug review process who reports wrongdoing; such people should have the right to report anonymously and directly to an independent whistle-blower agency.

Notes

1. Abby Hoffman, head of Health Canada's Therapeutics Access Strategy, made this comment in her address to the June 10, 2004 Health Canada public consultation.
2. See also a report from the U.S. Center for Science in the Public Interest, which revealed that a new National Cholesterol Education Program, written largely by industry-funded researchers and based on industry-funded studies, contained guidelines for women and the elderly that were not supported by the studies' data (Center for Science in the Public Interest, 2004).
3. See also Kirsch et al. (2008). Drawing on meta-analyses of published and unpublished trial data on antidepressant medications, the authors conclude that "drug-placebo differences in antidepressant efficacy increase as a function of baseline severity, but are relatively small even for severely depressed patients" (para. 3).
4. The ISDB is an organization founded in 1986 with the support of the World Health Organization. It is comprised of independent bulletins that publish articles on drugs and therapeutics.

Chapter 7

Reporting Adverse
Drug Reactions
What Happens
in the Real World?

———◦•✦•◦———

Colleen Fuller

Introduction

When a drug first comes to market, relatively little is known about its less frequent or less common harmful effects. Before approval, drugs are generally tested on limited numbers of people and, typically, for short periods of time. However, a drug may be used by many millions of people and for far longer periods than those tested. Clinical trials of new drugs may exclude people who are ill, young, old, or female, even though these groups may represent a drug's intended market. As a result, even the most rigorous pre-market clinical trials cannot predict the harm a drug may cause once it is in use in the real world. It follows that the assessment of safety and effectiveness after a drug has been approved for sale, known as post-market surveillance, is one of the most important parts of the drug regulatory process. Health Canada is responsible for this surveillance, as it is for all other aspects of the regulation of prescription medicines in Canada.

It is our view that Canada's system of post-market surveillance is severely hampered by an infrastructure that is under-resourced and inadequate for the task of gathering, analyzing, and acting on information about harmful effects of approved medicines. The death of 15-year-old Vanessa Young in March 2000 is a case in point. Ms. Young was diagnosed with bulimia when she was prescribed Propulsid (cisapride), a drug approved for nocturnal heartburn in adults, but often prescribed off-label to children with stomach ailments (Pandolfini & Bonati, 2005). In fact, cisapride was contraindicated for use in patients with bulimia and was not indicated at all for children. At the time of Ms. Young's death from cardiac arrest, 44 cisapride-associated cardiac arrhythmias had been reported to Health Canada, four letters warning of cardiac arrhythmias had been issued to Canadian doctors by the manufacturer, and the U.S. Food and Drug Administration (FDA) had issued an advisory about fatal cardiac arrhythmias among patients taking the drug ("Editorial, Lessons from cisapride," 2001, p. 1269; Sibbald, 2001). None of this information was known to Ms. Young's family until after her death. In July 2000, cisapride was pulled from the U.S. market, but "Canadians could keep filling their prescriptions until Aug. 7, more than 6 months after the FDA warning" ("Editorial, Lessons from cisapride," 2001, p. 1269).

A coroner's inquest into Vanessa Young's death criticized the federal government for not acting sooner on the information it had about the cardiac risks associated with cisapride. Citing evidence that Canada's system of voluntary reporting of adverse drug reactions was inadequate, the jury made 14 recommendations regarding the collection of information about serious adverse drug reactions and its distribution to patients and health care providers. But many years and dozens of public consultations later, Canadians still know too little about harmful effects associated with the drugs prescribed to them, nor do they know what steps to take when an adverse drug reaction occurs.

This chapter will examine Canada's system of post-market surveillance, with a particular focus on the reporting of adverse reactions to prescription medicines. We will look specifically at whether the current system serves women's needs and at how the system could be improved.

What Is an Adverse Drug Reaction?

An adverse drug reaction (ADR) is an unintended and undesirable response to a prescription medicine. Other terms that are commonly (and often interchangeably) used to describe reactions to drugs include "adverse effect," "adverse drug event," "side effect," "toxic effect," and "complication." The main difference among these terms is whether the drug caused the harmful effect, or whether the harmful effect was due to medical error or inappropriate use.

In 2004, the Canadian Adverse Events Study, for example, defined the term "adverse event" as "an unintended injury or complication that results in disability at the time of discharge, death or prolonged hospital stay and that is caused by health care management rather than by the patient's underlying disease process" (Baker et al., 2004, p. 1679). The study found that among almost 2.5 million annual hospital admissions in Canada, about 185,000 resulted in an adverse event and approximately 70,000 (37 percent) were considered preventable (Baker et al., 2004, p. 1679).

The term "adverse drug reaction," on the other hand, refers to an event that is suspected to have been caused by the drug itself rather than by human error. One way to describe this is "harm directly caused by the drug at normal doses, during normal use" (V.A. Center for Medication Safety, 2006, p. 1). Canada has adopted the World Health Organization's (WHO) definition of adverse drug reaction in Canadian law, as outlined in Box 7.1.

Canada's System of Post-market Surveillance of Prescription Drugs

Background

Post-market surveillance has been defined as the proactive collection of information on the quality, safety, or performance of pharmaceutical products after they have been approved for the market, and the investigation of adverse events and incidents (Garcia, 2007). Elements of an effective post-market surveillance program should include:

- collecting and analyzing data on effectiveness and adverse reactions
- disseminating information about drug effectiveness, safety, and harms to consumers, government agencies, physicians, pharmacists, and other health professionals

---

Box 7.1: Adverse Drug Reaction

In Canadian law:

Adverse drug reaction means a noxious and unintended response to a drug, which occurs at doses normally used or tested for the diagnosis, treatment or prevention of a disease or the modification of an organic function.

Adverse event means any adverse occurrence in the health of a clinical trial subject who is administered a drug that may or may not be caused by the administration of the drug, and includes an adverse drug reaction.

Serious adverse drug reaction means a noxious and unintended response to a drug that occurs at any dose and that requires in-patient hospitalisation or prolongation of existing hospitalisation, causes congenital malformation, results in persistent or significant disability or incapacity, is life-threatening or results in death.

Serious unexpected adverse drug reaction means a serious adverse drug reaction that is not identified in nature, severity or frequency in the risk information set out on the label of the drug.

Source: Food and Drugs Act: Food and Drug Regulations (Schedule no. 844), November 7, 1995.

- taking steps to improve the quality and effectiveness of prescription medicines by influencing physician prescribing practices
- reviewing pre-approval data where indicated
- requiring further testing of drugs and/or conducting further analysis of existing administrative data, in some cases through user registries, where indicated
- issuing warnings and/or withdrawing drugs from the market when necessary

ADR monitoring has been a key component of post-market surveillance since 1965, when formal collection of adverse drug reaction reports began in Canada, largely in response to the thalidomide fiasco. Thalidomide was used by pregnant women in Canada for about three years, from 1959–1962, to prevent morning sickness. Its use in North America and Europe prompted a wave of regulatory reform after the drug was found to cause peripheral neuritis and severely malformed limbs in newborns (Robinson, 2001). Some 135–200 Canadian children were exposed to the drug until it was pulled from the market in March 1962, more than three months after it had been banned in Europe (Thalidomide Victims Association of Canada,

2002). In the wake of the disaster, Canada established a system of spontaneous adverse drug-reaction reporting, as well as more rigorous pre-market regulatory standards. Manufacturers were required to provide "full information" pertaining to "animal or clinical experience, studies, investigations and tests conducted by the manufacturer or reported to him by any person concerning that new drug" (War Amputations of Canada, 1989, pp. 74–75).

Canada's current ADR reporting system was launched in 1990, when Dr. Curt Appel, then chief of Health Canada's Adverse Drug Reaction Monitoring Division, implemented a new drug safety monitoring program. This move was part of a trend that was occurring internationally in which many countries within the Organisation for Economic Co-operation and Development (OECD), the Paris-based body representing the world's 30 most industrialized countries, were reorganizing their regulatory systems to facilitate standardization of testing procedures for drug safety, quality, and efficacy (Kaitin, 2002; Organisation for Economic Co-operation and Development, 1999). The scheme established a system of regional reporting centres, expert advisory committees, and a communications strategy, which included a newsletter with information about adverse drug reactions reported to Health Canada. But 12 years later, Dr. Appel would criticize the "paltry budgets to provide minimal service," the "all but abandoned" expert advisory committee, and the inability of the regulator, for financial reasons, to "use high-quality provincial databases" with a wealth of information about adverse drug effects. "Evidently," Dr. Appel wrote, "Health Canada does not understand that drug-induced illness is a major public health concern" (Appel, 2002, pp. 884–885).

The Impact of Shifting Public Policy

Three years after the ADR Monitoring Division was in place, Health Canada unveiled a Risk Management Framework to guide discussions and activities under the broad umbrella of "health renewal," a framework that was adopted in 2003. The now-defunct Council of Science and Technology Advisors (CSTA) described it as a process that wove together science, ethics, and economics to assess and reduce or mitigate risk. Risk management, according to the CSTA, represented a combination of two factors: "the probability that an adverse event will occur" and "the consequences of the adverse event" (Halliwell, Smith & Walmsley, 1999a, p. 57).

The risk management approach reframed the role of Canada's drug regulator. There was less emphasis on ensuring the safety of a drug before it was allowed on the market. Instead, drugs were approved unless there was evidence that they were not safe. A key goal of such an approach was "[t]o achieve health and safety objectives while promoting, where possible, enhanced Canadian competitiveness" (Halliwell, Smith & Walmsley, 1999b, p. 6). But there were drawbacks to the new approach. New drugs were being approved more quickly, which meant that Canadians would "no longer have access to existing international post-market information before authorizing a product to be sold on the Canadian market and [would] need to rely more on proactive post-market surveillance systems" (Health Canada, 2006, p. 37). (See chapters 3 and 8 for a fuller discussion of the risk management approach.)

Within this framework, monitoring adverse drug reactions fell to the Marketed Health Products Directorate (MHPD), established within the Health Products and Food Branch (HPFB) in 2002. The launch of the MHPD was billed as "part of the re-alignment efforts by the HPFB toward a strengthened and consistent risk management approach" (Gorman, 2002). The risk management model relies on the collection of ADR reports by seven Canada Vigilance Regional Offices. These are in addition to a national office (the Canada National Vigilance Office) in Ottawa. Regional centres perform an initial review of the quality and completeness of adverse drug reaction reports, which are then processed and further analyzed at the national office.

The Canadian ADR Monitoring Program (CADRMP) (now known as Canada Vigilance) maintains a computerized database—called the Canadian Adverse Drug Reaction Information System—with information about all reported adverse drug reactions. The CADRMP guidelines emphasize that the definition of an ADR "includes *any* undesirable patient effect suspected to be associated with health product use," but does not require that a causal link be established before a report is submitted (Marketed Health Products Directorate, 2005, para. 1).

The shift in emphasis to expedited drug approvals and post-market surveillance had many critics. A key concern was that post-market surveillance was being strengthened as a trade-off for speedier approvals, possibly based on less evidence of effectiveness and safety. However, once a drug is on the market, it is harder to detect uncommon or more subtle harms, particularly if inadequate resources are allocated to post-approval monitoring (Greener, 2008). Further, MHPD was not provided with enforcement powers. The ability to remove drugs from the market if they are found to be unsafe is a responsibility that falls to the Therapeutic Products Directorate, which is also responsible for drug approvals and is "heavily reliant" on manufacturers for funds (Health Canada, 2007). MHPD's ability to monitor adverse drug reactions, determine causality, and communicate risk information to physicians, health professionals, and consumers was also threatened by inadequate resources (Lexchin, 2004; Manzer, 2006).

ADR Data Collection
The method of collecting and analyzing data about safety and efficacy, used internationally since the mid-1960s, is called "spontaneous reporting" (van Grootheest, de Graaf & de Jong-van den Berg, 2003). While adverse drug reaction reports can come from a variety of sources, including directly from consumers, it is mainly physicians and pharmacists who report, and reports usually go to either the

drug manufacturer or to the national regulator. In Canada, drug manufacturers are required to report serious ADRs within 15 days, but reporting by all other sources is voluntary. Most Canadians are unaware that there is a system to monitor adverse drug reactions and most consumers, along with most physicians, pharmacists, and other health professionals, do not report adverse effects (Canadian Treatment Action Council, 2007; Reynolds, 2006). Over twice as many reports are sent to manufacturers compared to Canada Vigilance regional offices. Physicians are the most common source of reports, followed by consumers, pharmacists, and nurses.

In addition to information obtained through its ADR monitoring activities, MHPD receives more than 200,000 reports annually that originate in other countries and are submitted by manufacturers. It also relies on non-governmental sources, including academic and scientific literature (including published case reports), post-market clinical trials conducted by manufacturers or health care institutions, and epidemiological studies. Patient groups may also submit information to Health Canada about adverse reactions, although privacy legislation limits the information they can provide in order to protect the identity of the person who has had the experience.

Why Effective Post-market Surveillance Is So Important

As noted above, data collected during pre-market clinical trials have limitations, making it difficult to assess the potential for new prescription medicines to cause harm. This has less to do with the clinical trial as an experimental research tool than it does with the duration and scope of most of the studies undertaken for marketing approval. Once a new substance is on the market, actual population exposure to the drug differs significantly from that in clinical trials, both in terms of the number and diversity of people receiving treatment and the dose and duration of therapy. General population exposure may include children, the elderly (75-plus years), women in general, and women of child-bearing age in particular, and people with multiple medical conditions taking more than one medication. It is often the case that individuals from these groups are represented either inadequately or not at all in clinical trials. As a result, different experiences are likely to be observed post-market than were seen in pre-approval research conditions.

For women, who may be excluded or underrepresented during the clinical trial process, and who are at greater risk of exposure to unsafe medications and drug interactions, an effective early warning system about possible harms caused by drugs is essential (Martin, Biswas, Freemantle, Pearce & Mann, 1998). But even the most rigorous clinical trial and government approval process cannot catch all potential harms associated with prescription medicines.

While the duration of clinical trials varies, they are typically carried out over a period of three to six months. In a 2002 paper, Joel Lexchin, of the School of Health

Policy and Management at York University, found that many clinical trials for drugs intended for long-term use lasted for less than six months. "If drugs … are meant for episodic use, short trials are justified," he wrote, but "the lack of trials lasting longer than 6 months [for drugs used to treat chronic conditions] might mean the long-term safety and efficacy are unknown" (Lexchin, 2002, p. 1490). In addition, many clinical trials are designed and financed by pharmaceutical manufacturers, raising concerns about objectivity (Sismondo, 2008). Therefore, it is not possible to know what the full range of harmful effects of any given drug may be on the basis of pre-market clinical trials alone.

Harm can also result from the use of approved drugs to treat conditions for which they have not been authorized, known as "off-label" use. Health Canada reviews a drug's efficacy in relation to its use within an identified population. Approval is granted for treatment of specific conditions and sometimes only in a specified group. However, Canadian physicians are not legally constrained from broader or off-label prescribing of a drug once it has been approved for a specific use. In off-label use, doctors are prescribing drugs for people and for conditions either for which Health Canada has rejected evidence of efficacy or safety, or for which no evidence was submitted in the first place. (See Chapter 6 for more information on off-label prescribing.)

There have been many instances of drugs approved for therapeutic use that have subsequently been found to cause serious harm, including long-term illnesses and sometimes death. An editorial in the *Canadian Medical Association Journal* noted that both the FDA and Health Canada "were aware of the increased risk of cardiovascular adverse events long before [Vioxx] was withdrawn from the market" and that "email evidence" indicated that the manufacturer had downplayed risks associated with the drug. "Why did it take 4 years for the increased risk … to emerge?" the journal asked ("Editorial, Vioxx: Lessons for Health Canada and the FDA," 2005, p. 5). The Vioxx (rofecoxib) story underscores the failure, not only of Canada's drug approval system, but also of the post-market surveillance regime.

An effective system of adverse drug reaction monitoring within a comprehensive framework of post-market surveillance cannot and, indeed, should not replace rigorous and thorough pre-market study and investigation. The purpose of post-market monitoring is not only to detect harms associated with prescription drugs that may not have been detected during clinical trials, but, importantly, to influence physicians' prescribing behaviour and support informed consumer decision making about medicines and treatment options. A key component of post-market surveillance, therefore, is an effective communications strategy to alert the public, including prescribing physicians, of potential harms associated with prescription medicines. Such a system is not currently in place in Canada for a number of reasons, including inadequate funding and under-reporting.

Box 7.2: The Case of Medical Devices: Post-market Surveillance of Breast Implants

by Anne Rochon Ford

Discussions of adverse reactions generally focus on prescription drugs, but some medical devices merit attention in this regard as well. Silicone gel breast implants in particular present health risks that have been a concern to women's health advocates for some time.

Medical devices regulations, adopted in 1975, provided minimal protection for consumers, and these were only moderately improved in 1998. Concern about a poor track record of post-market surveillance of medical devices was the subject of an inquiry by the auditor general of Canada in 2004, at which time she noted:

> Health Canada does not have a comprehensive program to protect the health and safety of Canadians from risks related to medical devices.... Health Canada needs to have a more proactive inspection program at the post-market phase to verify that industry is complying with the Medical Devices Regulations. (Auditor General of Canada, 2004, pp. 3–4)

In 1992, both the U.S. and Canada imposed moratoriums on silicone gel-filled implants because of safety concerns. Two manufacturers, Mentor and Inamed, redesigned their implants and requested Health Canada's approval for the new products. As a result, Health Canada undertook a public forum on silicone gel breast implants in 2005. The forum's design included both external experts and the general public. Unfortunately, the process was flawed with respect to both the public input component and the composition of the expert advisory panel (see Chapter 6). In October of the following year, Health Canada approved silicone gel breast implants for use in Canada by issuing a class IV licence with conditions to the manufacturers. Class IV is the most restrictive type of licence granted, indicating the highest risk category and problems that need close monitoring.

Because the 2005 public hearings were not very accessible, many of the women who had been harmed by silicone gel breast implants did not have an opportunity to tell their stories.

Research from the British Columbia Centre of Excellence in Women's Health has documented the growing costs to provinces as many women develop complications from breast implant surgery over time, and return continuously to the health care system for additional surgeries and other interventions and treatments related to implant rupture (Tweed, 2003, p. 40). Problems believed to be associated with the implants include questions about rupture rates and the potential migration of silicone into women's lymph nodes and organs. Rupture can be the result of normal deterioration, weakness in the shell or casing, and trauma to the breast. Some research points to an increased risk of autoimmune disorders, such as chronic fatigue, lupus, and fibromyalgia, in implanted women who have experienced a rupture of their devices (Katzin et al., 2005, p. 510).

Although non-essential breast implant surgery (which accounts for roughly 80 percent of all implants, with the remaining 20 percent being for reconstruction after cancer or prophylactic mastectomy) is paid for privately, when complications develop, women enter the publicly funded system for their care. The British Columbia research revealed that implanted women use the health care system seven to 10 times more frequently than other women, and are hospitalized four times more often. This is not surprising, given that a Mayo Clinic study in the U.S. found that 25 percent of women with breast implants suffered local complications requiring additional surgery within five years (Gabriel et al., 1997, p. 677).

A Health Canada round table on silicone gel breast implants, held in 1994, concluded with proposals for long-term follow-up and pointed to the need for a breast implant registry that would allow health care professionals or researchers to track women who receive breast implants and to follow up with patients should problems be identified. Unfortunately, between the time of that round-table discussion and the public hearings in 2005, not only was there no concerted follow-up by the Health Protection Branch on morbidity-related issues such as autoimmune reactions, but efforts to establish a national registry (including a private member's bill introduced by MP Judy Wasylycia-Leis in 2004) have been thwarted.

Given the history of documented and suspected problems caused by implants, the known cost to the public health care system resulting from complications, and the fact that approval of the devices was not based on any long-term studies, it seems logical that post-market surveillance of silicone gel breast implants would have been a major focus of the licence granted by Health Canada to the manufacturers in 2006. While the conditions for licensing stipulate that long-term research must be carried out by the manufacturer, Health Canada did not include a national mandatory registry as part of the plan. The manufacturers have committed to including implant registration cards with the devices and women can voluntarily return these cards to the manufacturer.

But voluntary registries in other jurisdictions (e.g., Great Britain) have been shown to be much less effective than mandatory ones (Pederson & Tweed, 2003), and recruitment to voluntary registries can be very problematic. It is unlikely that credible conclusions can be drawn from the data derived from voluntary registries due to participant bias. A mandatory registry would be a much clearer indication that Health Canada's health protection mandate is given priority over support for the cosmetic surgery industry, and that a key part of that mandate is collecting the information necessary to properly monitor adverse reactions.

Issues in the Current System

Funding

Post-market surveillance is the poor cousin within Canada's system of drug regulation: the Marketed Health Products Directorate (MHPD) has the lowest budget and the smallest staff complement within the Health Products and Food Branch. In 1999, the budget allocation for post-market surveillance of pharmaceutical drugs was $2.7 million, with 37 full-time positions dedicated to the task (HDP Group, 1999). When MHPD was created, it received an expanded mandate to monitor pharmaceuticals, biologics, vaccines, medical devices, natural health products, radiopharmaceuticals, and veterinary drug products. Its range of responsibilities has grown to include monitoring and collecting adverse reaction and medication incident data, reviewing and analyzing marketed health product safety data, conducting risk/benefit assessments of marketed health products, communicating product-related risks, and monitoring regulated advertising activities. Despite these expanded responsibilities, the MHPD was initially provided with only 35 scientific and 15 support staff. In its announcement of the new directorate, the Health Products and Food Branch announced that MHPD's budget would total $10 million annually (Gorman, 2002).

But two years later, while the directorate had increased its staff to 90, its budget was reported to be $8 million (Progestic International Inc., 2004). During the same period, the four directorates within the Health Products and Food Branch had 931 staff and received $84 million in 2004, with the greatest share of both staff (423) and funding ($38 million) going to the Therapeutic Products Directorate (TPD). Within its staff complement, TPD dedicated 182 people to reviewing drug submissions, compared with the MHPD's allocation of only 15 people to review and analyze ADR reports and medication incident data. By 2006, MHPD's staff complement had increased to 120 and its budget was reported to be $13 million, compared to the TPD, whose staff increased to 525 and its funding to $42 million (Manzer, 2006).

Beginning in 1994, regional monitoring centres, contracted to large health institutions such as hospitals, were established to educate the public and health professionals about the ADR reporting program, and to collect, evaluate, and provide feedback on reports (Motl, Timpe & Eichner, 2004). By 1998, when five regional reporting centres were up and running, the annual operating budget allocated to each centre for staff, space, administrative services, and program activities, such as promotions, was approximately $35,000 (HDP Group, 1999), with only one half-time staff position in each centre. By 2006–2007, the number of monitoring offices had been boosted to seven, with an annual budget for all offices of $1.2 million, including salaries and benefits for staff. Today each of the Canada Vigilance regional offices in Atlantic Canada, BC/Yukon, Alberta/NWT, Manitoba, and Saskatchewan have 1.5 full-time staff, while Ontario has three staff and Quebec has two (C. Saindon, Media Relations, Health Canada, personal correspondence, November 7, 2007).

Under-reporting

Underfunding has hampered efforts within the MHPD to raise public awareness about the importance and role of ADR reporting within Health Canada's drug safety strategy. One result is significant under-reporting by both the public and health professionals. Poor reporting rates make it difficult for MHPD to identify harm caused by drugs, resulting in delays in appropriate follow-up actions, such as providing additional information and warnings to health professionals and consumers, revising or adding information to a product's label, restricting use, or withdrawing a product from the market.

While the actual number of reports received by Health Canada each year increased from 4,000 in 1996 to 10,518 10 years later, an increase of over 150 percent ("Adverse reaction reporting—2006," 2007), the reporting rate remains low. The U.S. Food and Drug Administration has estimated that between 1 percent and 10 percent of actual adverse events are reported, and that those that are reported are unlikely to be representative of consumer experiences (General Accounting Office, 2000). The situation in Canada may be even worse. A report in the *Canadian Medical Association Journal* in 2001 noted that only 7,000 reports of adverse drug reactions were received by Health Canada annually, compared to 258,000 reports to the FDA in 1999. The article concluded that if reporting rates in Canada matched U.S. levels during the period, "there would have been roughly 25,000 reports here" (Sibbald, 2001, p. 1370).

Under-reporting of both serious and severe ADRs is widespread, both within Canada and internationally. A systematic review by Lorna Hazell and Saad Shakir estimated the median under-reporting rate of serious ADRs by physicians and hospitals in 37 countries was 94 percent (Hazell & Shakir, 2006). Put another way, only 6 percent of serious and severe ADRs are estimated to be reported to national regulators. An editorial in the *Canadian Medical Association Journal* pointed to "psychological and behavioural barriers to reporting [that] are not difficult to surmise," including the need for the physician to recognize that the reaction may be caused by the drug, to judge that the event is worth reporting, and to be willing to admit their own or a colleague's mistake if the event is due to physician error (Editorial, "Postmarketing drug surveillance," 2001, p. 1293). Others have cited similar attitudes, including one study that suggested that many physicians believe "really serious adverse drug events are well documented by the time the drug is marketed" and that "one case an individual physician might see cannot contribute to medical knowledge" (Figueiras, Tato, Fonatinas & Gestal-Otero, 1999, p. 810).

Canadian estimates of the number of ADRs and deaths linked to adverse reactions vary widely. In 1999, Duncan Hunter and Namrata Bains, in the *Canadian Medical*

Association Journal (*CMAJ*), estimated that an average of 16,344 Ontario hospital admissions each year were for adverse drug reactions (Hunter & Bains, 1999). In a study published by the *Journal of the American Medical Association*, researchers estimated that in 1994, more than 2.2 million patients in the United States had serious adverse drug reactions, excluding medication errors, either as the cause of admission to or while in hospital, while an additional 106,000 ADRs were fatal (Lazarou, Pomeranz & Corey, 1998). In a published interview, the researchers estimated that, based on a comparison of populations, the number of deaths in Canadian hospitals would be roughly one-tenth the U.S. figure, or 10,000 deaths each year (Abraham & Taylor, 1998). One report published in *CMAJ* estimated approximately 1,825 Canadian deaths a year could be attributed to adverse drug experiences (Bains & Hunter, 1999).

According to David Rosenbloom and Christine Wynne (1999), the annual number of deaths due to adverse drug reactions in Canada, using a 1:10 ratio of the population of Canada to that of the U.S., would total 7,600 annually. "This estimate would rank adverse drug reaction fatalities as the 7th leading cause of death in Canada, after cancer, heart disease, stroke, pulmonary disease and accidents, using 1995 Statistics Canada data," they said, adding that "adverse drug reactions prolong hospital stays by an average of 4.6 days, costing Can$300 million annually" (Rosenbloom & Wynne, 1999, p. 247). In 1999, Joel Lexchin offered an estimate of 2,925 deaths annually in Ontario alone due to adverse drug reactions (Lexchin, 1999). Another study, based on Health Canada data, found only 1,417 drug-related deaths—about 2.3 percent of all reported ADRs—nationwide between 1984 and 1994 (Mittman et al., 1997).

Lexchin has also noted that the great variance in the estimates is partially due to complexities associated with recognizing and reporting ADRs (Lexchin, 1991). These include difficulty in discerning whether the death was caused by a pre-existing condition or a drug, multiple medications taken by many hospitalized patients, lack of practical definitions on the appropriate information to collect, and the lack of a standard approach to reporting ADRs.

Thus, while the estimates regarding how many deaths due to adverse reactions are experienced each year in Canada vary widely, what is known with certainty is that adverse drug reactions are under-reported by all groups—physicians, pharmacists, and consumers. This was evident in a 2003 survey conducted by Decima Research for Health Canada in which "more than one in three (37 percent) consumers claim to have personally experienced an ADR, in most cases resulting from a prescription drug" (Decima Research, 2003, p. 5). The survey also found that reported ADRs were higher among women, the elderly, and low-income earners, but cautioned that "since these ADRs could not be independently validated, they cannot be interpreted as the true incidence of ADRs in the population." Nonetheless, the survey provided a powerful signal that the experiences Canadians have with prescription medicines are not adequately reflected in the data collected by the regulator.

Why Post-market Surveillance Is of Particular Concern to Women

Gender Differences

There is mounting evidence that sex and gender are significant risk factors for adverse drug reactions, which occur in women at a higher rate in both hospital and community settings. This may be due to physiological differences between men and women that might influence their reactions to drugs. Early studies by the U.S. Food and Drug Administration have found biological differences between men and women that suggest women may process drugs differently at the molecular level. The FDA found the same number of ADR reports for men and women in the U.S., but female reactions were more serious (Miller, 2001).

A number of studies indicate that female patients are 50–75 percent more likely to develop an adverse reaction to a drug, including adverse skin reactions, compared with male patients (Rademaker, 2001). A 1998 British study of ADR patterns across age and sex concluded that "suspected adverse drug reactions to newly marketed drugs are recorded more often in adults aged between 30 and 59 years of age and are 60 percent more common in women than in men. The sex difference occurs in all age groups over 19 years of age" (Martin et al., 1998, p. 510). A study by the Danish Medicines Agency of consumer ADR reporting in Denmark noted that 66 percent of all reports submitted by health professionals concerned adverse reactions experienced by women (Danish Medicines Agency, 2004).

The reasons for these differences between men and women are not wholly understood; however, the differences cannot be attributed solely to patterns of use. An important study published in 2004 by Monica Gandhi and colleagues found that "More and more examples of sex-related differences in pharmacokinetics and pharmacodynamics are emerging" (Gandhi, Aweeka, Greenblatt & Blaschke, 2004, p. 513). Evidence indicates, for example, that women experience more severe adverse reactions to typical antipsychotic medications than do men and "suffer from a greater number of adverse events, such as neuropathy, pancreatitis, and toxicity-driven regimen changes" on antiviral drugs used to treat HIV (Gandhi et al., 2004, p. 512). "Despite these increased reports of sex-based differences in adverse drug reactions for drugs already on the market," the authors concluded, "the evaluation of new drugs in development for differences in efficacy and toxicity by gender has not been fully instituted" (Gandhi et al., 2004, p. 513).

Thus, among certain groups—for example, those with HIV/AIDS—women may be at increased risk because they are using multiple drug therapy, one known risk factor, and because they are female, another possible risk factor. Although it is not known if sex/gender-based drug interactions are responsible for the increased adverse reactions associated with drug therapy in women, it is very clear that much more research is needed to determine the effects that usage patterns may have.

Women Are Not Served by Canada's Current System

Research on the effects of usage patterns is made more difficult in Canada because the reporting system that collects, organizes, and maintains data does not require that the sex of the patient be identified. At the very first step in the reporting process, regardless of who is reporting, there are barriers to developing a gender-based analysis of the experience Canadians have with prescription medicines. The information in filed ADR reports is required to identify:

- that a patient existed
- the suspect product
- the suspect reaction
- the reporter

While the identification of sex in ADR reports may be—and often is—submitted, it cannot be required because of the voluntary nature of the reporting system. However, a protocol of rapid follow-up could capture missing data and add an important dimension to our ability to analyze signals and identify trends. The most recent Canadian study of gender-related differences in adverse drug reactions examined patient data from the Sunnybrook Health Science Centre ADR Clinic covering the period from April 1986 to May 1996. The study found that being female is a risk factor for the development of adverse drug reactions, but concluded that "Further work is required to elucidate the mechanisms explaining the differences observed between male and female patients" (Tran et al., 1998, p. 1008). In order for such work to be conducted in Canada, there must be a more systematic and purposeful collection of data.

As of August 2008, the collection of sex-disaggregated data and gender analysis was not integrated into Health Canada's system of post-market surveillance (see Chapter 5).

Three years after Health Canada released its Guidance Document on the inclusion of women in clinical trials (see Chapter 5), it made public its Women's Health Strategy. The strategy identified four objectives, the first being "to ensure that Health Canada's policies and programs are responsive to sex and gender differences and to women's health needs." It commits Health Canada to "effective post-market surveillance and adverse events monitoring systems that safeguard women's health" (Health Canada, 1999, p. 15).

According to Susanne Reid, a manager in the Active Surveillance Division at MHPD, "No specific guidelines for the evaluation of gender, gender-related differences, and other sub-population differences have been developed" within the health protection system (personal correspondence, August 6, 2002). Similarly, she said, "the Therapeutic Products Directorate's pre-market pharmaceutical review bureaus do not look systematically at the ADR reports from a gender point of view." Reid said the directorate expected to develop guidelines to evaluate gender-related differences in adverse reactions to prescription drugs in the future. As of 2008, the post-market drug-surveillance system still did not provide adequate data to monitor and analyze sex and gender differences in ADRs, an important component of the 1999 commitment in the Women's Health Strategy.

In 2005, Health Canada initiated another round of public consultations aimed at "modernizing" the regulatory system. The resulting *Blueprint for Renewal* described a "life cycle approach" to prescription drug safety that would "encompass all stages of product development and use" (Health Canada, 2006, p. 16). At the core of the *Blueprint* was a "Progressive Licensing Framework" (PLF) that promised to manage risks and benefits more effectively, including a commitment to "a more proactive, post-market evaluation strategy" (Health Canada, 2006, p. 21) (see Chapter 8 on progressive licensing). The direction outlined in the Progressive Licensing Framework currently being proposed by Health Canada does not promise greater resources within the post-market arena to undertake this important task. And while some of the consultations concerning progressive licensing have identified the need to include considerations of sex- and gender-based analysis, it remains to be seen whether and in what ways gender-based analysis might be integrated into the PLF.

The primary purpose of collecting reports of adverse drug reactions is to "learn from experience" (Leape, 2002, p. 1633). The lack of a strategy to collect and evaluate data on women and adverse drug reactions raises concerns for a number of reasons, including that serious information gaps undermine our ability to develop evidence-based strategies designed to meet the needs of consumers. But, just as importantly, Canadian consumers have a right to be warned about drugs that may harm them and women have a right to learn from the experiences of other women. Health Canada has both a mandate and a responsibility to ensure this happens, and that the commitments in its 2000 Gender-Based Analysis Policy (see Chapter 1) and in the Women's Health Strategy, which includes post-market surveillance and monitoring of adverse drug reactions, are acted upon.

The Case for Consumer Reporting

Prior to 1997, consumers were not identified as a category among those reporting ADRs. In 1998, only 7.1 percent of ADR reports originated with patients/consumers, increasing to 9.1 percent in 1999, 13.7 percent in 2000, and 24.2 percent in

2006. Today, consumers are one of the most frequent sources of reporting after physicians, as indicated in the annual reports published in the *Canadian Adverse Reaction Newsletter*. The significant increase in the number of reports originating with consumers (identified as "consumer/patient" by CADRMP) has taken place in spite of the absence of an effective communications strategy to inform the public about the importance of reporting adverse reactions; that consumers can report directly to government; and how to go about doing so.

Table 7.1: Number of ADR Reports by Type of Reporter

Reporter	No. (%) of Cases* 1997	No. (%) of Cases* 2006
Physician	1,265 (27.1)	3,077 (29.2)
Pharmacist	1,751 (37.6)	2,396 (22.8)
Nurse	291 (6.2)	806 (7.7)
Health professional+	757 (16.2)	1,281 (12.2)
Consumer/patient	331 (7.1)	2,544 (24.2)
Other	268 (5.7)	414 (3.9)
Total	4,663 (100.0)	10,518 (100.0)

* Cases result from the merge of initial, follow-up, and duplicate reports.
+ Type not specified in report.

Sources: (1) Adverse drug reaction reporting—1998. (1999). *Canadian Adverse Reaction Newsletter (CARN), 9*(2), 5–6. Retrieved October 26, 2008, from: www.hc-sc.gc.ca/dhp-mps/alt_formats/ hpfb-dgpsa/pdf/medeff/carn-bcei_v9n2_e.pdf; (2) Adverse reaction reporting—2006. (2007). *Canadian Adverse Reaction Newsletter (CARN), 17*(2), 3–4. Retrieved September 9, 2008, from: www.hc-sc.gc.ca/dhp-mps/alt_formats/hpfb-dgpsa/pdf/medeff/carn-bcei_v17n2_e.pdf

Some evidence suggests that a majority of consumers who report adverse drug reactions are female, and some of their reports concern other family members (Miller, 2001). The Danish Medicines Agency study of consumer ADR reporting in Denmark found that, although only 7 percent of all ADR reports were submitted by consumers from July 2003 to June 2004, 71 percent of them were from women (Danish Medicines Agency, 2004).

Similar results were found in a study of a free patient-drug information service in The Netherlands. The service includes a toll-free telephone line funded by the Dutch Ministry of Health, as well as an Internet site that is a private sector initiative. The study compared the characteristics of those who used the telephone and the Internet, as well as the type of information both sets of users were seeking. It found that 68.9 percent of callers who used the direct-dial service were females, and 31.8 percent were between the ages of 20 and 40 years. Among those who accessed information on their computers, 59.5 percent were females, and 50.8 percent were between 20 and 40. In addition, a significant majority of those who used the phone were reporting or seeking information about adverse drug reactions, while those who used the Internet wanted more general information about diseases and groups of drugs. The authors of the report concluded that the differences in the two groups were probably related to differences in age and sex distribution among both populations, pointing to strategies that might be employed by regulators seeking information about adverse events (Bouvy, van Berkel, De Roos-Huisman & Meijboom, 2002).

In Canada, the sex of the reporter is not identified, but reporting patterns may be similar. *Hospital Quarterly* reported in 2002 that women were significantly more likely to report an adverse reaction than men, and were more likely to seek help in a hospital or from a health professional. The journal was unclear about the reasons for these gender differences, but suggested three possible factors: "one is that women take more medication and are therefore more likely to suffer an ADR; another is that women are more attuned to their bodies and recognize an ADR, or are more willing

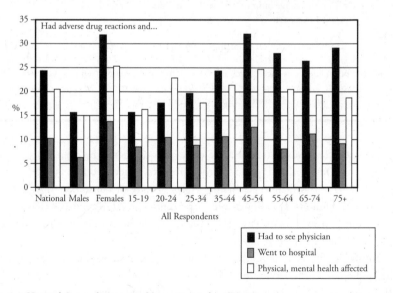

Figure 7.1: Adverse Drug Reactions: Reporting of ADRs Varies by Gender and Age

Source: Hospital Quarterly (now Healthcare Quarterly), 6(2), 95.

to acknowledge both that they are experiencing an ADR and that they should see someone about it; and the third is that there is a subjective aspect to the reporting of ADRs" ("Quarterly index: Adverse drug reactions," 2002, p. 95).

Consumer reporting was not part of the spontaneous ADR reporting system until very recently, and there continues to be debate, both in Canada and internationally, about the merits of information provided directly by those who experience adverse effects. A paper adopted at the WHO's First International Conference on Consumer Reports on Medicines in 2000 cited the continuing prominence of "medical mysticism" in some countries, a phenomenon "characterized by a desire to maintain secrecy around medical facts and thinking" that could inhibit more robust consumer reporting. "Improved public education and information services," the authors wrote, "coupled with more modern attitudes on the part of professionals, can do much to remedy such problems" (Finer, Albinson, Westin & Dukes, 2000, pp. 119–120).

Many have suggested that consumer ADR reports may be of a lower quality than reports made by health professionals and that the "usefulness of reports that have not been medically validated might be less because patients may misattribute symptoms [of illness] to an ADR" (Blenkinsopp, Wilkie, Wang & Routledge, 2006, p. 154). Even where attribution is correct, some felt that consumers would report a higher proportion of non-serious or known adverse reactions and that such "additional noise" might distract regulators and "result in system overload" (Blenkinsopp et al., 2006, p. 154).

Concerns about the potential contribution of non-professionals to post-market surveillance have been addressed in a growing number of studies about direct-from-consumer reporting (Blenkinsopp et al., 2006). A report from the Netherlands argued that "Consumer reporting is in line with the striving for quality in the healthcare system," concluding that more research is needed to accurately assess the value of this source of information (van Grootheest et al., 2003, p. 215). Others have found that "None of the countries with patient reporting systems has reported poor quality of patient reports to be an issue" (Blenkinsopp et al., 2006, p. 155). The work of Britain's Social Audit has shown that significant media and regulatory attention to a particular drug can substantially increase the number of consumer reports of harm (Medawar, Herxheimer, Bell & Jofre, 2002). Medawar and Herxheimer cite the case of Paxil (paroxetene) as a specific example, noting that "the overall quality of professional reporting and interpretation of data seemed poor, providing intelligence that was in some ways inferior to that provided in spontaneous reports from patients" (Medawar & Herxheimer, 2003/2004, p. 5).

A number of consumer groups have emerged in Canada and internationally to support a larger role for consumers in ADR data collection. Among the first was Kilen, the Swedish Consumer Institute for Medicines and Health. Founded in 1978, Kilen has provided effective leadership in a growing international movement to increase the role of consumers in the regulation of prescription medicines generally, and in post-market monitoring specifically. Kilen's experiences in consumer ADR reporting have been closely watched by women's health activists. In 2001, PharmaWatch was established in Canada to encourage consumer advocacy and raise public awareness about ADR reporting. Two years later, Health Canada began accepting ADR reports directly from consumers, but has yet to actively encourage such reporting (Blenkinsopp et al., 2006).

Women health activists are key advocates of direct-from-consumer reporting (as articulated by DES Action Canada, Women and Health Protection, and PharmaWatch), in part because it supports women acting as their own agents within the health system, an important goal of the women's health community (Murtagh & Hepworth, 2003). In some cases, physicians or manufacturers may not view an adverse drug reaction as serious enough to report, thereby contributing to low reporting rates generally, while undervaluing the opinion of the person who experiences the event.

Consumer reporting has the potential to be an important early warning system about problems associated with prescription drugs. A monitoring system that encourages consumers to play a role can increase knowledge about medicinal drugs and thereby reduce drug-related adverse effects and injuries. Expanding the source of information to include consumers empowers them in an environment in which manufacturers exercise almost total market control, including over information about safety and efficacy.

While MHPD does not actively encourage consumers to report adverse drug reactions, recent improvements have been made to the directorate's website. In August 2005, after extensive cross-country consultations, the directorate launched Medeffect, a web-based communication strategy to provide Canadians with information about prescription and over-the-counter (OTC) drugs, natural (herbal) medicines, and medical devices. The website provides public access to a broad range of information, including legislation and policies; a guide to reporting adverse drug reactions online, by telephone, or in writing; and drug advisories and warnings. Consumers and health professionals can also obtain information about ADR reports through CADRMP's database on the Medeffect website.

But the lack of a proactive strategy to encourage consumer reporting undermines efforts to raise public awareness about the ability of consumers to report directly to MHPD any adverse drug reactions that they or family members may experience. An effective strategy proposed by the Canadian Treatment Action Council (CTAC) in 2007 would encourage independent consumer groups to act as "community sentinels"—that is, groups that would collect consumer reports of adverse side effects and work within their own constituencies to raise awareness about the importance of ADR monitoring (Canadian Treatment Action Council, 2007).

Strategies to increase direct-from-consumer reporting are not only appropriate but, within the overall system of post-market surveillance, can provide key information about the safety of prescription medicines. A strategy that aims to increase public awareness will have to consider the higher reporting rates among females across all age groups, and the fact that women are also more likely to report on behalf of other family members. A strategy that addresses the specific socio-economic and cultural characteristics of different groups within the population at large will be more effective than one that ignores these factors.

Conclusion

The current system of post-market surveillance does not serve Canadians well, regardless of their sex. Women, however, are particularly affected because of their greater reliance on prescription medicines and their greater vulnerability to adverse effects caused by prescription drug use. Despite a number of strong and positive initiatives within Health Canada to develop strategies that support women's health, the regulations in place to ensure that women are protected once drugs are on the market are very weak. Existing programs and policies might have a positive influence on the system of post-market surveillance if that system were adequately funded. In addition, there must be a stronger political will to ensure that Canada's prescription drug surveillance is effective, and that information about drug safety and experiences flows both to and from consumers.

Chapter 8

Questioning Modernization
Legislative Change at Health Canada[1]

—————⟡—————

Anne Rochon Ford

The relationship between the regulator and the regulated … must never become one in which the regulator loses sight of the principle that it regulates only in the public interest and not in the interest of the regulated.

—Justice Krever,
Commission of Inquiry on the Blood System in Canada, 1997

Introduction

In 1997, the Canadian government issued a call for feedback on a document aimed at "modernizing" federal health protection legislation, a proposal that would see the existing *Food and Drugs Act*, along with 10 other acts of Parliament, replaced by new legislation. A number of women's health groups, academics, and health care workers felt compelled to respond to this initiative because of concerns that the federal government's duty to protect the health and safety of the people of Canada was being undermined.

Their concerns were based in a perceived weakening of regulators' authority over the pharmaceutical industry's activities. Examples from recent history, such as the tainted blood scandal of the 1980s, had not helped to instill confidence that the federal government was wholly adhering to its duty to put health protection above other objectives. More recent events, such as the withdrawal of the arthritis medication, Vioxx (rofecoxib), and the approval of silicone gel breast implants have only fuelled this fear.

This chapter looks at Health Canada's legislative "renewal" initiatives over the past 10 years, as well as the responses to these initiatives from health and social justice groups, including Women and Health Protection (WHP). While legislative change is not an issue specific to women only, women's health organizations became involved in this process because of the legacy of drug and device harms specific to women elaborated elsewhere in this book. Inherent in WHP's understanding of health protection issues is the belief that society's less powerful groups need an especially strong voice advocating on their behalf.

This story—a series of government proposals and actions, and corresponding community-based reactions—has evolved in important ways since 1997. However, a number of repeated threads are evident and continue to cause concern. Foremost is the question of the motivation behind the proposed changes, and the particular interpretation given to the words "modernize" and "renewal" in this context. Health Canada's shift in approach and methodology, from one based on the precautionary principle to a risk management framework (concepts addressed in chapters 3 and 7), is examined for its impact on health protection, with reference to how this discussion relates to women.

This account of legislative renewal in drug regulation is a slice of an ongoing process. Over 10 years have passed since the first initiative in 1997 and for the first time in the process, the federal government released new draft legislation in 2008. The writing of this chapter coincides with the release of Bill C-51, which is intended to amend the existing *Food and Drugs Act.* This chapter does not attempt to summarize the many responses to Bill C-51, and timing does not permit the author to report on the ultimate conclusion of the bill's movement through Parliament. For updates on the status of the bill, refer to the websites provided at the end of this chapter.

The Dawning of the "Smart Regulations" Era

A series of events in the federal government throughout the 1990s led to a concerted push for industrial expansion and innovation as a means of boosting the Canadian economy. While not a negative force in and of itself, tensions arose and continue to arise when this agenda bumps up against long-held Canadian values of health protection, values that include ensuring that the health of individual Canadians and the social health of Canadian society take precedence over commercial interests. One arena where this tension has played out most vividly is in drug regulation at Health Canada, where federal regulators are caught between the push from government to boost the economy through innovation and the long-standing imperative to protect the people of Canada from harms caused by new drugs and devices. Health Canada's proposals for "renewal" provide clear evidence that protection of the public is being subsumed by the move toward industrial and economic expansion in the pharmaceutical sector. WHP's summary of concerns in 1998 spoke of a growing public perception of an agency that increasingly viewed the pharmaceutical industry, and not the public, as its main client (Women and Health Protection, 1998).[2]

In 1994, Industry Canada revealed its strategy for economic and industrial expansion in its report, *Building a More Innovative Economy*, in which it spoke of the need for "regulatory reform to release business energies." In language apparently intended to reassure the public that it had its best interests at heart, the authors noted that: "Regulations help us to keep our markets competitive, our products safe and our environment clean." The document also stated that one of the six sectors where they hoped to "improve[e] regulations ... [to] help create jobs" and growth was that of health, food, and therapeutic products, the sector regulated by Health Canada (Industry Canada, 1994, pp. 4, 5).

There were signs in the document that the move to "smart regulations" was on the horizon. The authors note that "Business has told us that one of the most effective steps the government can take to encourage jobs and growth is to regulate smarter. We agree" (Industry Canada, 1994, p. 4). In other words, government regulation was seen to be inhibiting economic expansion and development, and so the tools used to regulate needed "modernizing." Health Canada's early presentations to the public, designed to explain the need for legislative "renewal," often included an image of a clearly outdated, older vehicle or a tool box without the proper tools in it, with references to an "outdated regulatory toolkit." These were intended as illustrations of how incontrovertibly outdated the legislation was, and why it needed to be overhauled.

This shift toward "smarter" regulating has been part of a larger international move toward adopting more flexible regulatory regimes and conforming to international norms set by organizations focused on market values, such as the World Trade Organization, the Organisation for Economic Co-operation and Development, the International Conference on Harmonization, the Tripartite and Trilateral Committees, and the Codex Alimentarius Commission, the international organization charged with developing standards for international trade in food. The process of harmonizing regulations in order to remove the barrier of national regulations that may not favour corporate interests has been a growing and persistent trend of the late 20th century and the early 21st century. This move toward globalization of the health care sector, in part through harmonization of related regulations, has been presented to the public by Health Canada as inevitable, with anything but this direction being simply "out of date," like the older car referred to above. In practice, harmonization with other countries can mean the lowering of Canadian health protection standards and demonstrates that Health Canada is allowing industrial competitiveness to share the stage with public health.

This historical context provides an important backdrop to any discussion of legislative renewal.

What's So Important about the *Food and Drugs Act*?

Canada's *Food and Drugs Act* and the regulations made under it were written in an era when the government was entrusted with and accepted the duty of protecting the public from harmful drugs, medical devices, and food. It was first passed in Parliament in 1920, and most recently amended in 1985. Its focus is on the production, import, export, and transport of food, drugs, contraceptive devices, and cosmetics. It addresses, as well, the conditions of sale, advertising, packaging, labelling, and inspection of these products. The act and its regulations are in place to ensure that approved drugs and medical devices are safe, that their ingredients are fully disclosed, and that they are effective and are not marketed in a misleading way.[3] Part C of the act pertains specifically to drugs. Despite the evolution of therapeutics since the legislation was originally passed, the basic public health values on which the act is based still remain valid.

In July 1998, Health Canada released a discussion paper entitled *Shared Responsibilities, Shared Vision: Renewing the Federal Health Protection Legislation*. Following on a series of proposals, which dated back to 1992, for changes to the structure and functioning of what was then known as the Health Protection Branch (reorganized and renamed, in 2000, the Health Products and Food Branch [HPFB]), this paper called for a significant overhaul of the *Food and Drugs Act*. One of the central issues for groups monitoring this process was whether it was either wise or necessary to open up and dismantle this critical piece of legislation.

Health Canada held a series of public consultations in major Canadian cities in the fall of 1998 to discuss the changes they were proposing and solicit public input into a series of recommendations relating to the regulation of drugs and devices. The need for sensitivity to sex and gender issues was raised throughout Health Canada's discussion paper, but it remained to be seen whether the implications for women's health or rights would be fully considered in this process. As noted elsewhere in this volume, women bring particular concerns to such tables of discussion. Women and Health Protection pressed for a gender-based analysis of any proposed changes to the legislation (Women and Health Protection, 1998).

In its presentation to the government consultation, Women and Health Protection maintained that the existing legislation still allowed Health Canada to achieve its health protection mandate effectively and that it was not necessary to dismantle the act: WHP argued that improved enforcement of the legislation, through a series of amendments to the regulations, would best further the goal of health protection without compromising the values in the legislation. As one example, WHP pointed out that a better post-marketing surveillance system and improved information to consumers about safety issues did not require legislative change. The group had a strong concern that the reference to modernization was simply a euphemism for making regulation more palatable to industry.

This concern about doing away with existing legislation is not unique. A decade ago, when the National Forum on Health[4] was carrying out its investigation of ways to improve the health system and the health of Canadians, it asked if the *Canada Health Act* adequately met current needs or whether there were deficiencies that needed to be addressed. The conclusion of this review was clear: although the act was imperfect, the risks of opening up the act outweighed any potential benefits (National Forum on Health, 1997).[5]

While proposals from the Health Products and Food Branch (HPFB) of Health Canada outlined what was missing in the existing legislation, and why "modernization" was needed to address various societal changes and drug-related tragedies, Health Canada has yet to make a convincing argument that dismantling the existing act and creating an entirely new one is necessary. For example, giving the government the authority to require additional testing of drugs once they are on the market, something many saw as a necessary change, could be achieved by regulation. The Krever Commission Report (1997) was cited in the 2004 proposal from HPFB as a reason for needing to replace the existing act. But while Justice Krever called for many changes to the current regulatory system, replacing the existing act with a new one was not specifically one of them; rather, the report called for improved and updated regulations.

Other critics of the legislative change process have argued that regulations are the most effective instruments for achieving policy objectives, such as safety, openness and transparency, and accountability. The Canadian Environmental Law Association (2004b), for example, offers to the debate that "adequately-resourced and enforced regulations have proven to be the best instrument for protecting public goods [because] … individual and corporate actors wish not to suffer the public disrepute, cost and other disadvantages of prosecution or penalty." They add further that "surveys of corporate leaders show that the existence and enforcement of regulations give the strongest motivation for compliance" (p. 3).

While the current legislation is not perfect, it does address many important health protection functions that are essential to preserve. For instance, the legislation makes it clear that it is the minister of health who has the final responsibility for enforcing the Act and therefore the government is accountable if there is a problem. The department was originally created to protect Canadians from harmful products, not to help market drugs and devices, nor to partner with industry. In all of Health Canada's literature about legislative change, there appears to be no mention of the department's duty to protect Canadians.

The concerns that have been expressed about opening up the act echo concerns expressed during the debate on health care privatization about opening the *Canada Health Act*: that the wishes of industry (the pharmaceutical industry in the case of the *Food and Drugs Act* and the purveyors of private health care in the case of the *Canada Health Act*) will predominate and will trump public health. WHP and others have argued that the current problems with Canada's health protection system have more to do with a lack of enforcement authority (or will) than with faults in the current legislation. Nowhere is this more true than in the laws respecting direct-to-consumer advertising (DTCA) (see Chapter 2). In fact, there is no lack of enforcement authority in the current law, but rather lack of bureaucratic and political will to enforce it.

Early Concerns about Legislative Renewal: What Was behind the Critiques?

> If industry takes on more responsibility for product safety and standards, Canadians want assurance that public health interests will continue to be the first priority.
> —*Health Protection for the 21st Century: Renewing the Federal Health Protection Program* (Health Canada, 1998a)

The shift from a focus on public health to a focus on industrial expansion has been gradual, and the push to "modernize" has been part of the discourse of Health Canada publications for more than a decade. Significant funding cuts to the Health

Protection Branch occurred in the early 1990s. In 1993–1994, the branch budget was $237 million; by 1999–2000, it was down to $118 million, with money from user fees imposed on industry replacing parliamentary appropriations. In the intervening years, in-house drug research laboratories, which were responsible for investigating drug quality, toxicity, bioequivalence, and clinical applications, were effectively dismantled. Whereas most health protection functions were once integrated within one area, some discrete functions were moved elsewhere, such as transferring food inspectors to the Canadian Food Inspection Agency and the Laboratory Centre for Disease Control, now under the aegis of the Public Health Agency of Canada. On the surface, these types of transfers may seem reasonable, but the Food Inspection Agency, for instance, is now part of Agriculture and Agri-Food Canada, which also has a mandate to support agribusiness.

In 2000, Health Canada undertook to "strengthen its health promotion and health protection activities" by "realigning" these functions into three newly created branches: Health Products and Food, Environmental and Product Safety, and Population and Public Health, with the Health Products and Food Branch assuming the activities related to drug regulation (Health Canada, 2000). While there may have been legitimate reasons for the name change and the above-noted reorganization,[6] these changes served as indicators to concerned citizens of a gradual erosion of the government's protective function. A Health Canada media release about the realignment spoke of this being "part of ongoing efforts to respond to challenges identified in consultation" (Health Canada, 2000). It is fair to ask whether the challenges referred to were those raised by industry or those raised by concerned citizens.

Also in 2000, members of Women and Health Protection met with legal counsel from the Office of Legislative Renewal to discuss their concerns and followed up in writing with a series of recommendations. First and foremost was the following: "That the stated objective of the new legislation must be the protection of the health and safety of Canadian women, men, and children, rather than the modernization of health protection statutes. The goals of modernization may not always put the health and safety of Canadians in the primary position it must occupy" (Women and Health Protection, 2000, p. 1). On a rhetorical level, Health Canada representatives agreed with the position of WHP; on a practical level, little seemed to change as new proposals for legislative renewal echoed the themes in previous versions.

Into the 21st Century: Where Are We Now?

Following consultations held by Health Canada in the late 1990s, a new phase of activity around health protection occurred in 2003 when a legislative proposal was prepared by the Office of Legislative Renewal. The proposal held up for review four major acts (the *Food and Drugs Act*, the *Hazardous Products Act*, the *Quarantine*

Box 8.1: The 4 Ds of Government and Corporate Response to Opposition (as explained at numerous public presentations over the past 10 years by Dr. Michèle Brill-Edwards, former staff scientist at Health Canada)

DENY for as long as possible that there is a problem even though it has been clearly spelled out.

DELAY any response to the claims by setting up committees, calling for more research, claim the problem is being dealt with.

DIVIDE those who are bringing forward complaints by telling the more easily appeased that they'll get what they want, while

*DISCREDIT*ing the more hard-line opponents by calling them "difficult" or "unreliable."

Source: Brill-Edwards, M. (1999). Canada's Health Protection Branch: Whose health, what protection? In M.L. Barer, K. McGrail, K. Cardiff, L. Wood & C.J. Green (Eds.), *Tales from the other drug wars (Papers from the 12th Annual Health Policy Conference held in Vancouver, BC, November 26, 1999)* (pp. 51–52). Vancouver: Centre for Health Services and Policy Research, University of British Columbia.

Act, and the *Radiation Emitting Devices Act*) with a recommendation that they be consolidated into a Canada Health Protection Act. (The other six acts mentioned in the 1997 proposal were being dealt with by alternate means.) Language that had been used to describe the previous phase of proposals for legislative change—"the HPB Transition"—was gone, but talk of the need to "modernize" was still very much present. "Health, safety, openness, and accountability" were repeated as the guiding principles of the document, and in response to calls in the previous round of consultations for adherence to the precautionary principle, this new proposal referred to "the concept of precaution."[7] Also new in this phase was the introduction of a "General Safety Requirement." This consisted of a proposed series of obligations that would be placed on manufacturers, importers, and suppliers and that, when violations occurred, would incur after-the-fact criminal prosecutions, rather than instituting policies that would prevent harm in the first place. It is worth noting that the term "General Safety Requirement" is not a legislative term and is not found in the proposed Bill C-51. As noted in a Health Canada background policy document entitled *The Role of the General Safety Requirement in Canada's Health Protection Regime*, "The legal and political *raison d'être* of the GSR is internal trade" (Health Canada, 2006a).

In its evaluation of the 2003 proposal from Health Canada, the Canadian Environmental Law Association (CELA) suggested that it took "a minimalist view of the role and responsibilities of Health Canada in the protection of people's health" (Canadian Environmental Law Association, 2004a, p. 5). Although CELA was speaking in the context of the environmental protection and health aspects of the proposal, its criticisms are equally relevant to the issues that concerned WHP. For example, CELA noted that the Government of Canada Regulatory Policy, which governs all departments, lists trade agreements that Canada has signed, but not any of the international health, human rights, or environmental treaties to which Canada is a party.

Many of the proposals in the 2003 draft of the legislation were not acted upon and, with the formal legislative "renewal" process becoming the lightning rod for much of the criticism of the drug regulatory system, changes that would lead to legislative change in a more indirect way began to happen within the Health Products and Food Branch.

Eliminating the Backlog

By the early 2000s, Health Canada had been experiencing growing pressure for some time from industry, supported by people from disease groups, to speed up the drug approval process. Canada's track record was compared to other countries and found wanting. Delays became an important consumer issue during the HIV/AIDS crisis, when AIDS groups fought for faster approval of life-saving drugs. The industry was able to take advantage of this groundswell of activism to push through policies designed to bring all drugs to market faster.

By 2001, movement on the legislative change front took the form of dealing with the backlog of drugs awaiting approval. Over half of the time between when a company filed a new drug submission and when a decision was made was taken up waiting for the review process to actually start. This prolonged delay was a particular sore point for the brand-name pharmaceutical industry, since it shortened the amount of patent-protected time their products had on the market. For consumers, in some cases, faster drug approvals have also meant faster exposure to unnecessarily harmful drugs.

As the goals of the industry and Health Canada became more aligned, Health Canada adopted some of the industry's goals and the elimination of the approval backlog became a major priority, with a corresponding significant investment of money and personnel. So it was partially in response to industry's call for faster approval of their products that the Health Policy Branch of Health Canada launched the Therapeutics Access Strategy in 2003. The strategy succeeded, over the following four years, in eliminating the backlog of reviews in pharmaceuticals and biologics, but the benefit mostly accrued to the pharmaceutical industry, not the consumers of the more rapidly approved medications. For example, in their analysis of the increase in drug withdrawals in the U.S. and U.K. between 1971 and 1992, Abraham and Davis concluded that "it is likely that acceleration of regulatory review times in the U.S. and the U.K. since the early 1990s is compromising drug safety" (Abraham & Davis, 2005, p. 881).

Opening the Medicine Cabinet

In the early 2000s, public hearings on prescription drugs again took place, this time for the all-party Standing Committee on Health. In 2004, the committee issued its report, *Opening the Medicine Cabinet*, based on findings from the hearings. The report made strong recommendations about some key issues: the need for increased transparency in how clinical trials are conducted; increased resources for post-marketing surveillance of adverse drug reactions; and an immediate prohibition of all industry-sponsored advertisements of prescription drugs to the public, including reminder ads and help-seeking messages.

Box 8.2: Key Points from the Report (Standing Committee on Health, 2004)

"The Committee strongly supports the development of accreditation and oversight for research ethics boards responsible for assessing clinical trials. It also wants a full and open public discussion about confidentiality agreements that currently prevent disclosure concerning negative outcomes in clinical trials. In particular, it feels that information on all serious adverse drug reactions observed during clinical trials and reported to Health Canada should be made publicly available" (p. 4).

"The Committee wants to ensure that the observations made by consumers about adverse drug reactions are taken seriously; that they are reported, recorded, reviewed and made publicly available" (p. 7).

"The Committee has multiple concerns about direct-to-consumer advertising of prescription drugs. It feels that such advertising contributes to increased health care costs; does not provide balanced and unbiased information; is potentially harmful to consumers; and has no ongoing scrutiny. The Committee therefore seeks strict measures to ensure that the existing prohibition is actively enforced" (p. 10).

Unfortunately, given the lag between activity at the parliamentary level and activity at the bureaucratic level of government, and with standing committee reports being subject to the desires of the government of the day, action by Health Canada on these recommendations proved to be less than one might have hoped. The recommendations on DTCA and increased resources for post-marketing surveillance were largely ignored, and the only significant action on increasing transparency has been the creation of a document called *Summary Basis of Decision* for new drugs (see Chapter 6). While there is some useful data in these documents, overall the amount of information released is too limited to allow people to look for safety and effectiveness issues that manufacturers and regulators may have ignored (Lexchin & Mintzes, 2004).

Box 8.3: When the Left Arm Is Confronted by What the Right Arm Is Doing

The following discussion, which occurred at the public hearings held by the Standing Committee on Health, aptly illustrates the information gap between parliamentarians and the federal bureaucracy. It raises questions about whether the legislative authority of elected officials is taken seriously by those in the civil service mandated to implement government policy. The following excerpted exchange occurred at the hearings in Toronto in October 2003 between the author and the member of Parliament chairing the Standing Committee at the time:

ARF: Can I just ask a question as to what the relationship is between this and the whole legislative renewal process that's going on? Will you feed into it—the recommendations?

The Chair: What do you mean by the legislative renewal?

ARF: Well, the whole process that's taking place within the legislative renewal office, the hearings across the country in response to proposals they've put forward about the changes, from the *Food and Drugs Act* to the new Canada Health Protection Act.

The Chair: What is the legislative renewal office? I have no idea. Our relationship is to the Minister of Health. We advise her. She does not control the notice of compliance regulations and the automatic injunction business.

ARF: Within Health Canada, there is an office of legislative renewal that has been set up in order to specifically transform and change the many acts that come under the *Food and Drugs Act*. They're proposing a new health protection act.

The Chair: … It is sheerly a bureaucratic exercise, and I'm actually a little bit annoyed they're calling it "legislative" renewal, seeing as they are not legislators. It should have been called "administrative" renewal because they are administrators. I will speak to the minister about that. It's ridiculous to call what bureaucrats are doing on their own at the request of their minister legislative renewal. That's why, obviously, it's natural for you to ask us about that because we're legislators. But as far as I know, they are not doing anything that has to do with legislation.

ARF: They're proposing legislation that will then go before you. That's the process.

The Chair: They are now preparing legislation on what subject?

ARF: On the *Food and Drugs Act*.

The Chair: Oh, the *Food and Drugs Act*. I wouldn't call that legislative renewal. I would call it a review of the *Food and Drugs Act*, the preparation of a new act or amendment.

ARF: It would be extremely beneficial if what you hear going across the country could be fed into that. There is a series of public hearings going on across …

The Chair: Into what?

ARF: Into that bureaucratic process that's happening as well. Because many of the same people are appearing at these same hearings on these very same issues. So, just in terms of the optics, it's difficult for us as consumers and citizens of Canada to not feel frustrated that we're being asked multiple times to get up and say the same things about what the issues are around prescription drugs from our particular perspectives. It would be extremely beneficial if there were discussions between the two processes that are going on. The legislative renewal office is headed by Len Kuchar in Health Canada.

The Chair: He is the top bureaucrat in charge of that process? Oh, I can't wait to get back there and phone him. I am absolutely enraged that they are holding hearings on the same topic. Is it on the topic of prescription drugs? And are they travelling as well?

ARF: Yes. It includes broader … the other acts, the Quarantine Act and the others that come under that jurisdiction, but prescription drugs is one of the main issues that's being discussed. They've put out a document called *Health and Safety First*, which contains the recommendations for what the change in legislation should look like. It includes things like direct-to-consumer advertising. All the things we've been talking about today are in there.

The Chair: We are completely and totally unaware of that exercise, despite the fact that officials from Health Canada were among our first witnesses as we began this study. So needless to say, there will be a slight fuss raised back in Ottawa next week because of what you told me.

Source: Excerpted from Standing Committee on Health, 2003. 37th *Parliament, 2nd Session, Standing Committee on Health, Evidence /Content, Wednesday, October 29.* Retrieved August 17, 2008, from: cmte.parl.gc.ca/cmte/CommitteePublication.aspx?SourceId=67157

Smarting from Smart Regulations

In keeping with the earlier-noted government directive on "smarter regulations," then Prime Minister Jean Chrétien established an External Advisory Committee on Smart Regulation (EACSR) in 2003. Although there was one consumer representative on the committee, there was no one there specifically representing health interests. The majority of the members, including the chair, came from the corporate sector. Not surprisingly, when the committee released its report in 2004, it called for deeper integration with the United States to enhance "greater international regulatory co-operation."[8] It spoke of the ability of "smart regulations to be both protecting and enabling," a notion that some found, at best, perplexing and, at worst, disturbing (External Working Group, 2004, p. 12).

Another key part of the EACSR report was its emphasis on risk management as an essential tool in building business confidence in the Canadian market and regulatory system. A risk management approach makes good sense where economic considerations are the primary concern. When applied to drug regulation, however, risk management involves weighing potential harmful effects of drugs against their potential health benefits. Since all pharmacologically active substances have multiple effects on the body, some of which are harmful, every drug-approval decision has an element of risk management associated with it and requires balancing potential benefit against potential harm. However, a precautionary approach to drug approval would dictate that greater emphasis be placed on the need for significant health benefits that clearly outweigh potential harm, putting the health of the drug consumer, not economic considerations, front and centre.

Management of the "smart regulation" process was taken up by the Privy Council Office, which called for public hearings to respond to the Smart Regulations Initiative and a draft directive to be produced for the purpose of consultation. In 2005, with leadership provided largely by the Canadian Environmental Law Association, WHP participated with a number of other non-governmental organizations (NGOs) in the preparation of a joint response to the draft directive. In hearings across Canada in 2005 and early 2006, many citizens' organizations concerned with safety and protection of health and the environment brought forward the message, earlier articulated by CELA, that government should build "government science, regulatory and enforcement capacity, not dismantle it through entrenchment of risk-based strategies and reliance on the free hand of the market" (Canadian Environmental Law Association, 2004b, p. 4).

This process of consultation ultimately resulted, in 2007, in a Cabinet Directive on Streamlining Regulations, a directive that, regrettably, does not include many of the key elements that advocacy and citizen groups were asking for in the consultations. The website where the consultations are summarized does, however, acknowledge the concerns that consultation participants had with the process and the draft directive:

> Generally speaking, participants from the public advocacy sector felt strongly that the draft Directive subscribed to a business/economy-first paradigm and therefore did not break with approaches in the past. They expressed disappointment that the draft Directive did not emphasize and prioritize respect and protection for the environment, human health and safety over economic concerns. They pointed out that this bias was reflected in the sections of the draft Directive that require: regulatory initiatives to comply with international trade obligations (such as the World Trade Organization (WTO) Agreement and the North American Free Trade Agreement); departments to conduct economic impact analyses of regulatory proposals, especially the reference to measuring costs and benefits; and, requirements to analyze and manage risks. In particular, they felt there was an excessive

emphasis in the draft Directive on fulfilling international obligations (lines 259 to 305; lines 291 to 343 in the French version), particularly those with a trade component. Suggestions were made for removing these references or at least rewriting the section to convey the idea that the need for protection of health, safety and environment supersedes economic factors, including Canada's international trade commitments (Privy Council Office, 2006, para. 11).

Blueprint for Renewal

In 2006, legislative reform re-emerged when the Health Products and Food Branch released its *Blueprint for Renewal: Transforming Canada's Approach to Regulating Health Products and Food*. The plan spoke of a continued need for "modernization," with a new focus on a "life cycle approach" that would "encompass all stages of product development and use" (Health Products and Food Branch, 2006, p. 3). The life cycle of a product is understood to include "research and development, through to clinical trial Phases I, II and III (where applicable), regulatory approval and market authorization, and use in the real world" (p. 16). The *Blueprint* was rooted in "a transformation of current business practices to increase efficiency, effectiveness, transparency and responsiveness" (Health Products and Food Branch, 2006, p. 27). The phrase "business practices" is especially noteworthy as it echoes the central theme in the Business Transformation Strategy (BTS) that was initiated in 2003. BTS "builds on the commitments made by the Government of Canada to 'speed up the regulatory process for drug approvals,' to move forward with a smart regulations strategy to accelerate reforms in key areas to promote health and sustainability, to contribute to innovation and economic growth, and to reduce the administrative burden on business" (Therapeutic Products Directorate, 2004, p. 1). Once again, the shift to corporate values, while subtle, was evident.

Women and Health Protection presented a brief to then assistant deputy minister in the Health Products and Food Branch, Neil Yeates, elaborating on its concerns about the *Blueprint for Renewal*:

> We are disappointed to see that many of the concerns that we and others have been raising for almost a decade continue to go unanswered. We come away from reading this document with a sense that the essence of the precautionary principle for drug and device regulation has been lost, only to be replaced by notions of "managing risk." With a legacy of problems that have arisen because precaution was not exercised (DES, HRT, Vioxx, etc.), it is distressing to see this ethic not being more wholeheartedly embraced by our regulators. Instead we read that "… science and management capacities are defined by the business processes that support the gathering of evidence,

generation of new knowledge and a rigorous approach to decision-making."
(Women and Health Protection, 2006, p. 1)

Progressive Licensing Framework
A critical component of the *Blueprint for Renewal* is the Progressive Licensing
Framework. The initial discussion paper on the framework noted: "The central
concept of Progressive Licensing is that, over time, there is a progression in knowledge
about a drug ... rather than placing the focus primarily upon pre-market assessment
... [t]he new proposed model is that a drug should be evaluated throughout its
life-cycle for its benefit-risk profile" (Health Canada, 2006b, p. 4). The framework
pointed to a "greater emphasis on pharmacovigilance and risk management" (lines
190–191), and acknowledged the difference between regulating drugs for different
situations (emergency situations, life-threatening conditions, minor conditions, etc.).
A key component of the proposed model was that it would allow for the collection,
analysis, and communication of information about a drug throughout the product's
life cycle. While a life cycle approach is potentially very valuable, its effectiveness
would depend on the way it is implemented. Unfortunately, Bill C-51, introduced
by the Conservative government in the spring of 2008, does not bode well for
implementation.

One concern is that progressive licensing would intensify an existing trend to
release drugs onto the market based on intermediate benefits, such as increasing bone
density, rather than their effect on people's actual health, such as a reduction in the
rate of symptomatic fractures. There are already concerns about existing standards
for measuring drug effectiveness, and that the public is, in fact, being used as trial
subjects without the benefit of proper informed consent. The Progressive Licensing
Framework would make the situation worse by relying on strengthened post-market
surveillance—one of the weakest, most understaffed and underfunded areas of the
Health Products and Food Branch.

Canada already has a policy in place, the "Notice of Compliance with conditions"
(NOC/c), which allows Health Canada to approve new drugs for serious illnesses
with only incomplete data. In return, manufacturers agree to perform additional tests
to validate the initial promise that these drugs show. However, some drugs have been
sold for up to nine years without these studies having been completed, and Health
Canada does not release any information about the status of these studies. As a result,
doctors continue to prescribe, and patients continue to take, drugs of unproven
effectiveness and about which there is limited safety information (see Chapter 6).

As of this writing, the directorate within the Health Products and Food Branch
responsible for post-marketing surveillance receives about one-fifth the amount of
money and has one-fifth the number of staff as compared to the directorate that
approves new drugs (Progestic International Inc., 2004, p. 24). If Health Canada is

going to effectively engage in post-marketing surveillance as Bill C-51 anticipates, there will have to be a massive investment in that area, an investment that has not been forthcoming to date.

Table 8.1: Allocation of $40 Million for Improvements in the Drug Regulatory System, Fiscal 2003–2004		
Program Area	Percent of Money	Dollars ($000,000)
Improved regulatory performance	78	31.2
Enhanced post-marketing safety	6.5	2.6
Optimal drug therapy	6	2.4
Price review capacity	1.25	0.5
Therapeutic access strategy	8.25	3.3

Source: Health Canada. (2003). *Improving Canada's regulatory process for therapeutic products: Building the action plan.* PowerPoint presentation to the multi-stakeholder session of the Public Policy Forum consultation, "Improving Canada's Regulatory Process for Therapeutic Products," Ottawa, November 2–3, 2003.

Finally, under Bill C-51, Health Canada would be given additional authority to issue market authorization for a drug, subject to additional terms and conditions, and to suspend the authorization if the company does not follow through on its obligations to conduct post-marketing studies regarding safety and effectiveness. While, in theory, this additional information would be valuable in assessing where new products should fit into the therapeutic armamentarium, in reality there are serious concerns about relying on industry-funded studies. A qualitative systematic review has shown that commercially sponsored research is much more likely to result in positive outcomes for the drug being studied than research funded from any other source (Sismondo, 2008).

Direct-to-Consumer Advertising

Also significantly influencing the direction of Health Canada's work on legislative change was the news in 2006 that CanWest Media had filed a lawsuit against the federal government, charging that Canada's prohibition of direct-to-consumer advertising (DTCA) of prescription drugs is an unjustified infringement of the company's freedom of expression, as guaranteed under Section 2(b) of Canada's Charter of Rights. Because it is Health Canada's responsibility to defend the current law prohibiting DTCA—a critical piece of the *Food and Drugs Act*—legislative changes relating to DTCA are indefinitely on hold. It therefore remains to be seen whether Health Canada will change the legislation to make it more favourable to industry or whether it will tighten enforcement of the current law as health advocates have been calling for. However, a clause in Bill C-51 may be a forerunner of what the government has in mind. Section 15.1 (2) of the bill states that "No person shall advertise a prescription therapeutic product to a person other than a practitioner *unless they are authorized by the regulations to do so*" (emphasis added). In the past, key shifts in health policy have required parliamentary debate, thus making the process more public. In more recent history, this power has been taken over by Cabinet. With a business-friendly government in power, there is a concern that the regulations will be used to further relax the rules on DTCA. (For more on DTCA, see Chapter 2 in this volume.)

Ongoing Key Issues

Going Public on Public Consultation and Input

The original Health Canada document calling for public input on legislative renewal was issued in 1998. The title, *Shared Responsibilities, Shared Vision*, raised a red flag for some. The document includes statement such as "Health Protection is everybody's business. All Canadians share the responsibility for safeguarding and improving health, just as all Canadians share the benefits of having a healthy population and work force" (Health Canada, 1998b, p. ii). Why was Health Canada interested in *sharing responsibilities* for issues and decisions that carry a high level of legislative authority? Was this a case of the minister of health possibly abdicating his or her responsibility as set out in the Department of Health Act?[9] WHP argued that in responding to requests for input, citizens needed reassurance that the minister of health would be no less accountable or liable for decisions made by Health Canada, or for its actions or inactions. As of this writing, these concerns have not been adequately answered.

The *Blueprint for Renewal* also proposed "promoting a culture of openness and transparency" (Health Canada, 2006b, p. 4), noting that "engagement and collaboration with stakeholders will be part of doing business" (Health Canada, 2006b, p. 30). Throughout the years of consultation since 1998, WHP has welcomed Health Canada's continued reference to the need for public input and the establishment of the Office of Consumer and Public Involvement (OCAPI). Often, however, the enthusiasm was tempered by questions of who the public was, what was done with the input, and why the public was being consulted when it sometimes seemed that decisions had already been made.

Public involvement in government decision making is a cornerstone of democracy, but there are grounds to question whether the call for public input into the decisions made at Health Canada has been genuine. One area of concern is whether Health Canada should be viewing members of the private sector on the same footing as members of the general public. The *Blueprint for Renewal* noted that Health Canada would "engage all concerned stakeholders regarding the roles and responsibilities of each participant—from industry to practitioner to consumer" (Health Products and Food Branch, 2006, p. 31). In its recommendations to the Office of Legislative Renewal in 2000, WHP noted that a distinct role needed to be formulated for each sector. It further recommended that in order to put citizens on a level playing field with industry, it was necessary to allocate budgets and resources for citizen participation, maintaining that citizens must be able to participate from the beginning of the process, when standards are established.

In a brief to Health Canada from the Maritime Centre of Excellence for Women's Health, Dalhousie professor Susan Sherwin offered this reflection on Health Canada's legislative renewal consultation process:

> We are worried that all "stakeholders" are not equally well situated to participate in this process.... Where industries may have significant resources at their disposal to ensure that new regulations shall not impinge on their profits, affected citizens are unlikely to be as well organized. (Sherwin, 1998, p. 4)

She added further that:

> Such a process must be broadly inclusive and fairly balanced to ensure that the perspectives of the most marginalized groups are not eclipsed by the well-organized voices of more privileged members of society or by the special interests of industry. (Sherwin, 1998, p. 9)

In recent documents, OCAPI also seems to have taken on the industry orientation reflected in other parts of the Health Products and Food Branch. A 2007 document on public input into the review of regulated products makes reference to the need to protect "confidential business information" and then appears to go on to define confidential business information as "Periodic Safety Update Reports issued under the Canadian Adverse Drug Reaction Monitoring Program; summary safety reports; relevant clinical ... data" (Health Products and Food Branch, 2007). Simply put, OCAPI appears to regard information about the safety and effectiveness of prescription drugs as information that must be kept secret unless the company that submitted the data agrees to their release. This contrasts with Michèle Brill-Edwards's statement that "instead of saying everything is secret unless you can get it through a freedom of information request, we need to move closer to 'everything is open unless there is a good reason to keep it under wraps'" (Brill-Edwards, 1999, p. 53).

Hidden Costs of the Cost-Recovery Model

The Therapeutic Products Directorate (TPD), the directorate within the Health Products and Food Branch that is in charge of approving new drugs, currently relies on industry user fees to meet about 32 percent of its operating costs (Health Canada, 2006b, Annex 5, p. 37). In other words, government relies on millions of dollars in fees collected from the pharmaceutical industry in order to carry out the work of regulating, licensing, and carrying out post-market surveillance of that industry's products. These costs were previously covered by general tax revenues. (Like the TPD, other public agencies have also moved to getting part of their operating budgets from the industries that they regulate.) This is known as the cost-recovery model. There is a concern that, by covering the costs of the approval process, industry may have a freer hand to pressure government to push products through the approval process more quickly and with less rigorous attention to safety. This system allows for the perception that the TPD views industry, rather than ordinary citizens, as its primary client. In fact, this view was confirmed in a memo from the director general of the predecessor to the TPD where he explicitly said that "the client is the direct recipient of your services. In many cases this is the person or company who pays for the service" (Michols, 1997). WHP and other citizens groups have maintained a conviction that such fees collected from industry should not be directly tied to the TPD, but should be channelled to general revenues within the federal government.

When regulatory agencies rely on drug companies for part of their funding, they also make implicit or explicit agreements to approve new drugs within a certain period of time or else suffer a financial penalty. Evidence from the United States, published in the *New England Journal of Medicine* in early 2008, shows drugs that are approved close to that deadline are much more likely to go on to have safety problems compared to drugs approved at other times (Carpenter, Zucker & Avorn, 2008). It appears that, as the deadline approaches, the Food and Drug Administration may rush drugs through the approval process in order to avoid a subsequent loss in revenue. New changes in Canada will also impose financial penalties on the regulator should it exceed its commitments in terms of the time taken to approve new drugs. This does not bode well for protection of the public.

Again, in their recommendations to the Office of Legislative Renewal in 2000, WHP recommended that if a cost-recovery system for financing drug approvals was to be implemented, it must operate through a "blind trust" to minimize the industry's direct influence on the drug approval process. They also argued that funds received through a cost-recovery system should be in addition to adequate public funding, not a replacement for public funding (Women and Health Protection, 2000).

In December 2006, at a meeting with senior officials from the Health Products and Food Branch, WHP presented an analysis showing that as the percentage of funding for the TPD that came from industry increased, there was a corresponding increase in the percent of applications that were approved and a decrease in the time taken for those approvals (Lexchin, 2006). The response from the officials in the minutes that they distributed was to characterize the analysis as "views" and not to debate the merits of the analysis.

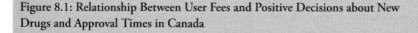

Figure 8.1: Relationship Between User Fees and Positive Decisions about New Drugs and Approval Times in Canada

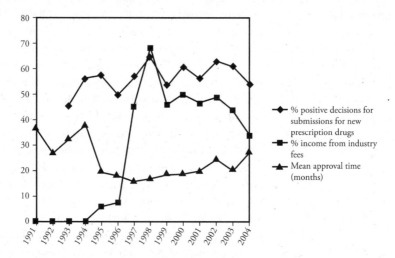

Source: Lexchin, J. (2006). Relationship between pharmaceutical company user fees and drug approvals in Canada and Australia: A hypothesis-generating study. *Annals of Pharmacotherapy, 40*(12), 2218. Retrieved from: doi 10.1345/aph.1H117

Concerns raised by WHP and others were echoed in the *2000 Report of the Auditor General*:

> The study of cost recovery by the Standing Committee on Finance raises a concern for the effect of cost recovery on the priorities of health and safety regulatory programs. The concern is that the government's policy on cost recovery to fund regulatory efforts may be creating a potential conflict between the public interest and the interest of private organizations that are paying fees to help fund regulatory programs. For example, the committee was told about concerns regarding the effect of cost recovery on the drug review process. The Auditor General told the committee that "as there is a greater dependency on fee recovery, a client-provider relationship could be established, and in some areas that may not be entirely healthy." (Auditor General of Canada, 2000, para 24.90)

Conclusion

In January 2008, journalist David McKie prepared a report for CBC's "The National" on the failure of Health Canada to successfully reach Canadian doctors with its drug safety warnings. McKie describes what he heard from some of the doctors he interviewed in a way that sums up what some would call the current state of affairs with drug regulation in Canada:

> The frustration that [they] experience is that no one seems to be accountable: Health Canada approves a drug if a company can demonstrate that its product works better than a sugar pill and doesn't kill anyone; the provinces actually pay for the drugs, many times even if there are cheaper and safer versions already on the market; doctors are free to treat their patients by, among other things, prescribing medications off-label; and drug companies promote their drugs, but say it's up to the other players to determine how the products are used [while] patients have been trained to rely on medications to treat a "a pill for every ill." (McKie, 2008)

McKie's quote reflects the ongoing disquiet that health advocates interested in drug regulation have felt in their dealings with Health Canada over more than a decade. At its best, the relationship has consisted of polite meetings where WHP expresses its concerns, officials from Health Canada or one of its many divisions listen, and then little happens in the way of subsequent action. At its worst, the government actively follows a "deny, delay, divide, and discredit" strategy (see Box 8.1) as it aligns the drug regulatory system more closely with the interests of the pharmaceutical industry and away from a focus on protection of the public.

In regulating pharmaceuticals, applying the values of commerce is antithetical to the health of women and men because those values speak to the need to earn a profit, not to the protection of public health. Competition and the profit motive may be the best way to get newer and better computers or washing detergents. Medications, however, are not ordinary consumer products and government is intimately and necessarily involved with almost all aspects of medicinal drugs because of their potential for harm and misuse, as well as their importance in health care. When government adopts the values of private industry in drug regulation, it is in essence telling the people of Canada that the needs and values of the private sector take precedence over the public's health. Within the Canadian drug regulatory system, democratic values such as openness, safety, and objective information must take precedence.

Notes

1. The author would like to thank Joel Lexchin and Patrick Orr for their comments on this chapter. However, the views expressed herein are solely those of the author.

2. Any publications of Women and Health Protection that are not available online at the time of reading can be requested by sending an e-mail to whp.apsf@gmail.com.

3. A noteworthy part of the act that has received a good deal of attention is Sub-section 3 (1) and 3 (2) of Section 3, which prohibits the labelling and advertising to the general public of food, drugs, cosmetics, or medical devices for the prevention, treatment, or cure of any of the diseases, disorders, or abnormal physical states listed in Schedule A of the act. Recently, however (March 14, 2007), Project 1539 was introduced, proposing the exemption of non-prescription drugs and natural health products from the prevention prohibitions in Section 3. Additionally, Project 1539 proposed revisions to the list of diseases in Schedule A.

4. The National Forum on Health was an advisory body established by the prime minister of Canada in October 1994 to advise the federal government on innovative ways to improve Canada's health system and the health of Canadians. The forum consisted of the prime minister as chair, the federal minister of health as vice-chair, and 24 volunteer members. Membership consisted primarily of academics, medical personnel, and members of NGOs.

5. "The public does not want to see any significant changes which would alter the fundamental principles of our publicly administered health care system. They have an abiding sense of the values of fairness and equality and do not want to see a health system in which the rich are treated differently from the poor. The Forum supports this view and supports necessary changes to our health system only if we preserve the essence of Medicare—universal coverage based on need, without financial barrier, portable across the country, to a comprehensive array of publicly administered health care services" (National Forum on Health, 1997).

6. Name changes occur for many different reasons, sometimes political, sometimes purely practical, and sometimes a mix of both. For example, the realm of health protection encompasses a range of health issues beyond drug regulation, including food and other product safety, immunization, pandemics, and emergency preparedness, so the decision to change to a name that more closely defined the territory that was covered could be seen as a logical one. Just the same, the optics of removing "protection" from the name of the branch that deals with drug safety were not good and probably not advisable.

7. For more on the precautionary principle and a critique of the risk management framework, see "Placing Limits on Health Protection by Managing Risks" in the "Further Readings" section of this chapter, as well as several publications on the Canadian Environmental Law Association website (www.cela.ca/), in particular "Implementing Precaution" (Canadian Environmental Law Association, 2002).

8. In response to a Health Canada document on progressive licensing, Joel Lexchin summarized a key concern about international harmonization: "Global harmonization has the potential to increase the efficient use of resources by regulatory agencies but it also has the potential to reduce the transparency of their work. Different regulatory agencies have different standards regarding transparency. When Health Canada reaches agreements regarding the use of material developed by other agencies it must ensure that the highest standards of transparency are adopted so that the public understands the genesis of the material and how it is being used" (correspondence from Joel Lexchin to the Health Products and Food Branch in response to their call for feedback on the Progressive Licensing Framework website, October 2007).

9. Section 4 of the Department of Health Act (retrieved August 18, 2008, from: laws.justice. gc.ca/en/showdoc/cs/H-3.2/bo-ga:s_4//en#anchorbo-ga:s_4) sets out the duties of the

minister, specifically under the heading called "Powers, Duties, and Functions of the Minister." The section reads, in part, as follows:

> ... the Minister's powers, duties and functions relating to health include the following matters:
>
> (a)   the administration of such Acts of Parliament and of orders or regulations of the Government of Canada as are not by law assigned to any other department of the Government of Canada or any minister of that Government relating in any way to the health of the people of Canada;
>
> (a.1)   the promotion and preservation of the physical, mental and social well-being of the people of Canada;
>
> (b)   the protection of the people of Canada against risks to health and the spreading of diseases;
>
> (c)   investigation and research into public health, including the monitoring of diseases;
>
> (d)   the establishment and control of safety standards and safety information requirements for consumer products and of safety information requirements for products intended for use in the workplace.

Chapter 9

Full Circle
Drugs, the Environment, and Our Health

———◆———

Sharon Batt

Introduction

Previous chapters have detailed the serious public health concerns raised by the ubiquitous nature of pharmaceuticals in our society and how they are regulated. Since the mid-1990s, news headlines about "drugs in the water" have alerted the public to an even more unsettling public health risk. Trace amounts of pharmaceuticals have been detected in Canada's lakes, rivers, streams, and tap water. Other chemicals from food and drug products—including food additives and the ingredients of personal care products, such as shampoos and perfumes—have also been detected, as have veterinary and agricultural chemicals. New biologics, genetic therapies, and genetically modified foods are more recent elements that could end up in this "chemical soup." As analytic methods for detection are developed, the number of drugs identified worldwide has grown, rising from 20 in 1998 (Ternes, 1998) to more than 200 in 2008 (Donn, Mendoza & Pritchard, 2008a).

There is no certainty about the health impacts on humans, but effects on marine life show that some drugs contaminating the environment are not benign, despite the very low concentrations that have been detected. Male fish downstream from sewage-treatment plants whose effluent includes estrogenic compounds become "feminized"—they begin to develop eggs in their testes (e.g., Desbrow, Routledge, Brighty, Sumpter & Waldock, 1998; Jobling & Tyler, 2003; Kavanagh et al., 2004). These "she-male" or intersex fish lose interest in spawning and their biological capacity to reproduce may be impaired. Indeed, when a team of researchers added low concentrations of the synthetic estrogen contained in birth control pills to a lake in northern Ontario, they not only detected changes to the reproductive systems of male and female fathead minnows, the species became virtually extinct within a few years (Kidd et al., 2007). An Environment Canada study found that effluent from a sewage-treatment plant entering the St. Lawrence River was toxic to drug-metabolizing cells in rainbow trout (Gagné, Blaise & André, 2006). Other research has demonstrated that effects can travel up the food chain: starlings who fed off earthworms polluted with estrogenic sewage contaminants sang more complex songs than control birds, and the area of their brain that controls song complexity was significantly enlarged (Markham et al., 2008); vultures in Asia that feed on the carcasses of livestock treated with an anti-inflammatory drug died of kidney failure (Oaks et al., 2004; Prakash et al., 2003; Swan et al., 2006). Some effects may be caused by a specific drug; others may be the result of chronic exposure to low levels of multiple bioactive substances (Jørgensen & Halling-Sørensen, 2000).

Such findings add another dimension to the evidence throughout this book that we need to rethink our relationship to pharmaceutical drugs. Taking a drug is not simply a personal decision that affects one individual's health. Drugs alter the ecosystem on which all living things depend. And, far from vanishing into the environment after use, these substances may travel full circle—into lakes and streams, and back into our bodies, via the water we drink and the foods we eat.

This chapter looks at this neglected form of environmental contamination from a public health perspective, with particular attention to its impact on women's health. The analysis evaluates federal government initiatives designed to protect the health of Canadians and the Canadian ecosystem from pharmaceutical and personal care products (PPCPs). We argue that reducing inappropriate pharmaceutical use is the most health-promoting, cost-effective strategy for reducing exposures to these substances. Similarly, reducing the vast quantities of unused drugs and disposing of any unavoidable excess safely is more ecological, economical, and socially just than trying to filter them from the water after the fact; improvements to water-treatment systems inevitably privilege wealthier communities and may bypass poor ones altogether. Reduced drug use remains oddly absent from most discussions of this issue, however.

The Problem in Context

Although policy initiatives in this area are recent, pharmaceuticals have very likely been present in the environment as long as they have been commercially marketed (U.S. Environmental Protection Agency, 2008). The bellwether scientific study appeared in the literature in 1977, documenting pharmaceutical drugs in Kansas City sewage (Hignite & Azarnoff, 1977). Little notice was taken for 20 years when, using more sensitive detection methods, researchers monitoring aquatic pesticide contaminants in Germany accidentally discovered the cholesterol-reducing drug clofibric acid in the drinking water in Berlin (Heberer & Stan, 1997). Clofibric acid is a chemical cousin to the weed killer 2,4-D; its presence in the tap water spurred researchers in Germany, Denmark, and Sweden to look for clofibric acid throughout Europe. They documented measurable quantities in the North Sea, the Danube River, and the Po River (e.g., Buser, Müller & Theobald, 1998; for an overview, see Montague, 1998). In 1999, the U.S. Geological Survey began an extensive, ongoing testing program that discovered dozens of PPCPs throughout the United States, in groundwater, surface water, streambeds, and tap water (U.S. Geological Survey, 2008). Nine years later, a five-month investigation by Associated Press found drugs in the water supplies of 24 major American metropolitan areas (Donn et al., 2008a).

Tests in Canada have been more limited. We now know, however, that our waterways also contain traces of antibiotics, painkillers, anti-inflammatories, hormones, tranquilizers, chemotherapy drugs, and drugs used to treat epilepsy and blood cholesterol (Stevenson, 2002). Nor has our tap water escaped contamination. Tests conducted by a laboratory in Ottawa for the *Globe and Mail* and CTV News found trace amounts of drugs in the tap water of four out of 10 Canadian communities sampled (Mittelstaedt, 2003). Waste-treatment systems are not designed to remove PPCPs, nor do municipalities routinely test for them. Testing is expensive and so far is limited to research. The City of Ottawa announced plans to begin testing in 2008

Table 9.1A: Some Effects of Drugs on Wildlife (Selected Samples from Literature)

Wild Fish Species	Habitat	Exposure	Effects Observed
Male rainbow trout	Laboratory study with graded exposures	Synthetic estrogen (EE2) used in oral contraceptives	Decreased fertility (50% fewer eggs fertilized from harvested semen reached maturity)
Male fathead minnow	Laboratory study	Minnows exposed to a mixture of five estrogenic chemicals in environmentally relevant concentrations	Chemicals acted additively to induce vitellogenin (egg yolk proteins indicative of feminization)
Male fathead minnow	Chemicals added to a pristine lake in northern Ontario	Synthetic estrogen used in oral contraceptives	Reproductive changes in males and females; virtual species extinction within a few years
Prawn	Natural waterway in Beijing, China, contaminated by water from a pharmaceutical plant	Pharmaceutical waste water from antibiotic production line	Acute dose-dependent toxicity causing death
Atlantic salmon	Laboratory study	Synthetic estrogen	Effects on gene transcription in brain and head kidney*
Adult male zebra fish	Laboratory study	Synthetic androgen methyltestosterone	Low concentrations significantly increased vitellogenin production and decreased endogenous ketotestosterone

* The head kidney is the definitive excretory organ of primitive fishes

Sources: Andersen, L., Goto-Kazeto, R., Trant, J.M., Nash, J.P., Korsgaard, B. & Bjerregaard, P. (2006, March 10). Short-term exposure to low concentrations of the synthetic androgen methyltestosterone affects vitellogenin and steroid levels in adult male zebrafish (Danio rerio); *Aquatic Toxicology, 76*(3–4), 343–352; Brian, J.V., Harris, C.A., Scholze, M., Backhaus, T., Booy, P., Lamoree, M. et al. (2005). Prediction of the response of freshwater fish to a mixture of estrogenic chemicals. *Environmental Health Perspectives, 113*(6), 721–728; Gerhardt, A., de Bisthoven, L.J., Mo, Z., Wang, C., Yang, M. & Wang, Z. (2002). Short-term responses of *Oryzias latipes* (*Pices adrianichthyidae*) *Macrobrachium nipponense* (*Crustacea: Palaemonidae*) to municipal and pharmaceutical waste water in Beijing, China: Survival, behaviour, biochemical biomarkers. *Chemosphere, 47*(1), 35–47; Kidd, K.A., Blanchfield, P.J., Mills, K.H., Palace, V.P., Evans, R.E., Lazorchak, J.M. et al. (2007). Collapse of a fish population after exposure to synthetic estrogen. *Proceedings of the National Academy of Sciences, 104*(21), 8897–8901; Lyssimachou, A. & Arukwe, A. (2007). Alteration of brain and interrenal StAR protein P450scc, and Cyp11β and mRNA levels in Atlantic salmon after nominal waterborne exposure to the synthetic pharmaceutical estrogen ethynylestradiol. *Journal of Toxicology and Environmental Health, Part A, 70*(7), 606–613; Schultz, I.R., Skillman, A., Nicolas, J.M., Cyr, D.G. & Nagler, J.J. (2003). Short-term exposure to 17-alpha ethynylestradiol decreases the fertility of sexually maturing male rainbow trout (Oncorhynchus mykiss). *Environmental Toxicology and Chemistry, 22*(6), 1272–1280.

Table 9.1B: Some Effects of Drugs on Wildlife (Selected Samples from Literature)			
Bird Species	**Habitat**	**Exposure**	**Effects Observed**
Three species of vultures found in Indian subcontinent	Vultures in their natural habitat ingest chemicals when they feed on livestock carcasses	Suspected cause: veterinary use of diclofenac (an anti-inflammatory)	Kidney failure causing death and near-extinction of all three bird species
Studies of non-threatened Eurasian and African species of Gyps vultures	Controlled laboratory studies confirm causal link between diclofenac and vulture deaths	Diclofenac (veterinary anti-inflammatory, also used in humans)	Death from kidney failure
Wild-caught European starlings	Controlled laboratory studies matched exposures to those observed in birds foraging in sewage treatment sites	Estrogenic contaminants found in sewage	Birds sang more complex songs and brain changes were observed

Sources: Markman, S., Leitner, S., Catchpole, C, Barnsley, S., Müller, C.T., Pascoe, D. et al. (2008). Pollutants increase song complexity and the volume of the brain area HVC in a songbird. *PLoS ONE, 3*(2), e1074. Retrieved October 7, 2008, from: doi: 10.1371/journal.pone.0001674; Oaks, J.L., Gilbert, M., Virani, M.Z., Watson, R.T., Meteyer, C.U., Rideout, B.A. et al. (2004). Diclofenac residues as the cause of vulture population decline in Pakistan. *Nature, 427*, 630–633. Retrieved October 7, 2008, from: doi:10.1038/nature02317; Prakash V., Pain D.J., Cunningham, A.A., Donald, P.F., Prakash, N., Verma, A. et al. (2003). Catastrophic collapse of Indian white-backed *Gyps bengalensis* and long-billed Gyps indicus vulture populations. *Biological Conservation, 109*(3), 381–390; Swan, G.E., Cuthbert, R., Quevedo, M., Green, R., Pain, D.J., Bartels, P. et al. (2006). Toxicity of diclofenac to Gyps vultures. *Biology Letters, 2*(2), 279–282.

for PPCPs in the city's water supply, at a cost of $20,000 for eight water samples (Vaidyanath, 2008).

As consumers, we excrete PPCPs into sewers; we flush unused medications down the toilet or sink; and we rinse soaps, shampoos, and cosmetics down the drain when we bathe. Even posthumously, the drugs administered in the last years of our lives likely leach into cemeteries and groundwater (Daughton, 2003c, p. 777). Consumer use may account for the majority of trace pollutants in the environment, although the available information is insufficient to prioritize sources (Daughton, 2003c, pp. 775–785). Other contributors are hospitals and long-term care facilities, veterinary drugs (including large amounts of antibiotics), fish farms, drug-contaminated sewage sludge sold as farm fertilizer, and industrial waste disposal at plant sites (see Figure 9.1).

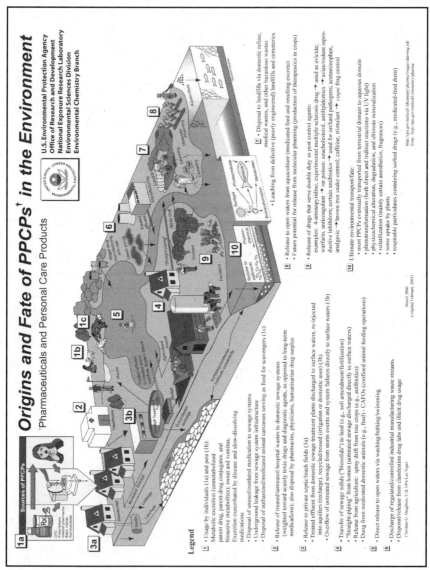

Figure 9.1

Source: Daughton C.G. (2006, March). *Origins and fate of PPCPs in the environment* [illustrated poster]. Las Vegas: U.S. Environmental Protection Agency. (Updated from an original work published in February 2001.) Retrieved September 14, 2008, from: www.epa.gov/ppcp/pdf/drawing.pdf

The concentrations detected in water are typically between 20 parts per billion (ppb) and less than one part per trillion (ppt); however, drugs are designed to have an effect in small quantities. Furthermore, recognizing that drugs in environmental waterways are highly diluted does not mean that quantities are small. In their study of clofibric acid in the North Sea, Buser, Müller, and Theobald (1998) estimated that one or two parts per trillion of the chemical in the sea volume of 12.7 quadrillion gallons translated into 48–96 tons of colfibric acid. The evidence is now indisputable that biological effects occur at these very low levels.

Some drugs (e.g., anti-epileptics) are persistent—that is, they do not break down. Others are "pseudo-persistent"—they break down, but are continually replaced by widespread use. Some drug compounds dissolve in water, but others dissolve only in fat, which enables them to enter cells and move up food chains, becoming more concentrated. A study by the Royal Danish School of Pharmacy found that more than 30 percent of all medical substances developed from 1992–1995 were lipophilic (fat-soluble) (Halling-Sørensen et al., 1998). The risks to both aquatic organisms and humans are largely unknown, but could include resistance to antibiotics and the disruption of endocrine systems.

Box 9.1: PPCPs Ranked of Greatest Concern to Human and Ecosystem Health

- antibiotics
- antidepressants, tranquilizers
- anti-epileptic drugs
- anti-inflammatory agents
- antimicrobials (e.g., used for parasite control in animals)
- calcium channel blockers
- estrogenic steroids
- genotoxic drugs (e.g., cancer treatments)
- multi-drug transporters (efflux pumps)
- musk fragrances

Sources: Health Canada. (2003). *Issue identification paper: Environmental assessment regulations:* Ottawa: Health Canada. Retrieved October 31, 2008, from: www.hc-sc.gc.ca/ewh-semt/alt_formats/hpfb-dgpsa/pdf/contaminants/iip-dde-eng.pdf ; U.S. Environmental Protection Agency. (2007, December). *Pharmaceuticals and personal care products: Frequent questions.* Retrieved March 11, 2008, from: www.epa.gov/ppcp/faq.html; Collier, A.C. (2007). Pharmaceutical contaminants in potable water: Potential concerns for pregnant women and children. *EcoHealth, 4*(2), 164–171.

Women, Health Products, and Environmental Pollution

Ecosystem contamination with PPCPs has the potential to affect flora and fauna, fish and fowl, women and men. However, there are some ways in which women are particularly affected by PPCPs.

Biologically, women have different vulnerabilities to chemicals than men at certain points in the life cycle. Pregnancy is the most obvious example. The diethylstilbestrol (DES) and thalidomide tragedies shattered the long-held rule of toxicology that "the dose makes the poison." Minute quantities of a drug taken by a pregnant woman at a particular stage in fetal development can cause deformities, cancer, and subtle cognitive effects. DES is now recognized as a member of a class of chemicals that disrupt the endocrine (hormonal) system. Some specialists believe no dose of synthetic hormones is safe for the developing embryo and fetus (Colburn, Dumanoski & Meyers, 1996; DES Action Canada, 2001). Emerging research on endocrine disruptors suggests that the male fetus may be more sensitive than the female fetus to many effects of these chemicals (Canadian Partnership for Children's Health and the Environment, 2007). Indeed, epidemiological studies show a small but steady reduction in the proportion of boys born in Japan and the U.S. over the past four decades. Evidence that the "missing boys" phenomenon is the result, in part, of *in utero* exposure to endocrine-disrupting chemicals comes from communities where chemical exposures are exceptionally high. A 1976 explosion of dioxin from a chemical plant in Seveso, Italy, was followed by an immediate loss of males: 46 females and 28 males were born in the next seven years. The First Nations community of Aamjiwnaang, situated in Sarnia, Ontario, the heart of Canada's petrochemical refining industry, has shown a startling 40 percent decline in the ratio of males to females over more than a decade (Van Larebeke et al., 2008).

Abby C. Collier, a pharmacologist at the University of Hawaii, used published dose-response data and clinical prescribing guidelines to estimate the risk that pharmaceuticals commonly identified in drinking water might pose to pregnant women and children (Collier, 2007). She analyzed 26 pharmaceuticals found in measurable quantities in various studies of drinking water systems and estimated cumulative drinking water exposures for these vulnerable populations. She concluded that five drugs were of greatest concern for pregnant women: ethinyl estradiol (a synthetic estrogen), norethindrone (a contraceptive), diazepam (a tranquilizer), invermectin (widely used for parasite control in livestock), and the NSAIDs ibuprofen and diclofenac (anti-inflammatory agents). She ranked these same five drugs, plus the anti-cancer drug methotrexate, as the substances of greatest concern for the pediatric population, with the safety of an additional four not yet established (Collier, 2007, p. 169).

Based on her calculations, a pregnant woman drinking 2 litres (64 ounces) of water per day would ingest 13 percent of a minimum dose of ethinyl estradiol over a nine-month pregnancy, approximately 1.5 percent of a minimum clinical dose of norethindrone, and almost 5 percent of a minimum clinical dose of diazepam. For invermectin, ibuprofen, and diclofenac, the estimated percentages of a minimum clinical dose were 4 percent, 3 percent, and 2 percent respectively. Despite being lower than levels used in clinical treatments, Collier expressed concern about exposures to these drugs since they may not show linear dose-response relationships when causing birth defects (i.e., doubling the dose may mean more than twice the risk). "Because drinking water is considered healthy and positive in pregnancy, exposure of pregnant women to these five drugs through drinking water is a public health concern," she concludes (2007, p. 169). As noted earlier, drugs in combination may interact so that estimated exposures to individual substances don't tell the whole story.

To date, most research on the effects of chemical exposures to the developing fetus and to young children has focused on industrial toxins in the environment, such as pesticides, dioxins, lead, arsenic, and mercury. Evidence is mounting that these exposures affect both boys and girls, but the health effects manifest differently in the two sexes. Boys are at greater risk for cancer, asthma, learning disorders, certain birth defects, and testicular dysgenesis syndrome (Canadian Partnership for Children's Health and the Environment, 2007). Girls are at greater risk for premature puberty, which is associated with a variety of psychopathologies in adolescence, including depression, eating disorders, drug abuse, cigarette smoking, and alcohol use. Early puberty in girls is also associated with a higher risk of breast cancer later in life (Steingraber, 2007). At present, there is a lack of research to specifically link these trends with pharmaceuticals in the environment. However, as Danish researchers Jørgensen and Halling-Sørensen (2000) argue, drugs are "in principle not different from other chemicals" so "to distinguish between drugs and other chemicals when they are discharged into the environment is preposterous" (p. 695).

Chemical contamination of breast milk is another women's health issue linked to environmental contamination. Aromatic amines—used to make pharmaceuticals, dyes, plastic foams, and pesticides—have been detected in human milk and are known to cause cancer in mammary rat tissue (DeBruin, Pawliszyn & Josephy, 1999; Steingraber, 1999).

Pregnancy and lactation are not the only windows of vulnerability in a woman's life cycle. Puberty, menstruation, and menopause are all the result of hormonal fluctuations. The cells in women's breasts appear to reach full maturity only at a first full-term pregnancy, when they become more resistant to cancer-causing chemicals and radiation. Women of any age who have not had children may therefore have increased susceptibility to carcinogenic chemicals in the environment compared to women of the same age and health status who have had children (Steingraber, 1997). Furthermore, women have more fatty tissue, on average, than men so they store more endocrine disruptors in their bodies. Women also have adverse reactions to drugs more often (see Chapter 7). This difference is only in part because women use more drugs than men and tend to weigh less. A report by the U.S. General Accounting Office (now called the Government Accountability Office) concludes that "Greater health risks for women may be due to physiological differences that make women differentially more susceptible to some drug-related health risks" (Heinrich, 2001).

Another consideration is that older women have had more years to absorb bioaccumulative drugs from the environment and reduced immunity could make them more sensitive to some effects of environmental chemicals in the water.

Health protection policies should be designed to protect all members of society, especially the most vulnerable. Despite the evidence of the particular damage chemicals can have on women's health, safety standards for chemicals have often been based on healthy, White, adult males.

Canada's Approach to PPCPs: The Environmental Assessment Regulations Project (EARP) and the Environmental Impact Initiative (EII)

In September 2001, under the auspices of its Office of Regulatory and International Affairs, Health Canada launched a project to address the health and environmental effects of PPCPs. Called the Environmental Assessment Regulations Project (EARP), the program had three components: (1) regulations to protect the environment from PPCPs; (2) a scientific research program; and (3) best practices and public education programs (Health Canada, 2003).

The project did not meet its targeted completion date of 2003 and work continued for several more years. In 2006 it was relaunched with a new name (the Environmental Impact Initiative or EII), under a new director (Gordon Stringer), with a new target date, 2011. The EII will continue developing regulations, best management practices, and consumer education programs. A multi-stakeholder working group drawn from government, industry, and consumer and public interest groups oversees the EII process and meets several times a year. At the time of writing, insufficient information was available about the Environmental Impact Initiative to assess its import or progress. The analysis that follows is based on documentation produced under EARP and the author's attendance at multi-stakeholder consultations held in 2002, 2003, and 2006.

EAR Project documentation suggests a vision that meets many of the criteria for a model public health initiative. The project was to interpret health protection broadly, including harmful effects on the environment or its biological diversity, as well as direct human health impacts (Health Canada, 2003, p. 4). The proposed decision-making strategy would incorporate the precautionary principle, which means protective action can be taken before harm has been demonstrated with scientific certainty (Health Canada, 2003, pp. 15, 40). Prevention would take precedence over mop-up, "avoiding the creation of pollutants rather than trying to manage them after they have been created" (Health Canada, 2003, p. 38). A commitment to open discussion invited the public's participation in solving the problem (Health Canada, 2003, p. 43).

Much of the work conducted under EARP fell short of these ideals. The project highlighted toxicological research on specific substances and meetings with industry stakeholders about potential trade impacts. Discussions with public interest groups, including environmental, women's health, and consumer groups, which took place in the years 2002, 2003, and 2006, were limited.

The Regulations

Central to EARP was a project to develop regulations that would limit the environmental impact of PPCPs. Drug safety data submitted by companies under the *Food and Drugs Act* (F&DA) regulations are designed to evaluate drug safety only for the individual consumer taking a drug. These data do not take the environment into consideration, nor are they concerned with health problems arising from environmental contamination by PPC products. A separate regulatory framework, the Canadian Environmental Protection Act (CEPA), is designed to protect Canada's environment. CEPA, which came into force in 1988 and was revised in 1999, is administered by Environment Canada.

According to an EAR document, when CEPA was enacted both Health Canada and Environment Canada were under the mistaken belief that the substances regulated under Canada's *Food and Drugs Act* were exempt from CEPA, so Health Canada did not require environmental safety data in the information packages manufacturers submitted for review (Health Canada, 2003). The purpose of developing new regulations is, therefore, to expand and define the data required of food and drug manufacturers. When the regulations are complete, manufacturers will have to include environmental safety assessments demonstrating that their products conform to CEPA. In addition to assessing safety and efficacy for the immediate user, Health Canada will review all new PPCP submissions for their environmental impact. In the meantime, new products that fall under the *Food and Drugs Act* are to be screened under existing CEPA regulations (the New Substances Notification Regulations), while the tens of thousands of PPCPs already on the market are to be included in a gradual review of existing products taking place under CEPA.

Science and Research

A second key component of EARP was its national science agenda. While a science agenda is essential to an action program, the EARP's research priorities were tied to its toxicological regulatory agenda. For example, a workshop that Health Canada and

Environment Canada sponsored in February 2002 to discuss PPCPs in the Canadian environment included as its main objectives "identifying major scientific knowledge gaps and establishing risk assessment and risk management needs in Canada" (Health Canada, 2002a, p. 11). Not surprisingly, research priorities identified by workshop participants reflected this agenda (e.g., obtain scientific data on exposure and effects of PPCPs in the Canadian environment; foster development of a Canadian regulatory framework in harmonization with international organizations).

Making toxicological assessment research the centrepiece of the science agenda excludes or marginalizes other, equally important, scientific research that would support immediate and medium-term action. For example, research to determine the best ways to reduce inappropriate drug use would explore ways to modify behaviours and would draw from the social sciences. Although EARP included behavioural change in its third prong (discussed in the next section), the framework for social science research could be greatly expanded, as the discussion of the Green Pharmacy approach (see p. 199) argues.

Public Education

The third prong of EARP comprised public education and public participation initiatives (Health Canada, 2003, p. 5). A Benchmark Survey, conducted for Health Canada in 2002, assessed consumer attitudes to waste disposal, including the disposal of pharmaceuticals and other PPCPs (Health Canada, 2002b); however, a patchwork of provincial waste-removal practices has stalled a national take-back program. Increasingly, the public is encouraged to take unused drugs back to the pharmacy, rather than disposing of them in the toilet or sink. Unless pharmacists in a province or municipality have an organized system to dispose of the drugs safely, however, the pharmacist may simply make bulk deposits into the sewage, as one Ontario pharmacist was discovered doing in September 2003 (Environmental Commissioner of Ontario, 2005, p. 184). Canadian pharmacists recommend take-back programs as a model standard of practice (Campbell, 2007, p. 29) and such programs have been in effect in British Columbia since 1996; however, as of this writing, only British Columbia, Alberta, Nova Scotia, and Prince Edward Island have province-wide pharmacy-based programs for the return and safe disposal of unused drugs. A non-profit association funded by pharmaceutical industry groups, the Post-consumer Pharmaceutical Stewardship Association (PCPSA) provides information about programs across the country and supports these programs on a cost-sharing basis (Post-consumer Pharmaceutical Stewardship Association, 2008). A truly national take-back program would be a first step, but educational programs to instill best practices also need to actively promote reduced use of PPCPs (Daughton, 2003a, p. 762).

Assessing Environmental Assessment Regulations

As we have seen throughout this book, the regulation of drugs always requires a delicate process of weighing potential health benefits against potential health risks, with economic drivers the unacknowledged elephant in the room. In other chapters, the authors express concerns about Health Canada's drug review processes, including government-industry conflicts of interest, the worrisome move toward fast-tracking of drugs, excessive secrecy in decision making, lack of public consultation, and evidence that Canada's trade objectives often override health protection concerns. One question underlying the critique that follows is whether trade and economic considerations are similarly impeding the environmental regulation of PPCPs. Already the years of inaction on this dossier suggest a process stalled by corporate lobbying.

The spectre of contaminated water can be frightening, instilling a sense of helplessness over shrinking resources necessary to life. We can, however, act responsibly, based on our present knowledge about inappropriate and excessive drug use. Some medication is necessary to good health, but there is growing evidence to show that some is not and causes harm. Corporate practices designed to promote drug use that is not scientifically based need to be curtailed. Examples are direct-to-consumer advertising (see Chapter 2) and commercially sponsored seminars to encourage off-label prescribing (Berenson, 2008).

Substituting non-toxic complementary and alternative medicine (CAM) approaches for conventional pharmaceutical interventions, and the replacement of synthetic ingredients in personal care products with others made of biodegradable substances, could have considerable impact, says Dr. Warren Bell of the Canadian Association of Physicians for the Environment. "Many CAM interventions have no effect on the ecosystem (e.g., manual therapies, body/mind therapies); others have minimal effects (e.g., homeopathy, lifestyle alterations). Many others probably have limited effects, or at least involve simple redistribution of known components of the biosphere (e.g., plant remedies, Epsom salts compresses, vitamin and mineral supplementation and therapy), often themselves considered to be broadly beneficial or at least neutral in effect," says Dr. Bell (personal communication, June 26, 2003).

Much thought needs to be given to the framing of educational messages and programs so that risks are neither downplayed nor sensationalized. Educating the public about PPCPs in the drinking water presents some of the same difficulties as educating nursing mothers about chemical contaminants in breast milk. Apprehension about drugs and other chemicals in the water could drive people to avoid their necessary intake of water, or to purchase expensive home filtering systems and bottled water, which may be no less contaminated. Penny Van Esterik, in an analysis of communicating risks about infant feeding, notes the importance of placing the issue in a broad environmental health context, so that the goal is reducing pollution rather than avoiding breastfeeding (Van Esterik, 2002). Public education about drugs in the water requires a similarly broad focus. Questions for public debate include: What is the full range of remedies? What solutions will be emphasized? When parties disagree, who decides? Furthermore, as Sandra Steingraber points out in her discussion of chemical contaminants in breast milk, educating the public to make "safer" lifestyle choices avoids the central question, namely, what political action can be taken to eliminate these contaminants (Steingraber, 2001, pp. 274–280).

Public Participation and the EARP Consultation Process

Beginning with the 2001 Notice of Intent (Health Canada, 2001), Health Canada stated its commitment to a process of consultations with stakeholders in the development of the new environmental assessment regulations. This process included meetings to explain EARP to government employees, industry stakeholders, and members of non-governmental organizations concerned about health and the environment. A benchmark survey of 1,512 Canadians was conducted to determine prevalent attitudes and product disposal habits. Passive methods of communication with the public included a website, newsletters, and an information line to disseminate information and register reactions.

However, despite the stated commitment to public participation in EARP, the consultations were geared to industry players and failed to engage the public or non-governmental organizations (NGOs). Rather than enlisting the public as full partners in debating the "big picture," discussions with the public were narrowly focused on the proposed regulations for reviewing drugs. The agendas at these meetings were pre-set, with PowerPoint presentations and guided discussion of an Issue Identification "workbook" on the regulatory proposals. The opaque language of risk assessment and regulation set up barriers to NGO participation by framing the problem and the process in terms meaningful only to industry and government.

The industry groups' domination of the consultation process is reflected in the concerns that stakeholders most often expressed: that the regulations would slow down the introduction of new substances onto the Canadian market, affect international trade (Health Canada, 2002c, p. 2), or prevent new drugs from entering the Canadian market "solely for environmental factors" (Health Canada, 2006, p. 20). The adequacy of the proposed regulations for health and environmental protection—ostensibly the purpose of the exercise—was not even mentioned in the account of stakeholder responses. As well, a key discussion paper issued in 2003 excluded non-specialists from the dialogue with technical language and a legalistic emphasis on a regulatory framework (Health Canada, 2003).

If health and environmental protection are to take precedence over trade issues, the participation of health and environmental advocacy groups in framing policy approaches is vital. However, for NGOs working with tight budgets and staff cutbacks, EARP public consultations from 2002 through 2006 were not a priority.

NGOs were invited to only three meetings and were expected to study, on their own, documents that appeared to have been written for industry lawyers by their government counterparts. No funds were provided to assist groups that wanted to brief themselves on the implications of EARP for public health, or to meet among themselves to develop a public health perspective on EARP issues. Industry representatives, by contrast, had more than 40 meetings with government as of May 2002. Not surprisingly, few non-profit groups in Canada have taken up the issue of PPCPs.

The Green Pharmacy: A Holistic Program for Change

An interesting counterpoint to the Canadian government's strategy for addressing PPCPs is the Green Pharmacy Stewardship Program proposed by Christian Daughton, a scientist at the U.S. Environmental Protection Agency. Much like the goals of EARP on paper, Daughton envisions a broad, holistic program. His "blueprint" is more detailed and programmatic than EARP, however, proposing a broad spectrum of actions to be jointly overseen by the health care industry and consumers. Three goals shape the Green Pharmacy concept: protect the environment, reduce medical expenses for the consumer, and improve patient and consumer health (Daughton, 2003a, 2003b).

In contrast to EARP, Daughton questions how useful a risk assessment approach can be in controlling PPCPs in the environment given the pitfalls of trying to track and regulate potential chemical stressors. "The spectrum of pollutants typically identified in an environmental sample represents but an unknown portion of those actually present (possibly very small), and they are of unknown overall risk significance," he asserts (2003b, p. 758). Daughton also argues that the traditional chemical-by-chemical approach to pollutant tracking and regulation needs to give way to an approach based on probable cumulative exposure, "understanding the ramifications of entire classes [of chemicals] that share a common MOA [mechanism of action]" or a common physiological or behavioural end point (Daughton, 2003b, p. 759). He notes that any approach that uses "predicted" environmental concentrations fails to account for three major factors: (1) geographic variability in drug usage; (2) sources other than legal sales (e.g., physician samples and black market sales); and (3) interactions between chemical stressors (Daughton, 2003b, pp. 760–761).

Daughton notes that curtailing some uses of medication can improve health outcomes. He proposes a multidisciplinary approach based on a cohesive, scientifically sound set of principles that would guide changes to packaging, distribution, and purveyance of PPCPs, many of which could be implemented rapidly (Daughton, 2003a, p. 9). One example of such a change is lowering drug dosages. Some studies show that the effective doses of some drugs can be lower than previously realized. Cutting doses could reduce adverse drug reactions, including deaths, while lessening the potential for environmental effects (Daughton, 2003b, pp. 41–42).

Another area for change with a potential for immediate impact is reducing the amount of medication wasted. A survey of drug disposal in Ontario estimated the annual cost of wasted medication in the province at over Can$40 million (Boivin, 1997). Drug shelf life is a third case in point. Research has shown that shelf lives for some drug formulations exceed the duration indicated by the expiry dates (under ideal storage conditions), providing the basis for substantial savings without compromising health (Daughton, 2003a, p. 54).

Despite this comprehensive plan developed by a government agency, the U.S. government's response to the PPCP issue as of early 2008 has been as disappointing as Canada's. An American media analysis (Donn, Mendoza & Pritchard, 2008b) observed that regulators in the U.S. had never rejected a drug on the basis of its environmental impact, and concluded that drugs in the environment were not a government priority.

Gender Affects Purchase and Use

Effective policies designed to reverse this form of pollution need to consider cultural (gender) differences between the sexes. Because of cultural influences, women are the family members most often responsible for health, including purchase of drugs and food, food preparation, caring for sick family members and disposal of home-use products. Many drugs are gender-specific (e.g., birth control, menopausal hormone therapy) or are prescribed more often to women than to men (e.g., antidepressants). Women are also the main users of cosmetics, perfumes, and hair products, many of which have been found to contain phthalates, a family of industrial chemicals linked in animal studies to permanent birth defects in the male reproductive system (Houlihan, Brody & Schwan, 2002). Some phthalates have been detected in drinking water, as have synthetic musk fragrances from perfumes and other toiletries (Daughton, 2003b, p. 766).

Strategies to reduce use of particular drugs or ingredients in cosmetics and toiletries will be most effective if they recognize the gender dynamics underlying promotion and use of PPCPs.

Women predominate in two demographic categories for which PPCP use may have a particular impact: the elderly and the poor. Elderly women constitute a large and growing segment of the population. The elderly ingest more drugs than the young, and use them more often. Geriatric medicine has been shown to result in particularly high wastage, for a number of reasons, including frequent physician alterations in dosage and prescribing new drugs, patient improvement, "silent symptoms" that provide the patient with no incentive for continuing medication, and patient death. Many drugs for geriatric patients have been found in environmental monitoring studies (Daughton, 2003c, p. 781). These factors argue for a gender-based, age-sensitive approach to research, education, and policies related to drugs in the environment.

Box 9.2: The Evra Patch: A Closer Look at One Product and Its Impact on the Environment

Evra, a birth control patch that transfers hormones through the skin, was approved for use in Canada in 2002. It is promoted for its convenience. The patch is no more effective than birth control pills in preventing pregnancy and it has more side effects, including an increased risk of blood clots (see Chapter 2). Each patch contains 6 mg of norelgestromin and 0.6 mg of ethinyl estradiol. Users are instructed to replace the patch after seven days. At that point, the patch still contains over 80 percent of the norelgestromin and over 75 percent of the ethinyl estradiol. According to Janssen-Ortho, the manufacturer of the patch, this high level of waste is necessary to ensure that adequate amounts of the hormones are absorbed. The large amount of synthetic hormone remaining in the patch when it is discarded has been found to feminize male fish. The hormone is persistent—that is, it does not break down over time. But in a birth control market crowded with many different types of pills, a patch can be marketed as something new. This marketing advantage comes at the expense of greater environmental risks because of the amount of hormone remaining in the patch when is discarded.

If the patch is folded in half and discarded with other household waste, as recommended by the manufacturer, the residual hormone may well find its way into the ecosystem and pollute our waterways. In Europe, the patch is distributed with its own disposal pouch. While this still doesn't guarantee that the hormones won't eventually leak out into the environment, it does illustrate an important point: disposal instructions are not based on what's good for the global ecosystem, but rather on what's required in each regulatory environment.

The impact that the disposal of drugs has on the environment is the responsibility of environment ministries, mostly at the provincial level. The actual disposal of hazardous drugs by individual households is the responsibility of municipal waste systems. Licensed medical/hazardous waste-disposal companies dispose of drugs from pharmacy take-back programs. This multi-level, multi-ministerial, public/private sector shared responsibility has created a jurisdictional gridlock. Unfortunately, most prescription drugs, including those containing synthetic hormones that are known to be endocrine disruptors,[a] are not classified as hazardous waste.

While the Canadian Environmental Protection Act (CEPA), passed in 1988 and revised in 1999 and administered by Environment Canada, does have a set of regulations intended to protect Canada's environment by preventing pollution, these regulations were designed with industrial chemicals in mind. A project to develop regulations under the *Food and Drugs Act*, which Health Canada administers, has been in bureaucratic limbo since September 2001. Until Health Canada's Environmental Impact Initiative is completed, CEPA regulations do apply to pharmaceutical products. The case of Evra suggests, however, that pharmaceutical products are not currently being restricted on the basis of environmental harm.

Every opportunity for a pharmaceutical chemical to leach into the water table allows a discharge into the natural environment. Although we are only beginning to understand the bioaccumulative[b] effect that these chemicals can have on the health of the ecosystem, the little we do know is enough to say that any discharge is unacceptable. We cannot control what happens once a chemical has been discharged into the ecosystem. Where we do have control is in reducing use.

Notes

a. *Endocrine disruptor:* Dr. Theo Colborn, a co-author of *Our Stolen Future*, defines an endocrine disruptor as "a compound that interferes with the production, release, transport, metabolism, binding action and/or elimination of hormones in the body."

b. *Bioaccumulative:* Toxic chemicals are isolated and stored in fatty tissue of living organisms. These toxins accumulate exponentially as they move up the food chain. Much like the greenhouse effect, this is known as a bioaccumulative effect—i.e., the end product of many chemicals interacting.

Source: Adapted from *Evra and the Environment*, written by Suzanne Elston for Women and Health Protection in 2004 and available on the WHP website.

Women are overrepresented among Canadians living in poverty. The poor are less able to afford technical solutions, such as home filter systems. Corrective programs that require costly individual initiatives could widen class-based health disparities.

Gender and Values

As a group, women are more willing to go out of their way to protect human health and the environment (Seager, 1993; Wyman, 1999). Women scientists, including Rachel Carson (1962), Sandra Steingraber (1997, 2001, 2007), Theo Colburn (Colburn, Dumanoski & Meyers, 1996), and Devra Lee Davis (2007) have been trailblazers in showing connections between chemical pollution of the environment and both human and ecosystem health. Feminist theorists have also challenged the assumption, embedded in much of Western philosophy, that humans have a right to dominate all other life forms (d'Eaubonne, 1974; Mies & Shiva, 1993; Warren, 2000). The women's health movement and the eco-feminist movement promote health protection and environmental protection respectively.

The survey conducted as part of the Environmental Assessment Regulations Project captures this gender gap in values.[1] Women were more likely than men to say they were interested in learning "all I can" about how to safely dispose of household products so they don't harm the environment (74 percent versus 66 percent); and women were more likely to say they would dispose safely of household products "all the time, even if it's inconvenient" (70 percent versus 62 percent). This commitment to health and the environment suggests women could be key players in programs for change. The gender values gap must also be considered when framing value-laden policies, such as risk assessment and the precautionary principle. More men hold decision-making positions in industry, government, and elected office, while more women are poor and have little political power. Whose values will prevail in deciding what level of risk is acceptable to a community? Who decides when scientific evidence is sufficient to trigger the precautionary principle?

Planning with Foresight

Clean water is so basic to human life that burbling brooks and waterfalls are enduring symbols of the life force. Fresh water is also an increasingly scarce and coveted resource. In the face of uncertainty about what effect PPCPs in the environment will have, the prudent course is to treat PPCPs in the water as an urgent issue for short-, medium-, and long-term action.

Under CEPA and, in turn, under EARP and the Environmental Impact Initiative, the federal government affirms Canada's commitment to the precautionary principle, a policy concept based on the German word meaning "foresight":

> The precautionary principle emerged during the 1970s in the former West Germany at a time of social democratic planning. At the core of early conceptions of precaution (or *Vorsorge*) was the belief that the state should seek to avoid environmental damage by careful forward planning. The word *Vorsorge* means foresight or taking care…. (Jordan & O'Riordan, 1999, p. 19)

Science often lags behind the ideal that would permit fully informed decision making. The precautionary principle calls on governments, when faced with partial scientific evidence, to tilt policies in favour of protecting health and the environment. Rather than requiring the government to demonstrate certainty of harm before curtailing a product's use, the precautionary principle shifts the onus to industry to demonstrate a product's safety before bringing it to market. The Canadian government has an "international commitment to implement the precautionary principle" (Health Canada, 2003, p. 40), yet a close look at the details in EARP documents reveals a compromise that blunts the principle's edge for protecting health and the environment.

Usually it is much easier to calculate the short-term economic benefits from introducing a product compared to the long-term economic harm from its introduction. Advocates of environmental protection and health protection have advanced the precautionary principle as a challenge to the risk management practices that now guide government decision making. The precautionary principle exhorts governments to curtail the use of potentially unsafe technologies, even if national economies could suffer some short-term losses as a result (Health Canada, 2003, pp. 40–41). EARP documents state that Canada promotes a precautionary approach, "distinctive within science-based risk management" (Health Canada, 2003, p. 38). Subsuming the precautionary principle within risk management tempers the precautionary imperative in the interests of economic goals. An alternative assessment strategy (O'Brien, 2000) would recognize that developing a "clean" technology industry is a way to realize direct and indirect economic gains. With vision, Canada could promote the development of ecologically sound PPCP policies and technologies, combining our well-established policy expertise in health promotion with a forward-looking "green science" agenda.

As the EARP "Issue Identification Paper" acknowledges, the precautionary principle is "ultimately guided by judgment, based on values (acceptable levels of risks)" (Health Canada, 2003, p. 41). Key questions then become: Whose judgments? Whose values? For a manufacturer eager to get a new product to market, zero contamination may seem too stringent; a pregnant woman may want no less.

Conclusion

By early 2008, the evidence that pharmaceuticals in the environment are disrupting aquatic life and other wildlife was so unequivocal and disturbing that scientists were calling for action. A five-month study reported in the American media quoted Steven Goodbred, of the U.S. Geological Survey, as saying, "The onus has been on the scientific community to provide the research, but at this point the evidence is conclusive. Now it's up to the public and policymakers to decide what they want to do about it" (Donn, Mendoza & Pritchard, 2008b, para 9).

As this chapter argues, we can begin by taking a hard look at the sheer quantity of drugs we use. The increase in pharmaceutical drugs, in humans, veterinary practices, agriculture, and aquaculture has been astonishing (Holtz, 2006, pp. 7–10). Materials prepared for EARP do not discuss policy tools that would reduce prescription drug use and therefore reduce environmental contamination. These could include tightening and enforcing the ban on direct-to-consumer advertising, taking drug-promotion regulation out of the hands of the pharmaceutical industry and voluntary bodies such as the Pharmaceutical Advertising Advisory Board, opening the drug approval process to public scrutiny, and adopting a more stringent interpretation of the precautionary principle. Many of these approaches would help curtail the medicalization of health.

The ubiquitous presence of chemicals from PPCPs in the environment extends the risks to the entire ecosystem, which we have a collective responsibility to protect. Our focus on testing individual drug and food products for toxicity could serve mainly to postpone action by deflecting attention and resources from initiatives that would curtail our excessive dependence on drugs. Human health, particularly the health of children and developing fetuses, may be in danger; the health of aquatic life and other non-human species certainly is. Can there be any question that it's time to "treat" our unhealthy addiction to prescription drugs?

Note

1. A total of 1,512 people completed the survey; half were males and half females. All differences reported were statistically significant, although the report does not specify levels of significance. The authors describe gender differences as "relatively small"; however, the pattern of difference is consistent.

Chapter 10

Finding a Way Forward

———◆◆◆———

The Steering Committee of Women and Health Protection

Medical drugs, when prescribed and taken appropriately, have the potential to save lives and improve their quality; each of us has seen evidence of this, whether it is a medicine we took or something that helped a friend or family member. It is perhaps because of these experiences with medical drugs that we tend to believe they will always help us. But what if this persuasive save-and-help story about drugs were not the only one? Does this focus on the "rescues" that drugs can offer mask the fact that drugs come with a price—a price both to the individual, with the potential for serious side effects, and to the environment, with a growing toll on our waterways? And does a collective "buying in" to the notion of drugs as solutions also provide a breeding ground for media exploitation, from direct-to-consumer advertising to manipulative first-person accounts of miracle cures?

Canadians, along with residents of other resource-rich countries, now consume medical drugs not only for real diseases, but for all manner of minor discomforts, for possible and sometimes imagined risks to our health, for things that might happen in the future, and for normal conditions related to various stages of life that are deemed inconvenient or unattractive. These patterns of consumption are evident both among the healthy and among those with actual diseases, and are not simply the result of human weakness or media exploitation. They could not have developed without an aggressive corporate push from the pharmaceutical, biotechnological, and public relations industries, as well as the willingness of some in the research and medical communities to buy in to the corporate model and federal regulators' lack of will to uphold the key principles of public health.

The preceding chapters have illustrated the various ways in which industry pressure has influenced, if not distorted, health policy in Canada. We have shown how direct-to-consumer advertising has led to inappropriate prescribing and fuelled a disease-mongering trend in our society. We have discussed how the industry's claim that it needs to keep information private (proprietary), and our regulators acceding to that claim, has contributed to a lack of transparency in our drug regulation system. We have shown how the growing presence of medications in the water system is creating an entire new set of problems that regulators had not anticipated. And throughout, we have pointed out how this has all been deleterious to women's health.

Examining drug policy and health protection through the lens of women's experience not only highlights the gendered nature of medicine use and regulation, but also provides a reminder of how we cannot understand the social determinants of health without specifically integrating women's health research into this work. The 2008 report of the World Health Organization (WHO) illustrates this point in their discussion of gender equity (World Health Organization, 2008). Moreover, this perspective reminds us that acting on the social determinants of health and protecting health requires that we look upstream at the conditions and situations that result in ill health and disease. Making significant improvements to the conditions under which women live and work and prioritizing environmental protection are prerequisites to sustained health promotion and health protection.

Good public policy is the key to ensuring the safety and accessibility of medical drugs for those who need them; it is also fundamental to controlling the activities of industry and promoting the kinds of social changes that will improve health and reduce the need for medical drugs.

Thus, we cannot discuss women's increased use of, for example, potentially unsafe antidepressants, or even problems in drug regulation, without also elaborating on the context of most women's lives. If the circumstances of some women make their lives unmanageable, is daily medication the answer or is systemic change required to give women equitable pay for their work, meaningful jobs, less violence in their homes, affordable daycare, and safe and affordable housing? Similarly, we cannot consider whether women should be routinely placed on cholesterol-lowering medications without also examining policies about the distribution and affordability of healthy foods. In terms of treatment options, if health insurance plans covered non-drug alternatives—such as swimming; yoga and fitness classes; or running, relaxation, and meditation programs—might it not be more "healthful" for a physician to prescribe these instead of a statin medication? (See, for example, Frisby et al., 2001.)

Unfortunately, the overhyping of some current trends in pharmaceutical use and regulation does not inspire hope or confidence that social and structural change is being favoured over industrial expansion and an increased reliance on technology. A few examples of these trends are:

- *Personalized medicine, wherein extensive blood and genetic testing is used to help determine the kind and dose of medicine appropriate for a specific individual:* This practice will not only be completely unaffordable to most people, but may further favour medication over alternative therapeutic approaches.
- *Brain imaging, using increasingly sophisticated diagnostic technologies:* This not only may lead to the blurring of "normal" and "abnormal," but by reinforcing the notion of the importance of early diagnosis, it diverts attention from what makes people sick in the first place.
- *Developments in the field of nanotechnology (the manipulation and use of materials on a molecular scale):* These are claimed to offer new approaches for diagnosis and treatment, but there are huge gaps in our knowledge of these particles and their impact on human health and the environment—and there are still no coherent regulatory mechanisms in place.
- *Direct-to-consumer advertising is expanding beyond prescription drugs and is now applied to marketing "do-it-yourself" at-home genetic testing kits:* In many countries, neither the advertising nor the use of these testing kits is appropriately regulated.

- *The proliferation of medications (e.g., human growth hormones), procedures (e.g., Botox injections), and devices (e.g., silicone gel breast implants) geared to "enhancement":* All of these play on fears of aging and promote an unattainable quest for perfection. Government sanctioning of these products and devices runs the risk of further institutionalizing this trend.

- *The expanding use of reproductive technologies leading to the "harvesting" of eggs from healthy women for use by other women seeking infertility treatments:* The risks of these procedures for the women involved, and the children who may be born, remain unmonitored, under-regulated, and understudied.

- *The continued tendency to medicalize normal bodily functions, such as the increasing promotion of drugs for menstrual suppression:* As a result, an ever-increasing number of healthy women are consuming drugs over extended periods—with unknown long-term consequences and risks.

These trends have the potential to directly harm women's health, and the absence of robust mechanisms to regulate them is troubling. They also raise substantial ethical and social concerns, and these concerns have not had the necessary public discussion that must underlie responsible policy-making.

Women's Health through Active Engagement

While these troubling trends are clearly cause for concern, there are also many examples of effective alternatives and solutions. Women's health activism in Canada has a long and commendable history (see Box 10.2), with some notable successes. This history holds important lessons, not the least of which is that collective action by women, rooted in their experience, can be an effective tool in protecting women's health.

After decades during which women's health activists raised concerns that menopausal hormone therapy had not been adequately tested to know whether claimed health benefits did, in fact, exist, the Women's Health Initiative (WHI) was launched to study the drugs' health effects. In 2002, the WHI was stopped early because of the finding that serious harm, mainly due to heart disease and breast cancer, outweighed benefit. This led to a large drop in the rate of prescriptions for estrogen/progestin combinations for menopausal women; a notable decline in cases of breast cancer in post-menopausal women followed (Kerlikowske, Miglioretti, Buist, Walker & Carney, 2007).

Emergency contraception offers a more recent example of effective collective action by women. Women's health organizations, including the Canadian Women's Health Network and Women and Health Protection, joined with researchers and clinicians from across the country to propose that emergency contraception should not require a physician's prescription. They provided evidence showing that the drug

Box 10.1: The Story of the Gardasil Vaccine

by Abby Lippman

The HPV vaccine, Gardasil, was first approved for use while this book was being prepared. Its story summarizes many of the themes we have raised, particularly those centred on the meaning of prevention, the limits of clinical trial data, direct-to-consumer advertising (DTCA) and marketing excesses, and the weaknesses of government regulatory mechanisms.

Gardasil is the brand name of a vaccine formulated to immunize recipients against four types of human papilloma virus (HPV); two of these have been associated with 70 percent of cervical cancer cases. In early 2007, the federal finance minister announced a $300 million budget allocation to fund a Gardasil vaccination campaign. This announcement was accompanied by an extraordinary marketing blitz for the vaccine, leading Canadian women's health advocates to wonder how and why cervical cancer had become the "poster child" for the government's concern about women's health in this country.

Cervical cancer is a serious and lethal disease worldwide; 80 percent of cases occur in the developing world. In Canada, there are about 400 deaths per year from cervical cancer; by contrast, 5,300 women die from breast cancer and 8,900 from lung cancer annually. Noteworthy is that these 400 deaths are concentrated among women who are marginalized in our society, women who often have not had the Pap testing needed to detect early, treatable cellular changes. Thus, deaths from cervical cancer in Canada result primarily from weaknesses in current prevention programs. This fact has been obscured in extensive media advertising by both pharmaceutical companies and provincial public health agencies. This marketing manipulates fears and parental guilt to encourage compliance with school-based HPV vaccination programs, implying that parents who do not have their daughters immunized are irresponsible. The success of organized, systematic Pap testing in preventing the development of, and reducing deaths from, cervical cancer in Canada is rarely, if ever, mentioned.

Government regulators approved Gardasil for use by girls and women aged nine to 26 years; the school-based programs in Canada target mostly nine- to 12-year-old girls. Although the international clinical trials of the product included over 20,000 women, only 1,200 of those were nine- to 15-year-olds and only 200 of those were nine- and 10-year-olds, raising concerns about how much we truly know about how this age group will react to the vaccine (Food and Drug Administration, 2006, p. 20).

These trials, all supported by the vaccine's manufacturer, were of limited length (at the time of approval, about five years). As a result, it is not known how long protection provided by the vaccine will actually last. This information, too, has been neglected in much of the educational material about the vaccine.

Moreover, the advertising campaigns tell only a very partial story about HPV infections, e.g., omitting how HPV is a necessary but not a sufficient cause of cervical cancer. In fact, most HPV infections are transient: of the many Canadian women who will contract this sexually transmitted virus, about 90 percent will clear it spontaneously from their system within one to two years. Only when the viral infection persists—and this is more likely to happen when women are immuno-compromised or are otherwise unable to maintain good health for a variety of socio-economic reasons—and Pap testing is either not done or is falsely negative, is there a chance that cervical cancer will develop. In other words, while almost all heterosexually active girls and women will probably have an HPV infection at some time in their lives, most will suffer no ill health effects as a result. Cervical cancer is concentrated among those at greater risk because they are marginalized (racially, geographically) and therefore fail to access health services. Advertising for the vaccine and vaccine programs does not even hint at this truth.

When the HPV vaccine was rushed to market, women's health advocates immediately raised questions: To what extent were political decisions fully informed by sound public health principles and, more specifically, what was known about the "real world" effectiveness of this product in Canada? These questions remain unanswered.

---

was safe and essential, and that the need to obtain a physician's prescription was inhibiting timely access to the medication when girls and women urgently needed it. Using research and education, this coalition succeeded first (2005) in having the drug's status moved from prescription-by-physician to prescription-by-pharmacist ("behind the counter"), and subsequently (2008) in having the drug's status changed so it would be available "in front of the counter," but still within a pharmacy. These changes demonstrate the ability of coalitions to secure policy changes. As well, these changes, which make emergency contraception more widely available, have had important health benefits for women by resulting in fewer unplanned pregnancies.

Another example of effective activism is evident in the increasing public awareness about water-quality issues. Individuals and groups in the women's health and environmental movements have brought their concerns about the environmental impact of medications and personal care products (PCPs) in the water to public and government attention. As we go to press, articles on the topic appear on a regular basis in the research literature, and federal candidates canvassing for the Fall 2008 election were faced with questions about the issue. Here again, community and academic research, presented through the lens of women's health protection and promotion, has shown its value.

Another counterbalance to current troubling trends is the existence of some alternative models in the drug world, such as independent research groups that

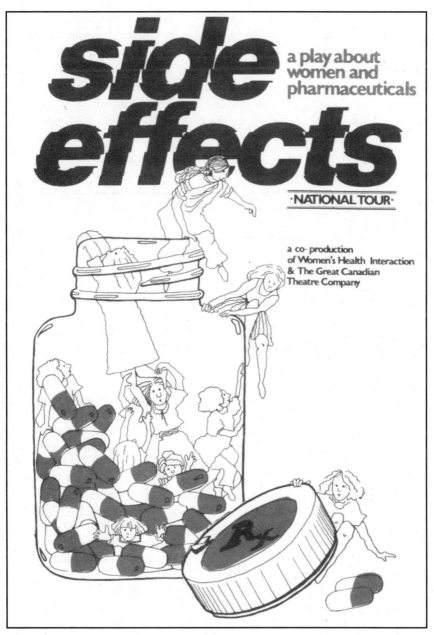

Figure 10.1: *Side Effects*, a play on women and pharmaceuticals, was originally developed and produced by Inter Pares and the Great Canadian Theatre Company for Women's Health Interaction. Poster by Heather Walters.

Source: Inter Pares and the Great Canadian Theatre Company for Women's Health Interaction.

provide unbiased comparative information on health and pharmaceuticals. One example is the Therapeutics Initiative (TI), an independent organization at the University of British Columbia dedicated to providing up-to-date, evidence-based, and practical information on rational drug therapy. The TI works at arm's length from government, the pharmaceutical industry, and other vested interest groups, thereby ensuring that its analyses of classes of drugs, such as osteoporosis medications, SSRI antidepressants, menopausal hormone therapy, and statins, are independent and based only on reliable data. The focus of many of their bulletins is on medicines used primarily by women.

Box 10.2: Canadian Milestones in Collective Action to Promote and Protect Women's Health

- Critical work on access to birth control and abortion done by the McGill Women's Press (1969)
- Ruth Cooperstock's pioneering research on psychotropic drug use and prescribing patterns of physicians, as well as on the medicalization of women's social problems (1960s and 1970s)
- The launch of DES Action Canada, which evolved out of the personal experiences of a mother and daughter affected by the hormone DES (1983)
- National theatre tour of *Side Effects*, a play about women and pharmaceuticals produced by the Great Canadian Theatre Company, Inter Pares, and a range of local women's groups across Canada, which spawned new women's groups nationwide focused on issues relating to women and drugs (1985)
- Publication of *Adverse Effects: Women and the Pharmaceutical Industry*, a co-production between Women's Press in Canada and the International Organization of Consumer Unions in Malaysia (1986)
- Collective action and advocacy work regarding the Dalkon Shield IUD and Depo-Provera (Canadian Coalition on Depo Provera), with a particular focus on use among women with disabilities and Aboriginal women (1980s)
- The Royal Commission on New Reproductive Technologies, the result of considerable lobbying by women's health academics and activists, amassed a substantial body of knowledge about prescription drugs used in assisted human reproduction (1989–1993)
- Canadian moratorium imposed on silicone gel breast implants as women with a host of problems associated with the devices came forward (1993)
- Creation of Women and Health Protection within the Centres of Excellence for Women's Health Program, with a mandate to respond to policy initiatives at Health Canada respecting the regulation of prescription drugs and devices and their impact on women's health (1998)

Effecting change is difficult and slow, but even the most troubling trends in how medical drugs and devices are developed, monitored, marketed, and used need not be inevitable. And certainly the excessive medicalization of women's lives can be contested and resisted. Our collective vision is of a universal health care system rooted in authentic and diverse sources of evidence.

Preparing this book has been a reminder for us, and we hope for our readers, that collective action and involvement in public policy development are both productive and essential ways to promote women's health. Moreover, it is our right and our duty as citizens living in a democracy to speak, act, and participate in the decisions that will affect us all. A more visionary approach by our federal regulators, one that is solidly grounded in the precautionary principle and where protection of the public's health and safety is the clear, unfettered goal, is necessary. The principles of health protection make it clear that the "smart regulation" approach increasingly favoured by the Canadian government over the last decade, whereby business interests are allowed to trump public health, is not in the public interest. Sound health protection principles further demand that our regulators develop, adopt, and enforce policies that support primordial prevention—prevention upstream where the root causes of ill health and disease are found.

Further Reading

Chapter 1

Cooperstock, R. & Hill, J. (1982). *The effects of tranquillization: Benzodiazepine use in Canada.* Ottawa: Minister of Supply and Services Canada.

This publication takes an honest and well-referenced look at the overprescription of benzodiazepines at the time it was written, incorporating some of the critical social factors that contribute to overprescribing. It raises brave questions about the inappropriate use of medication for "dulling social pain," and the inadequate training of physicians in helping people "cope with stresses without the aid of chemicals."

Cooperstock, R. & Lennard, H.L. (1979). Some social meanings of tranquilizer use. *Sociology of Health and Illness, 1*(3), 331–347.

This Canadian article was a landmark academic publication examining the relationship between medicines and women's health, and women's experience of medicines.

Hankivsky, O., Varcoe, C. & Morrow, M. (Eds.). (2007). *Women's health in Canada: Critical perspectives on theory and policy.* Toronto: University of Toronto Press.

This book is an excellent academic resource that explores many of the issues related to women's health in Canada covered in the present volume.

McDonnell, K. (Ed.). (1986). *Adverse effects: Women and the pharmaceutical industry.* Toronto: The Women's Press.

Initially published in Malaysia by the International Organization of Consumer Unions, this book discusses many of the issues relating to women and pharmaceuticals that are covered in *The Push to Prescribe*; reading it, one gets an astonishing sense that not much has changed in 20+ years. Authors in this volume are from several countries, including Canada.

Tickner, J.A., Kriebel, D. & Wright, S. (2003). A compass for health: Rethinking precaution and its role in science and public health. *International Journal of Epidemiology, 32*(4), 489–492.

In this article, the scientific and public health communities are urged to help define what precaution means in practice, including tools for its implementation. Interest in precaution provides an opportunity to move toward a more constructive view of environmental and health policy, reinvigorating the core values and preventive traditions of public health.

Van Doorslaer, E., Masseria, C. & Koolman, X., for the OECD Health Equity Research Group. (2006). Inequalities in access to medical care by income in developed countries. *CMAJ, 174*(2),177–183.

This article investigates the relationship between medical visits and income in developed countries. The findings: in most countries, general practitioner visits are equitably distributed across income groups and any significant inequity that emerges is often pro-poor. However, the picture is very different for medical specialist consultations. The rich are significantly more likely than the poor to see a specialist and, in most countries, will see them more frequently.

Chapter 2

Abramson, J. (2005). *Overdosed America: The broken promise of American medicine.* New York: HarperCollins.

Abramson describes the overmedication and overmedicalization of Americans due to the commercialization of health care, and debunks the myth that more expensive care means better care. *Overdosed America* includes examples of relevance to women's health, such as the marketing of cholesterol-lowering drugs and hormone replacement therapy.

Frosch, D.L., Krueger, P.M., Hornik, R.C., Cronholm, P.F. & Barg, F.K. (2007). Creating demand for prescription drugs: A content analysis of television direct-to-consumer advertising. *Annals of Family Medicine, 5,* 6–13. doi:10.1370/afm.611

This content analysis of a systematic sample of U.S. television advertisements looks at the methods these advertisements use to influence the public and the key messages in the advertisements about the drugs and the diseases they treat.

Gilbody, S., Wilson, P. & Watt, I. (2005). Benefits and harms of direct to consumer advertising: A systematic review. *Quality and Safety in Health Care, 14,* 246–250. doi:10.1136/qshc.2004.012781

This is a systematic review of the published research evidence, to late 2004, on the effects of DTCA on patient and physician behaviours, costs, and health. It provides a good overview of the types of research methods that can be used to examine effects of advertising, and what is and is not known about its effects.

Mintzes, B. (2006, January). *Direct-to-consumer advertising of prescription drugs in Canada: What are the public health implications?* Toronto: Health Council of Canada. Available at: www.healthcouncilcanada.ca/docs/papers/2006/hcc_dtc-advertising_ 200601_e_v6.pdf

This is a detailed report on DTCA policy developments in Canada. It also includes a review of the research evidence and discussion of policy in the European Union, the U.S., and New Zealand.

Moynihan, R. & Cassels, A. (2005). *Selling sickness: How the world's biggest pharmaceutical companies are turning us all into patients.* Emeryville: Avalon Publishing Group.

Selling Sickness describes the systematic way that drug companies widen the very boundaries that define illness, redefining mild problems as serious illness and common complaints as medical conditions requiring drug treatment. For example, premenstrual syndrome has been redefined as a psychiatric condition, premenstrual dysphoric disorder, and low bone density as osteopenia.

Chapter 3

Batt, S. (1994). *Patient no more: The politics of breast cancer.* Charlottetown: Gynergy Press.

Written by a Canadian woman after her breast cancer diagnosis, *Patient no more* provides a feminist's account of the many debates over cancer causality, detection, treatments, and research. The chapter "Hormones" (pp. 111–138) describes the clash of cultures between women's health activists and cancer research promoting the use of hormone-blocking drugs to prevent breast cancer. The chapter "Prevention" (pp. 187–209) discusses interventionist and environmental perspectives on breast cancer prevention.

Epp, J. (1986). *Achieving health for all: A framework for health promotion.* Ottawa. Available at: www.hc-sc.gc.ca/hcs-sss/pubs/system-regime/1986-frame-plan-promotion /index-eng.php

Also known as the Ottawa Charter on Health Promotion, this document was developed under the auspices of the World Health Organization and constitutes a revolutionary approach to health because it highlights *social* determinants of health ("peace, shelter, education, food, income, a stable ecosystem, sustainable resources, social justice, and equity") rather than medical care and individual "lifestyle" strategies.

European Environment Agency. (2002). *Late lessons from early warnings: The precautionary principle 1896–2000.* Environmental issue report no. 22. Copenhagen: Author.

This report by the European Environmental Agency uses 14 case histories to illustrate the precautionary principle. Several involve drugs, including DES and hormones, as growth promoters. Based on these historical studies, the authors challenge myths, such as the belief that use of the precautionary principle will stifle innovation or compromise science. The full report, or individual chapters, can be downloaded from: www.eea.europa.eu/publications/environmental_issue_report_2001_22/en

Krieger, N. et al. (2005). Hormone replacement therapy, cancer, controversies, and women's health: Historical, epidemiological, biological, clinical, and advocacy perspectives. *Journal of Epidemiology and Community Health, 59,* 740–748. doi:10.1136/jech.2005.033316

This article traces the ways in which menopause was medicalized through the various lenses of the authors contributing to this paper. It provides a good "case history" with lessons applicable to other aspects of women's health.

Lippman, A. (1998). The politics of health: Geneticization versus health promotion. In S. Sherwin (Coordinator) and the Feminist Health Care Ethics Research Network, *The politics of women's health: Exploring agency and autonomy* (pp. 64–82). Philadelphia: Temple University Press.

This essay critically analyzes the distinction between health promotion achieved by addressing the social determinants of health (see Batt's *Patient No More,* above) and the pursuit of health as the absence of disease. The author also discusses the links among health promotion, empowerment, bottom-up approaches to health, and feminist understandings of health as developed within the contemporary women's health movement and its precursors.

Moynihan, R., Doran, E. & Henry, D. (2008). Disease mongering is now part of the global health debate. *PLoS Medicine* 5(5), e106. Available at: www.medicine.plosjournals.org/perlserv/?request=get-document&doi=10.1371/journal.pmed.0050106

In this article the organizers of the inaugural conference on disease-mongering report briefly on the conference, discuss its subsequent impact, and raise possible directions for academic inquiry and policy reform.

Chapter 4

Brennan, T.A., Rothman, D.J., Blank, L., Blumenthal, D., Chimonas, S.C., Cohen, J.J. et al. (2005). Health industry practices that create conflicts of interest: A policy proposal for academic medical centers. *JAMA, 295*(4), 429–433.

The authors propose a policy under which academic medical centres would take the lead in eliminating the conflicts of interest that still characterize the relationship between physicians and the health care industry.

Chalmers, I. (2007, August 25). The Alzheimer's Society, drug firms, and public trust. *BMJ, 335*, 400; Furlini, L. (2007, September 26). Why I am no longer a member of the Alzheimer Society. *BMJ*; and Dudgeon, S. (2007, October 3). Alzheimer Society of Canada responds to Linda Furlini "Why I am no longer a member of the Alzheimer Society." *BMJ*. Dr. Chalmer's article and both letters are available at: www. bmj.bmjjournals.com/cgi/eletters/335/7619/541-a#176939

These letters are an exchange of views about disease charities, funding from the pharmaceutical industry, and the evaluation of drugs for inclusion on provincial formularies.

Delaney, M. (2005). AIDS activism and the pharmaceutical industry. In M.A. Santoro & T.M. Gorrie (Eds.), *Ethics and the pharmaceutical industry* (pp. 300–325). New York: Cambridge University Press.

In this chapter, a long-time American AIDS activist describes the sometimes antagonistic, sometimes collaborative relationship between AIDS activists and pharmaceutical companies in the U.S. He concludes that the AIDS movement needs funding from Big Pharma to provide the range of services the community needs, but acknowledges that conflicts of interest have become a major issue. He proposes a series of guidelines to help groups maintain their independence while accepting industry funds.

Ford, A. (1998) *A different prescription: Considerations for women's health groups contemplating funding from the pharmaceutical industry.* Toronto: Institute for Feminist Legal Studies at Osgoode Hall, York University. Available at: www.whp-apsf.ca/en/ documents/diff_prescrip.html

This booklet was written by a Canadian women's health activist to assist groups struggling with the pharma funding question. The booklet is structured as a series of arguments for and against accepting money from the pharmaceutical industry. Each question is followed by reflections that draw out the complexities of the point of view expressed.

Hoey, J. (2006). Guideline controversy. *CMAJ, 174*(3), 333.

The *CMAJ* editor introduces a series of articles that debate the relationship between clinical practice guidelines and industry influence with respect to the criticism by the Canadian Diabetes Association of the Common Drug Review for its decision not to recommend funding of a new long-acting insulin.

Howlett, M.C. & Little, D. (2006). The Canadian Diabetes Association guidelines: Putting the evidence first. *CMAJ, 174*(3), 333–334.

Laupacis, A. (2006). On bias and transparency in the development of influential recommendations. *CMAJ, 174*(3), 335–336.

O'Donovan, O. (2007). Corporate colonization of health activism? Irish health advocacy organizations' modes of engagement with pharmaceutical corporations. *International Journal of Health Services, 37*(4), 711–733.
    This article, based on a study of health advocacy groups in Ireland, describes their "modes of engagement" with the pharmaceutical industry. The groups' approach to industry varies along a continuum, from "corporatist" at one extreme, to "confrontational" at the other, with "cautiously co-operative" in between. The research provides evidence of a strong and growing cultural tendency in Irish health advocacy organizations to frame pharmaceutical corporations as allies in their quests for better health. The author cautions, however, against a simplistic conclusion that this is evidence of corporate colonization. The study provides an interesting cross-cultural comparison with the Canadian examples in this chapter.

Chapter 5

Caron, J. (2003). *Report on governmental health research policies promoting gender or sex differences sensitivity.* Prepared for the Institute of Gender and Health. Ottawa: Canadian Institutes of Health Research. Available at: www.cihr-irsc.gc.ca/e/pdf_25502.htm
    This report examines international health research policies and programs intended to promote gender/sex-difference sensitive research. In addition to reviewing these policies, it reports on texts discussing criteria essential to successful implementation of such policies.

Clarke, A., Shim, J.N., Mamo, L., Fosket, J. & Fishman, J.R. (2003). Biomedicalization: Theorizing technoscientific transformations of health, illness, and U.S. biomedicine. *American Sociological Review, 68*, 161–194.
    This is an excellent review of the ways in which the concept of "medicalization" has evolved and of the forces feeding this evolution. Adele Clarke and her colleagues' ideas about "biomedicalization" were developed at the same time as those about "neomedicalization" were emerging, and there are many parallels between the perspectives.

Epstein, S. (2007). *Inclusion: The politics of difference in medical research.* Chicago: University of Chicago Press.

Steven Epstein's most recent book charts the rise, and examines the consequences, of managing difference, including gender difference, in biomedical research in the U.S.

Institute of Gender and Health. *What's sex and gender got to do with it? Integrating sex and gender into health research.* Ottawa: CIHR IGH. Available at: www.cihr-irsc. gc.ca/e/pdf_25530.htm

This report is the outcome of an international think tank that brought together participants from a range of research disciplines to discuss ways in which sex and gender could be integrated into a program of health research. The think tank explored different conceptions of sex and gender, and provided a forum for discussing challenges and opportunities for integrating sex and gender and health research.

Mastroianni, A.C., Faden, R. & Federman, D. (Eds.), for the Committee on Ethical and Legal Issues Relating to the Inclusion of Women in Clinical Studies, Institute of Medicine. (1994). *Women and health research: Ethical and legal issues of including women in clinical studies* (vol. 1). Washington: National Academies Press.

Mastroianni, A.C., Faden, R. & Federman, D. (Eds.), for the Committee on Ethical and Legal Issues Relating to the Inclusion of Women in Clinical Studies, Institute of Medicine. (1999). *Women and health research: Ethical and legal issues of including women in clinical studies: Workshop and commissioned papers* (vol. 2). Washington: National Academies Press.

The papers collected in these two volumes provide essential background material relevant to issues about the inclusion of women in clinical trials.

Shah, S. (2006). *The body hunters: How the drug industry tests its products on the world's poorest patients.* New York: The New Press.

This is a very readable and extremely critical review of the ways in which the pharmaceutical industry conducts clinical trials in developing countries.

Wizemann, T.M. & Pardue, M.-L. (Eds.). (2001). *Exploring the biological contributions to human health: Does sex matter?* Washington: National Academies Press.

Frequently referred to in discussions of sex and gender influences on health, this book provides a useful overview of "sex" from the level of DNA to the entire organism.

Chapter 6

Dhalla, I. & Laupacis, A. (2008, February 12). Moving from opacity to transparency in pharmaceutical policy. *CMAJ, 178*(4), 428–431. doi:10.1503/cmaj.070799

This article posits that transparency in pharmaceutical policy-making would probably lead to increased confidence in the decision-making process and to better decisions. In addition to the pharmaceutical industry, researchers, governments, quasi-governmental agencies, payers, and medical journals need to make more information available to the public. The authors suggest that Canada could be a world leader in this area.

Health Canada. (2006). *Access to therapeutic products: The regulatory process in Canada.* Ottawa: Health Products and Food Branch, Health Canada. Available at: www.hc-sc.gc.ca/ahc-asc/pubs/hpfb-dgpsa/access-therapeutic_acces-therapeutique_e.html

This document outlines, from the government's point of view, the involvement of the regulator all the way from pre-clinical studies to post-market activities.

Hypatia. (2006, Summer). Special issue: Feminist epistemologies of ignorance, *21*(3).

This special issue of the feminist journal *Hypatia* is devoted entirely to the theme "feminist epistemologies of ignorance." Traditional scholarship of knowledge (i.e., epistemology) often assumes that ignorance is simply a lack of knowledge. Contributors to this volume argue that a liberatory scholarship will understand ignorance as the result of particular practices in the way knowledge is produced. Leading feminist scholars discuss the way practices of ignorance are often intertwined with practices of oppression and exclusion.

Lexchin, J. (2007). The secret things belong unto the Lord our God: Secrecy in the pharmaceutical arena. *Medicine and Law, 26*(3), 417–430.

This article argues that secrecy in the pharmaceutical arena has taken on more importance in the recent past as the pharmaceutical industry has assumed greater prominence in the funding of clinical research and has also become a funder of the agencies that are charged with regulating it. The author suggests that because regulators are now partially dependent on the pharmaceutical industry for their existence, regulators are unwilling to challenge industry.

Lexchin, J. (2007). Notice of compliance with conditions: A policy in limbo. *Healthcare Policy, 2*(4), 114–122.

Drugs approved under a Notice of Compliance with conditions (NOC/c) must undergo post-marketing trials to show clinical benefits. The reasons why some drugs receive a NOC/c are not always apparent and the Therapeutic Products Directorate releases only general information regarding the conditions that need to be fulfilled. Some drugs have fulfilled their conditions in under 1.4 years, but others had unfulfilled conditions after seven years. Doctors may not be aware that drugs are marketed with a NOC/c or that some drugs have had their NOC/c withdrawn and, as a consequence, may be prescribing inappropriately for their patients.

Lurie, P. & Zieve, A. (2006). Sometimes the silence can be like thunder: Access to pharmaceutical data at the FDA. *Law and Contemporary Problems, 69,* 85–97.

The article describes how small dents have been made in the imposing edifice of the confidential commercial exemption in the United States. The larger question remains: Why should trade secret law automatically trump public health concerns?

Chapter 7

Decima Research. (2003, December). *Public opinion survey on key issues pertaining to post-market surveillance of marketed health products in Canada. Final report to Health Canada.* Ottawa: Author. POR# 298-02.

This public opinion survey provides an interesting look at the public's experience of adverse drug reactions. The survey also looked at perceptions among health professionals of their patients' experiences and of their familiarity with the ADR reporting system. Both groups were also surveyed about their views on physicians' mandatory reporting of ADRs. Three different health products were included .in the survey: prescription drugs, non-prescription drugs, and natural health products. Some 37 percent of consumers surveyed reported they had experienced an adverse drug reaction at some time in the previous six months.

Healy, D. (2003). *Let them eat Prozac.* Toronto: Lorimer.

Healy's account of the marketing of depression includes a sharp critique of how post-market surveillance has failed to pick up warning signals of possible suicides linked to SSRI use in Britain. The book calls for a "separation of powers" within regulatory agencies between those who approve drugs and those who are responsible for detecting potential harms.

Medawar, C. & Herxheimer, A. (2004, February 17). A comparison of adverse drug reaction reports from professionals and users, relating to risk of dependence and suicidal behaviour with paroxetine. *International Journal of Risk and Safety in Medicine, 16*(1), 3–17. Available at: iospress.metapress.com/content/103162/

Medawar and Herxheimer are strong proponents of the value of direct-from-consumer reporting of adverse drug reactions. This report, available on the Social Audit website, compares reports from professionals with patients' reports of the same suspected adverse drug reactions. The goal of the study was to learn more about the effects of the SSRI antidepressant paroxetine (Paxil) and to evaluate the most effective sources of high-quality information about such ADRs. The authors concluded that "the overall quality of professional reporting and interpretation of data seemed poor, providing intelligence that was in some ways inferior to that provided in spontaneous reports from patients." The Social Audit is the publishing arm of the Public Interest Research Centre located in London, England.

Moore, T.J., Cohen, M.R. & Furberg, C.D. (2007, September 10). Serious adverse drug events reported to the Food and Drug Administration, 1998–2005. *Archives of Internal Medicine, 167*(16), 1752–1759.
This study charts the increase in the number of serious adverse drug reactions in the United States during the period under review. The authors found that "the overall relative increase [of serious ADRs] was four times faster than the growth in total U.S. outpatient prescriptions" during the same period.

Chapter 8

Abergel, E. (2000). *Placing limits on health protection by managing risks.* Unpublished report prepared for the Women and Health Protection Working Group, with edits by Madeline Boscoe, 2004. Toronto: WHP. Available upon request from WHP at: whp.apsf@gmail.com
The report is an academic appraisal of the creeping trend toward a risk management framework in the federal government.

Barer, M.L., McGrail, K., Cardiff, K., Wood, L. & Green, C.J. (Eds.). (1999). *Tales from the other drug wars (Papers from the 12th Annual Health Policy Conference held in Vancouver, BC, November 26, 1999).* Vancouver: Centre for Health Services and Policy Research, University of British Columbia.
In addition to Michèle Brill-Edwards's presentation of a behind-the-scenes look at the inner workings of the Health Protection Branch, other topics by Canadian health policy experts include a critical appraisal of lipid-lowering drugs, a tribute to a Canadian whistle-blower, uses and abuses of the research process, and how the Canadian government controls drug promotion.

Canadian Health Coalition. (2003). *Risk first: Safety last! A citizen's guide to Health Canada's "Health and safety first! A proposal to renew federal health protection legislation."* Ottawa: Author. Available at: www.healthcoalition.ca/safetylast.pdf
Following the release of Health Canada's *Health and Safety First!* the Canadian Health Coalition responded with this hard-hitting critique of the proposed changes.

Health Canada. (1998). *Shared responsibilities, shared vision: Renewing the federal health protection legislation: A discussion document.* Ottawa: Author. Available at: www.hc-sc.gc.ca/ahc-asc/pubs/cons-pub/shared-respon-partag-cp-pc_e.html

This is one of the original documents that mobilized Women and Health Protection and many other Canadian NGOs to bring forward concerns about the direction the federal government was taking in drug regulation.

Health Canada. (2003). *Health and safety first! A proposal to renew federal health protection legislation.* Ottawa: Author. Available through the Library of Parliament.
This 2003 document represents the government's thinking after a series of consultations with Canadians and puts forward proposals for changes to health protection legislation.

Chapter 9

Holtz, S. (2006). *There is no "away." Pharmaceuticals, personal care products, and endocrine-disrupting substances: Emerging contaminants detected in water.* Toronto: Canadian Institute for Environmental Law and Policy. Available at: www.cielap.org/pdf/NoAway.pdf
This paper by the Canadian Institute for Environmental Law and Policy covers some of the same ground as this chapter, but provides a different perspective on the issue of PPCPs in Canada. As a group with an environmental rather than a health focus, CIELAP's emphasis is on the environment-related effects rather than the implications of medical use. The paper also provides an extensive analysis of drugs used in Canada for veterinary and aquaculture purposes.

Khosla, P. & Pearl, R. (2003). *Untapped connections: Gender, water, and poverty: Key issues, government commitments, and actions for sustainable development.* New York: Women's Environment and Development Organization. This is available online and can be downloaded in pdf format: www.wedo.org/wp-content/uploads/untapped-eng.pdf
The Women's Environment and Development Organization (WEDO) is an international advocacy network that promotes a healthy planet and social, political, and environmental justice for all. This publication presents a framework for thinking about gender and the right to safe water as a public resource. Topics covered include gender differences in water use and management; international commitments on gender, poverty, and water; and lists of contacts and resources. Brief case studies from five countries illustrate the role women have played in managing local water supplies.

Rimkus, G.G. (Ed.). (2004). *Synthetic musk fragrances in the environment.* Berlin/Heidelberg: Springer.
Synthetic musk fragrances in the environment have been studied for over a decade and German scientist Gerhard Rimkus is a leading researcher in this area. While this chapter has focused on pharmaceuticals, musks are an important class of PPCPs

found in drinking water, lakes, streams, fish and wildlife, human fat tissue, blood, and breast milk. Synthetic musks are high-volume, lipophilic chemical compounds with poor degradability used in perfumes, cosmetics, soaps, and laundry detergents as substitutes for expensive musk extracts derived from musk deer, muskrats, and other animals.

Chapter 10

Armstrong, P. & Deadman, J. (Eds.). (2008). *Women's health: Intersections of policy, research, and practice*. Toronto: Women's Press.

This book incorporates work that has been produced from grassroots investigations of women's health issues and addresses specific health concerns, diversity issues, and a variety of issues previously unexplored. *Women's Health* highlights the work of women whose voices may not normally be heard or recognized in a way that stretches beyond the traditional parameters of knowledge-sharing practices.

Dua, E., Fitzgerald, M., Taylor, D. & Gardner, L. (Eds.). (1994). *On women healthsharing*. Toronto: Women's Press.

This contributed text includes essays about, and contributions from, 15 years of publishing of *Healthsharing: A Canadian Women's Health Quarterly*, published in Toronto between 1979 and 1994.

McBane, M. (2005). *Ill-health Canada: Putting food and drug company profits ahead of safety*. Ottawa: Canadian Centre for Policy Alternatives.

In this book, the author argues that Canada's political and industry elites are choosing to allow corporate profits to trump the protection of citizens' health. He presents evidence to indicate that the federal health and safety regulatory agencies have been captured by industry.

Sherwin, S. (Ed.). (1998). *The politics of women's health: Exploring agency and autonomy*. Philadelphia: Temple University Press.

The chapters in this edited volume by Canadian academics address many of the issues raised in *The Push to Prescribe*. Women's health status and health care delivery in different countries are examined, as are the assumptions behind the dominant medical model of solving problems without regard to social conditions. The book explores feminist health care ethics from the vantage point of women's experiences and concerns.

Related Websites

⸻⸻⸻

Chapter 1

Canadian Research Institute for the Advancement of Women (CRIAW)
www.criaw-icref.ca

"CRIAW is a research institute which provides tools to facilitate organizations taking action to advance social justice and equality for all women. CRIAW recognizes women's diverse experiences and perspectives; creates spaces for developing women's knowledge; bridges regional isolation; and provides communication links between/ among researchers and organizations actively working to promote social justice and equality for all women."

Committee on Women, Population, and the Environment (CWPE)
www.cwpe.org

CWPE is a multiracial alliance of feminist community organizers, scholarly activists, and health practitioners committed to promoting the social and economic empowerment of women in a context of global peace and justice, and to eliminating poverty.

DES Action Canada
www.web.net/~desact/

This is an excellent source of information about DES (diethylstilberstrol), which was withdrawn from the Canadian market in 1971 due to catastrophic side effects. These effects continue to impact the children and grandchildren of women who used the drug to prevent miscarriage over a period of 33 years. During the 1950s, studies found DES did not prevent, but rather increased the risk of, miscarriage. In 1971, DES was directly linked to the occurrence of vaginal cancer in daughters whose mothers were prescribed it. DES Action groups were formed around the world to educate the public about the ongoing risks related to the drug. This website is an outstanding example of the power of consumer evidence-based advocacy that aims to educate and reduce harms to the public.

Chapter 2

Canadian Health Coalition

www.healthcoalition.ca/dtca.html

The Canadian Health Coalition, founded by the Canadian Labour Congress, is a not-for-profit, non-partisan organization dedicated to protecting and expanding Canada's public health system for the benefit of all Canadians. Its website on DTCA includes updated postings of media reports and an overview of policy discussions in Canada, especially as they relate to equity in access to health care.

Healthy Skepticism

www.healthyskepticism.org

This is an international non-profit health organization, based in Australia, which aims to improve health by reducing harm from misleading drug promotion. Its website includes a library with references on direct-to-consumer advertising and AdWatch, which deconstructs the messages in drug advertisements.

No Free Lunch

www.nofreelunch.org

No Free Lunch is an organization of health care providers who believe that gifts from the pharmaceutical industry—even small ones—affect clinical practice. The website includes informational and educational materials on the effects of drug promotion on medicine.

PharmedOut

www.pharmedout.org

PharmedOut is an independent, publicly funded project that empowers physicians to identify and counter inappropriate pharmaceutical promotion practices. PharmedOut promotes evidence-based medicine by providing news, resources, and links to pharma-free CME courses.

Women's Health Action Trust

www.womens-health.org.nz/index.php?page=dtc-advertising

Women's Health Action Trust is a grassroots New Zealand women's health organization. As New Zealand is the only country with full public health care that allows direct-to-consumer advertising, its experience is relevant to Canada. The web page above includes links to New Zealand media and other reports on DTCA.

World Health Organization (WHO) Drug Promotion Database

www.drugpromo.info

This is a searchable database of research articles on the effects of drug promotion on attitudes, knowledge, behaviours, health, and costs. It was jointly developed by the World Health Organization and a non-profit organization, Health Action International.

Chapter 3

Canadian Environmental Law Association: The precautionary principle
www.cela.ca/coreprograms/detail.shtml?x=1329
    This site contains a collection of documents discussing the precautionary principle, including a detailed bibliography.

Center for Medical Consumers
www.medicalconsumers.org
    The Center for Medical Consumers is a member organization of Consumers United for Evidence-Based Healthcare (CUE), a pioneering effort started in 2003, which unites consumer advocates with a common interest in integrating understanding and interpretation of evidence-based health care (EBHC) into their advocacy activities.

Science and Environmental Health Network (SEHN)
www.sehn.org/index.html
    Founded in 1994, the SEHN is the leading proponent in the United States of the precautionary principle as a basis for environmental and public health policy. In 1998, the SEHN sponsored the Wingspread Conference on the Precautionary Principle, which resulted in an articulation of the precautionary principle, now in widespread use. This website includes the Wingspread statement on the precautionary principle, with its preamble and signatories, as well as subsequent related statements, such as the Vancouver Statement on Globalization and Industrialization of Agriculture (1998) and the Bemidji Statement on Seventh Generation Guardianship (2006). This website also includes include ecological medicine and law, ethical economics, public interest research, and news.

The Cochrane Collaboration
www.cochrane.org
    The Cochrane Collaboration's goal is to make widely available systematic reviews of evidence from randomized controlled trials of the effects of health care. Their website provides a portal to a significant body of research, catalogued in the Cochrane Library. It is designed to be broadly accessible.

Women's Health Initiative
www.nhlbi.nih.gov/whi/
    The Women's Health Initiative (WHI) is being conducted under the auspices of the U.S. National Institutes of Health heart, lung, and blood institutes with 15

participating centres and an initial budget of $115 million. The largest coordinated study of women's health ever undertaken, the WHI was designed to determine the major causes of death, disability, and frailty in post-menopausal women. The project combines clinical trials and observational methods. It was launched in 1992, at which time a coordinating centre was awarded funding for 15 years. Additional funding has permitted the study to be extended. Research bulletins and updates are posted on the WHI website on an ongoing basis, with links to studies in peer-reviewed journals. Although the most widely publicized aspect of the WHI was the clinical trial finding that hormone therapy (HRT) raises the risk of breast cancer and promotes rather than inhibits heart disease, the study is much broader than HRT effects and includes findings on low-fat diets for women, and the effects of calcium and vitamin D supplements.

Chapter 4

American Medical Student Association, AMSA Pharmfree Scorecard 2008
amsascorecard.org

The AMSA PharmFree Scorecard 2008 evaluates conflict-of-interest policies at the 151 medical colleges and colleges of osteopathic medicine in the United States. Using letter grades to assess schools' performance in 11 potential areas of conflict, the Scorecard offers a comprehensive look at the landscape of conflict-of-interest policies across American medical education, as well as more in-depth assessment of individual policies that govern industry interaction with medical school faculty and trainees.

Center for Media and Democracy
www.prwatch.org/cmd/

The Center for Media and Democracy (CMD) is a non-profit public interest organization that monitors and investigates the public relations industry with the intention of exposing spin and propaganda. Based in Madison, Wisconsin, the organization was founded in 1993 by an environmentalist writer and political activist, John Stauber. The CMD publishes a weekly newsletter on the public relations industry, *PR Watch*, which often includes articles on the pharmaceutical industry and on industry-funded groups. An index of topics includes "Pharmaceuticals," "Women," and "Public Relations" ("Astroturf" and "front groups" are subtopics of the latter).

Centre for Science in the Public Interest (Canada)
www.cspinet.org/canada

The Canadian branch of Centre for Science in the Public Interest seeks to educate the public, advocate government policies that are consistent with scientific evidence on health and environmental issues, and counter industry's powerful influence on public opinion and public policies.

HealthNewsReviews.Org
www.healthnewsreview.org/independentexperts.php
This website lists medical experts from a wide variety of disciplines who do not have financial ties to drug or medical device manufacturers.

Integrity in Science: A CPSI project
www.cspinet.org/integrity/disclosure.html
The Integrity in Science project promotes full disclosure of conflicts of interest when scientists publish in journals, are quoted in the press, or appear before legislative or regulatory bodies at all levels of government. The project and its allies in the scientific community believe total disclosure of conflicts of interest is mandatory if the public is to maintain its faith in the integrity of the scientific process, and the government is to remain a fair and impartial arbiter of scientific disputes that determine the laws and regulations that affect the health and safety of the American people.

Office of Consumer and Public Involvement (OCAPI)
www.hc-sc.gc.ca/ahc-asc/branch-dirgen/hpfb-dgpsa/ocpi-bpcp
Health Canada established the Office of Consumer and Public Involvement to provide opportunities for members of the public to become involved in decision-making processes at the Health Products and Food Branch, which regulates pharmaceutical products. In 2008, the office was given an expanded mandate. OCAPI's Voluntary Statement of Information for Public Involvement, a form that invites groups or individuals participating in government consultations to declare any funding they may have received from industry sources, is among the reports and publications available on the site.

The Society for Diabetic Rights
www.diabeticrights.ca
The Society for Diabetic Rights was founded in 2003 to represent the interests of people who need or want natural animal insulin products. It has raised awareness that some pork and beef insulins are available in Canada. Largely due to the society's efforts, Canada became the first industrialized nation to recognize that a significant minority of insulin-dependent diabetics require animal insulin to maintain their health and quality of life.

Chapter 5
Alliance for Human Research Protection (AHRP)
www.ahrp.org
This is a national network of lay people and professionals dedicated to advancing responsible and ethical medical research practices, minimizing the risks associated

with such endeavours, and ensuring that the human rights, dignity, and welfare of human subjects are protected.

Clinicaltrials.gov
clinicaltrials.gov
Clinicaltrials.gov is a registry of federally and privately supported clinical trials conducted in the U.S. and around the world. A service provided by the U.S. National Institutes of Health, this website has general information about clinical trials, as well as a search function to find information about specific trials.

Health Action International
www.haiweb.org
This is the website for Health Action International, an activist non-governmental organization that aims to engage civil society in advocacy about medicines policy around the world.

Health Canada's Gender-Based Analysis Policy
www.hc-sc.gc.ca/hl-vs/women-femmes/gender-sexe/policy-politique-eng.php
This website includes a link to a booklet that introduces the concept of gender-based analysis (GBA), looks at the issue of gender equality in health, and explains why Canada is adopting GBA. A key example outlined in the booklet is Canada's policy regarding the inclusion of women in clinical trials.

The James Lind Alliance
www.lindalliance.org
The James Lind Alliance website includes information on uncertainties and gaps in knowledge about the effects of treatments in health care. Established to encourage patient-clinician partnerships, this website has general information, as well as access to the *Database of Uncertainties about the Effects of Treatments (DUETs)*.

World Health Organization (WHO) International Clinical Trials Registry Platform (ICTRP)
www.who.int/ictrp
This very useful site lists all clinical trials registries meeting WHO criteria for listing and also has a newsletter that updates listings, links to recent announcements, events, and publications of interest that relate to clinical trials.

Chapter 6
Health Action International
www.haiweb.org

This is the website for Health Action International, an activist non-governmental organization that aims to engage civil society in advocacy about medicines policy around the world.

Health Canada
www.hc-sc.gc.ca/dhp-mps/index_e.html
Health Canada's Drugs and Health Products web page provides links to documents and particular subjects, such as adverse drug reaction reporting. However, this site can be difficult to navigate and the search function sometimes pulls up many individual documents, but not the main link to a subject area.

Public Citizen, Health Research Group
www.citizen.org/hrg/
This is the website for the Health Research Group of Public Citizen, a non-profit organization that is the leading watchdog of the U.S. Food and Drug Administration. The web page has links to alerts, publications, and a range of information about marketed drugs.

Therapeutics Initiative
www.ti.ubc.ca
This is the main web page for the Therapeutics Initiative at the University of British Columbia. The TI is useful for health care practitioners and citizens alike as it provides unbiased practical information on rational drug therapy.

U.S. Food and Drug Administration
www.fda.gov
The main web page provides links to information about clinical trials, drug approvals, and the Center for Drug Evaluation and Research.

Chapter 7

Committee on Women, Population, and the Environment (CWPE)
www.cwpe.org/initiatives/depodiaries
CWPE is a "multi-racial alliance of feminist community organizers, scholarly activists, and health practitioners committed to promoting the social and economic empowerment of women in a context of global peace and justice; and to eliminating poverty." Much of the group's work focuses on safe birth control for women. One feature of CWPE's website is "Depo Diaries," a unique pilot project designed to document the adverse effects of Depo-Provera from the perspective of the women who have used the synthetic hormone.

Drug Safety Canada
drugsafetycanada.com
A not-for-profit research foundation and advocacy group begun by Terence Young, father of Vanessa Young, a teenager who died as the result of an improperly prescribed medication.

Kilen
www.kilen.org/indexe.htm
One of the world's first consumer ADR reporting groups, Kilen, the Consumer Association for Medicines and Health, is based in Stockholm. It has been an effective voice advocating greater consumer involvement in efforts to "achieve safe and rational use of medicines." Kilen has established a well-earned reputation as a reliable source of knowledge about consumer experiences with medicine, and with the quality of consumer reports.

Medeffect
www.hc-sc.gc.ca/dhp-mps/medeff/index-eng.php
Health Canada conducted extensive consultations across the country prior to launching its new website, Medeffect, in 2005. The result is an improvement over previous attempts at communicating risk to Canadians. The website provides the public with access to information about drug and health products, safety advisories and warnings, a database of reported adverse drug reactions, and the *Canadian Adverse Reaction Newsletter (CARN)*.

Public Citizen/Health Research Group (HRG)
www.citizen.org/hrg/drugs/index.cfm
U.S.-based Public Citizen was founded by Ralph Nader in 1971 to work for increased consumer protection. The HRG was formed at the same time under the leadership of Dr. Sidney Wolfe, today an adjunct professor of internal medicine at Case Western Reserve University School of Medicine. The group is one of the most effective and informed voices on drug safety in the United States and internationally. In 1994, the HRG began publishing *Worst Pills, Best Pills*, initially a newsletter described as an "older adult's guide to avoiding drug-induced death or illness." Today, *Worst Pills, Best Pills* is a comprehensive guide to prescription medicines approved for use in the United States. It is available by subscription at www.worstpills.org.

SSRI Stories
www.ssristories.com
Subtitled "Anti-depressant Nightmares," this website provides media accounts of incidents, mostly criminal in nature, where the use of SSRI antidepressants is

implicated. The site's primary aims are to assist those attempting to safely wean themselves off antidepressants and to support people who have lost family members to SSRIs through suicide. They focus on exposing the harms of this class of drugs and their overuse in contemporary society. The site notes that they are *not* affiliated with The Church of Scientology or the Citizens Commission on Human Rights.

World Health Organization (WHO)
www.who-umc.org/DynPage.aspx
The WHO has been a leader in the collection and cataloguing of adverse drug reaction reports, working since the early 1960s to establish greater uniformity of standards among nations. Today, the WHO Collaborating Centre for International Drug Monitoring contains more than 2.5 million reports of suspected ADRs from nearly 60 participating countries. While each country has its own national system, the WHO has developed a common reporting form and guidelines for entering information, common technologies, and standardized classifications. It has also created compatible systems for storing and retrieving data, and for disseminating the data to member countries.

Chapter 8

Canadian Environmental Law Association
www.cela.ca
CELA has been very engaged for a number of years in federal issues related to regulation. While its primary focus is on regulation pertaining to environmental issues, CELA have produced a broad range of reports and submissions relating to regulation in general.

Canadian Health Coalition
www.medicare.ca
The CHC has had a long-standing interest in drug regulation at Health Canada and has produced several documents in response to federal government initiatives.

Government of Canada regulation website
www.regulation.gc.ca
This site provides an explanation of the role of regulation at the federal government level. Also found here is the outcome of the consultation process on "smart regulations." (See "Cabinet Directive on Streamlining Regulation" on the site.)

Health Canada's Health Products and Food Branch
www.hc-sc.gc.ca/ahc-asc/branch-dirgen/hpfb-dgpsa/index-eng.php

This site provides an understanding of the workings of Health Canada in the area of drug regulation, this is the site to go to. Current policies, reports, and guidelines related to the drug-approval and monitoring processes can be found here. Unfortunatey, historical documents are frequently removed from the site within a couple of years.

Chapter 9
Environmental Defence
www.environmentaldefence.ca
"Environmental Defence protects the environment and human health. We research solutions. We educate. We go to court when we have to. All in order to ensure clean air, clean water and thriving ecosystems nationwide, and to bring a halt to Canada's contribution to climate change."

Environmental Impact Initiative
www.hc-sc.gc.ca/ewh-semt/contaminants/person/impact/index-eng.php
This is the official Health Canada site for the government's initiative to protect the environment from pharmaceuticals and personal care products. At the time this book went to press, the site was still rudimentary and contained only historical material from the predecessor project, the Environmental Assessment Regulations Project.

Rachel's Democracy & Health News
www.rachel.org
Named for the ecologist and writer Rachel Carson, *Rachel's Democracy & Health News* was a weekly online publication of the Environmental Research Foundation. The foundation's mission is to promote social justice and prevent harm to the environment and human health. Since 1986, Rachel's has published thoughtful essays and news stories about the links between health and the environment based on the latest scientific research. By arming community groups with information, Rachel's aspires to build a movement for a just and sustainable society. Although they ceased publication in February 2009, an archive dating back to 1986 is maintained on the site.

The U.S. Geological Survey
www.usgs.gov/aboutusgs/
The U.S. Geological Survey was created in 1879 to provide America with reliable information about the earth, including types of contamination. In 1999, an extensive, ongoing program to test for PPCPs throughout the United States was begun. Under the topic file "Contaminants," see the subtopic "pharmaceutical contamination" where you will find photographs, maps, descriptions of geological methodologies used, and scientific findings related to PPCPs (www.usgs.gov/science/science.php?term=1693).

Chapter 10

Breast Cancer Action Montreal (BCAM)
www.bcam.qc.ca

BCAM is a non-profit activist/advocacy group directed by women who have been sensitized to the trauma of breast cancer (affecting themselves or someone close to them) and who have a long-term commitment to eradicating the disease. Their website provides a range of information on long-term breast cancer prevention strategies and is a good example of community-based, grassroots activism.

Canadian Women's Health Network (CWHN)
www.cwhn.ca

This bilingual website is the home page of the CWHN, created in 1993 as a voluntary national organization to improve the health and lives of girls and women in Canada and the world by collecting, producing, distributing, and sharing knowledge, ideas, education, information, resources, strategies, and inspirations. It houses an abundance of content relevant to issues presented in this book.

Centres of Excellence for Women's Health
www.cewh-cesf.ca

This website provides an overview of the Centres of Excellence Program funded by Health Canada, as well as links to each of the individual centres.

Fédération du Québec pour le planning des naissances
www.fqpn.qc.ca

This is a Quebec-based advocacy and information organization made up of individuals and interest groups concerned with women's reproductive and sexual health. Operating since 1972, the group's main areas of focus are: contraception, abortion, new reproductive technologies, family planning, sexual education, and the medicalization of women's reproductive health.

National Women's Health Network
www.womenshealthnetwork.org

The National Women's Health Network exists to improve the health of all women by developing and promoting a critical analysis of health issues in order to affect policy and support consumer decision making. The network aspires to a health care system that is guided by social justice and reflects the needs of diverse women. This website includes health alerts, as well as information on a broad range of information pertaining to women's health.

Our Bodies, Ourselves (OBOS)
www.ourbodiesourselves.org

OBOS, also known as the Boston Women's Health Book Collective, is a non-profit, public interest women's health education, advocacy, and consulting organization. Beginning in 1970 with the publication of the first edition of *Our Bodies, Ourselves*, OBOS has been an ongoing source of inspiration for the U.S. and global women's health movement. Their website provides a wealth of information on women's health issues and organizing.

Réseau Québécois d'action pour la santé des femmes (RQASF)
rqasf.qc.ca

This Quebec-based organization, established in 1997 with a focus on the improvement of the physical and mental health of women as well as their living conditions, works in concert with other networks, unions, professional and community-based organizations. Their aim is to improve the health of women through political action, research, and education. Recent dossiers have included: prescription drugs, body image, breast cancer, lesbian health, menopause, and reform of the health care system.

References

Chapter 1

Armstrong P., Lippman, A. & Sky, L. (1997). *Social change, women's health, and policy development*. A synthesis paper prepared under contract for the 5th National Health Promotion Research Conference, Halifax, July 4, 1997.

Bartlett, C., Doyal, L., Ebrahim, S., Davey, P., Bachmann, M. et al. (2005). The causes and effects of socio-demographic exclusions from clinical trials. *Health Technology Assessment, 9*(38). Retrieved November 2, 2008, from: www.hta.ac.uk/fullmono/mon938.pdf

Basen, G., Eichler, M. & Lippman, A. (Eds). (1993). *Misconceptions: The social construction of choice and the new reproductive technologies* (vols. 1–2). Hull: Voyageur Publishing.

Bunkle, P. (1993). Calling the shots? The international politics of Depo-Provera. In S. Harding (Ed.), *The racial economy of science: Toward a democratic future* (pp. 287–302). Bloomington: Indiana University Press.

Canadian Women's Health Network. (2004, November 19). *Significant bone loss associated with Depo-Provera use is sadly no surprise; We call for action to make sure this doesn't happen again*. Media release. Retrieved November 2, 2008, from: www.cwhn.ca/pr/11-19-04.html

Cassels, A. & Moynihan, R. (2005). *Selling sickness: How the world's biggest pharmaceutical companies are turning us all into patients*. New York: Nation Books.

Canadian Research Institute for the Advancement of Women. (2006). *Intersectional feminist frameworks: An emerging vision*. Ottawa: Author.

DisAbled Women's Network Ontario (DAWN). (n.d.). *Women with disAbilities and reproductive Rights*. Retrieved November 2, 2008, from: dawn.thot.net/wwd_reproductive_rights.html

Food and Drug Administration (FDA). (2004, November 17). *Black box warning added concerning long-term use of Depo-Provera contraceptive injection.*

Washington: Author. Retrieved November 2, 2008, from: www.fda.gov/bbs/
topics/ANSWERS/2004/ANS01325.html

Hankivsky, O., Varcoe, C. & Morrow, M. (2007). *Women's health in Canada: Critical perspectives on theory and policy.* Toronto: University of Toronto Press.

Hawaleshka, D. (2005, November 24). A shot in the dark? *Maclean's.* Retrieved August 18, 2007, from: www.macleans.ca/science/health/article.jsp?content=20051128_116635_116635

Health Canada. (2005, July 7). *Health Canada endorsed important safety information on Depo-Provera (medroxyprogesterone acetate).* Retrieved November 2, 2008, from: www.hc-sc.gc.ca/dhp-mps/medeff/advisories-avis/prof/_2005/depo-provera_2_hpc-cps-eng.php

Kalbfuss, E. (1987, July 29). IUD's victims wait for compensation. *The Gazette* (Montreal). Retrieved from Lexis Nexis database.

Leslie, B., Metge, C., Weiler, H., Young, K., Yuen, K. et al. (2002). *First Nations Bone Health Study (FNBHS).* Winnipeg: University of Manitoba Centre for Aboriginal Health Research. Retrieved August 18, 2007, from: www.umanitoba.ca/centres/cahr/cahr-research/present_research/research-firstnationbone.html

Library and Archives Canada. (2008). *Celebrating women's achievements: Elizabeth Bagshaw.* Retrieved August 19, 2008, from: www.collectionscanada.ca/women/

Littlecrow-Russell, S. (2000). *Time to take a critical look at Depo-Provera* (DifferenTakes series, no. 5, Summer). Amherst: Population and Development Program, Hampshire College. Retrieved November 2, 2008, from: popdev.hampshire.edu/projects/dt/5

Puil, L. (2006). *Depot medroxyprogesterone acetate (DMPA or depo-provera) and bone health in pre-menopausal women and adolescents.* Internal document commissioned by Women and Health Protection.

Regush, N. (1992, January–February). Toxic breasts: A *Mother Jones* investigation. *Mother Jones, 17*(1), 25–31.

Roberts, D. (1998). *Killing the black body: Race, reproduction, and the meaning of liberty.* New York: Pantheon Books.

Sarojini, N.B. & Murthy, L. (2005). Why women's groups oppose injectable contraceptives. *Indian Journal of Medical Ethics, 13*(1). Retrieved August 18, 2007, from: www.ijme.in/131di008.html

Shea, L. (2007). *Reflections on Depo Provera: Contributions to improving drug regulation in Canada.* Toronto: Women and Health Protection.

Smith, A. (2003, Spring). Not an Indian tradition: The sexual colonization of Native Peoples. *Hypatia, 18*(2), 70–85.

Tait, C.L. (2000). *A study of the service needs of pregnant addicted women in Manitoba.* Winnipeg: Prairie Women's Health Centre of Excellence. Retrieved August 18, 2007, from: www.gov.mb.ca/health/documents/PWHCE_June2000.pdf

Toronto Women's Health Network. (2002, January). The IUD. *TWHN newsletter, XXI*(5). Retrieved August 19, 2008, from: www.web.net/%7Etwhn/ IUD%20%28jan02%29.htm

U.S. court frees $2.5 billion fund for women injured by Dalkon Shield (1989, November 7). *Toronto Star.* Retrieved from Lexis Nexis database.

Williams, W. (1999, Fall). Gender-based analysis: Will it make things better for women? *Network, 2*(4). Retrieved January 26, 2009, from www.cwhn.ca/network-reseau/2-4/genderlens.html.

Woloshin, S. & Schwartz, L.M. (2006, April 11). Giving legs to restless legs: A case study of how the media helps make people sick. *PLoS Medicine, 3*(4), e170. Retrieved October 28, 2008, from: medicine.plosjournals.org/perlserv/ ?request=get-document&doi=10.1371/journal.pmed.0030170&ct=1&SESSID =d4e8415a7f5389566b9e29701ab99e46

Women's Health Action. (2005). *Fact sheet on Depo Provera.* Pamphlet. Auckland: Author.

Women's Health Interaction & Inter Pares. (1995). *Uncommon knowledge: A critical guide to contraception and reproductive technologies.* Ottawa: Author. Retrieved August 18, 2007, from: www.interpares.ca/en/publications/pdf/uncommon_knowledge.pdf

Zarfasm D.E., Fyfe, I. & Gorodzinsky, F. (1981, October). *The utilization of DMPA in the Ontario government facilities for the mentally retarded: A pilot project.* Toronto: Ontario Department of Community Services.

Chapter 2

Aikin, K.J., Swasy, J.L. & Braman, A.C. (2004). *Patient and physician attitudes and behaviors associated with DTC promotion of prescription drugs—summary of FDA survey research results.* Retrieved August 22, 2008, from U.S. Dept of Health and Human Services, Food and Drug Administration. Center for Drug Evaluation and Research: www.fda.gov/cder/ddmac/researchka.htm

Aldhous, P. (2008, March 31). U.S. wasted billions on ineffective cholesterol drugs. *New Scientist, 11,* 38. Retrieved August 22, 2008, from: www.newscientist. com/channel/health/dn13557-us-wasted-billions-on-ineffective-cholesterol-drugshtml

Bell, R.A., Kravitz, R.L. & Wilkes, M.S. (2000). Direct-to-consumer prescription drug advertising 1989–1998. A content analysis of conditions, targets, inducements, and appeals. *Journal of Family Practice, 49*(4), 329–335.

Bell, R.A., Wilkes, M.S. & Kravitz, R.L. (2000). The educational value of consumer-targeted prescription drug print advertising. *Journal of Family Practice, 49*(12), 1092–1098.

Brownfield, E.D., Bernhardt, J.M., Phan, J.L., Williams, M.V. & Parker, R.M. (2004). Direct-to-consumer drug advertisements on network television: An exploration of quantity, frequency, and placement. *Journal of Health Communication, 9*, 491–497.

Chitale, K.A. (2004, December 29). Consumer promotion analyst, Division of Drug Marketing, Advertising and Communication, U.S. Food and Drug Administration. *Untitled letter to J. Carrado, Barr Research, re: Seasonale.* Retrieved August 22, 2008, from: www.fda.gov/cder/warn/2004/12748.pdf

Code of Federal Regulations. (1997). Title 21, Food and Drugs, Chapter 1, Food and Drug Administration, Department of Health and Human Services, Part 201, Labeling 21. (CFR201.57). U.S. Government Printing Office via GPO Access, pp. 19–28. Retrieved November 11, 2008, from: www.fda.gov/cder/pediatric/21cfr20157.htm

Common Drug Review (CDR). (2004). *Recommendation on reconsideration and reasons for recommendation. Norelgestromin/ethinyl estradiol transdermal patch (Evra—Janssen-Ortho Inc.).* Ottawa: Retrieved August 22, 2208, from: cadth.ca/index.php/en/cdr/search

Correa-de-Araujo, R. (2005). Improving the use and safety of medications in women through sex/gender and race/ethnicity analysis: Introduction. *Journal of Women's Health, 14*(1), 12–15.

Curry, P. & O'Brien, M. (2006.) The male heart and the female mind: A study in the gendering of antidepressants and cardiovascular drugs in advertisements in Irish medical publication. *Social Science & Medicine, 62*(8), 1970–1977.

Donohue, J.M., Cevasco, M. & Rosenthal, M.B. (2007). A decade of direct-to-consumer advertising of prescription drugs. *New England Journal of Medicine, 357*(7), 673–681.

European Agency for the Evaluation of Medicinal Products (EMEA), Committee for Proprietary Medicinal Products (CPMP). (2003). *Summary information on referral opinion following arbitration pursuant to Article 30 of council Directive 2001/83/EC for Prozac and associated names.* London: Author. Retrieved August 22, 2008, from: www.emea.europa.eu/pdfs/human/referral/326303en.pdf

Evans, B.W., Clark, W.K., Moore, D.J. & Whorwell, P.J. (2007). Tegaserod for the treatment of irritable bowel syndrome and chronic constipation. *Cochrane Database of Systemic Reviews, 4*, Article CD003960.

Forgacs, I. & Loganayagam, A. (2008). Overprescribing proton pump inhibitors. *BMJ, 336*, 2–3.

Frosch, D.L., Krueger, P.M. & Hornik, R.C. (2007). Creating demand for prescription drugs: A content analysis of television direct-to-consumer advertising. *Annals of Family Medicine 5*, 6–13.

Gardner, D.M., Mintzes, B. & Ostry, A. (2003). Direct-to-consumer prescription drug advertising in Canada: Permission by default? *CMAJ, 169*(5), 425–427.

Graham, D.J., Campen, D., Hui, R., Spence, M., Cheetham, C., Levy, G. et al. (2005). Risk of acute myocardial infarction and sudden cardiac death in patients treated with cyclo-oxygenase 2 selective and non-selective non-steroidal anti-inflammatory drugs: Nested case-control study. *Lancet, 365*(9458), 475–481.

Grow, J.M., Park, J.S. & Han, X. (2006). "Your life is waiting!": Symbolic meanings in direct-to-consumer antidepressant advertising. *Journal of Communication Inquiry, 3*(2), 163–186.

Handlin, A. (2007). Gendered opportunities to enhance direct-to-consumer advertising of gender-neutral pharmaceutical brands: Factors arising from information processing, message content, and demographic change. *The Business Review, Cambridge, 7*(1), 33–39.

Hansen, F.J. & Osborne, D. (1995). Portrayal of women and elderly patients in psychotropic drug advertisements. *Women & Therapy, 16*(1), 129–141.

Hausken, A.M., Skurtveit, S., Rosvold, E.O., Bramness, J.G. & Furu, K. (2007). Psychotropic drug use among persons with mental distress symptoms: A population-based study in Norway. *Scandinavian Journal of Public Health, 35*(4), 356–364.

Health Canada. (2004, August 9). Advisory: Health Canada advises of potential adverse effects of SSRIs and other anti-depressants on newborns. Retrieved August 22, 2008, from: www.hc-sc.gc.ca/ahc-asc/media/advisories-avis/_2004/2004_44-eng.php

Health Canada. (2006, November 21). Health Canada endorsed important safety information on Evra (norelgestromin and ethinyl estradiol) transdermal system. Retrieved November 11, 2008, from: www.hc-sc.gc.ca/dhp-mps/medeff/advisories-avis/prof/_2006/evra_hpc-cps-eng.php

Health Canada, Health Products and Food Branch, Bilateral Meeting Program. (2007). *Record of decisions: NAPRA (National Association of Pharmacy Regulatory Authorities).* Retrieved November 11, 2008, from: www.hc-sc.gc.ca/dhp-mps/prodpharma/activit/assoc/2007-12-20-eng.php

IMS Health. (2002). *Therapeutic trends. Rise in anti-arthritic market: 35% increase since introduction of Cox-2 inhibitors.* Retrieved August 22, 2008, from: www.stacommunications.com/journals/cpm/cpmpdf/therapeutictrends.pdf

Kastelein, J.J.P., Akdim, F., Stroes, E.S.G., Zwinderman, A.H., Bots, M.L., Stalenhoef, A.F. et al. (2008). Simvastatin with or without ezetimibe in familial hypercholesterolemia. *New England Journal of Medicine, 358*(14), 1431–1443.

King, E. (1980). Sex bias in psychoactive drug advertisements. *Psychiatry, 43*(2), 129–137.

Kirsch, I., Deacon, B.J., Huedo-Medina, T.B., Scoboria, A., Moore, T.J. & Johnson, B.T. (2008). Initial severity and antidepressant benefits: A meta-analysis of data submitted to the Food and Drug Administration. *PLoS Medicine, 5*(2), e45.

Kravitz, R.L., Epstein, R.M., Feldman, M.D., Franz, C.E., Azari, R., Wilkes, M.S. et al. (2005). Influence of patients' requests for direct-to-consumer advertised antidepressants: A randomized controlled trial. *JAMA, 293*, 1995–2002.

Lacasse, J.R. & Leo, J. (2005). Serotonin and depression: A disconnect between the advertisements and the scientific literature. *PLoS Medicine, 2*(12), e392. Retrieved August 22, 2008, from: doi=10.1371/journal.pmed.0020392

Lexchin, J. (1995). Debating benzodiazepine use. *Canadian Family Physician, 41*, 1293–1295.

Lexchin, J. (2006). Bigger and better: How Pfizer redefined erectile dysfunction. *PLoS Medicine 3*(4), e132.

Main, K. (2008). Pharmacare: Should direct-to-consumer advertising be limited? No. The transforming health care landscape: The case for direct-to-consumer advertising. In J. Greenberg & C.D. Elliott (Eds.), *Communication in question: Competing perspectives on controversial communication studies* (pp. 240–248). Toronto: Nelson, Thomson Canada Ltd.

"Menopause? I said yes to HRT." (2002). Advertisement for Prempro. Retrieved November 11, 2008, from: store.vintagepaperads.com/servlet/-strse-9528/2002-Prempro-Ad-w-fdsh-/Detail

Mintzes, B. (2006). Disease mongering in drug promotion: Do governments have a regulatory role? *PLoS Medicine 3*(4), e198.

Mintzes, B. (2007). A pill for every ill—or an ill for every pill? *Visions: BC's Mental Health and Addictions Journal, 4*(2), 21–22. Retrieved August 22, 2008, from: www.heretohelp.bc.ca/publications/visions/medications/alt/2

Moynihan, R. (2003). The making of a disease: Female sexual dysfunction. *BMJ, 326*, 45–47.

Parry, V. (2007, October 15). Branding disease. *Pharmaceutical executive.* Retrieved August 22, 2008, from: pharmexec.findpharma.com/pharmexec/article/articleDetail.jsp?id=465561&sk=&date=&pageID=2

Patten, S.B. (2004). The impact of antidepressant treatment on population health: Synthesis of data from two national data sources in Canada. *Population Health Metrics, 2*(1), 9.

Payer, L. (1992). *Disease-mongers: How doctors, drug companies, and insurers are making you feel sick.* New York: John Wiley & Sons.

Peppin, P. (2003). Manufacturing uncertainty: Adverse effects of drug development for women. *International Journal of Law and Psychiatry, 26*(5), 515–532.

Peppin, P. & Carty, E. (2001). Semiotics, stereotypes, and women's health: Signifying inequality in drug advertising. *Canadian Journal of Women & the Law, 13*(2), 326–360.

Pfizer. (2004, August). Zoloft ad. *Shape* magazine, 23(12), 13.

Pfizer. (n.d.). *Recognizing depression and anxiety symptoms in others.* Retrieved August 22, 2008, from: www.zoloft.com

Piccinelli, M. & Wilkinson, G. (2000). Gender differences in depression: Critical review. *British Journal of Psychiatry, 177,* 486–492.

Rosenberg, H. & Allard, D. (2007, June). *Evidence for caution: Women and statin use.* Toronto: Women and Health Protection.

Schreiber, R. (2001). Wandering in the dark: Women's experiences with depression. *Health Care for Women International, 22*(1–2), 85–98.

Springuel, P. (2008, January). Transdermal norelgestromin-ethinyl estradiol (Evra): Myocardial infarction and thrombotic adverse reactions. *Canadian Adverse Reaction Newsletter, 18*(1), 3. Retrieved November 11, 2008, from: www.hc-sc.gc. ca/dhp-mps/medeff/bulletin/carn-bcei_v18n1-eng.php#4

Stockbridge, L. (1998, May 20). Regulatory review officer, Division of Drug Marketing, Advertising, and Communication, U.S. FDA. *Untitled letter to J.S. Sonk, Wyeth-Ayerst Laboratories, Re: Premarin (conjugated estrogen) tablets.* Retrieved August 22, 2008, from: www.fda.gov/cder/warn/may98/6663.pdf

Stockbridge, L. (2000, November 16). Regulatory reviewer, Division of Drug Marketing, Advertising, and Communication, U.S. FDA. *Untitled letter to G.T. Brophy, Eli Lilly & Co, Re: Sarafem (fluoxetine HCl) tablets.* Retrieved August 22, 2008, from: www.fda.gov/cder/warn/nov2000/dd9523.pdf

Therapeutics Initiative. (2005). Drugs for overactive bladder symptoms. *Letter no. 57.* Retrieved August 22, 2008, from: www.ti.ubc.ca/PDF/57.pdf

Toop, L., Richards, D., Dowell, T., Tilyard, M., Fraser, T. & Arroll, B. (2003, February). *Direct-to-consumer advertising of prescription drugs in New Zealand: For health or for profit?* Report to the minister of health supporting the case for a ban of DTCA. Dunedin: University of Otago.

United Nations. (1995). *The United Nations Fourth World Conference on Women: Platform for action.* Section C: Women and health, Article 106 (h). Retrieved November 11, 2008, from: www.un.org/womenwatch/daw/beijing/platform/ health.htm#object1

U.S. Food and Drug Administration. (2005, December 8). *FDA public health advisory: Paroxetine.* Retrieved August 22, 2008, from: 69.20.19.211/cder/drug/ advisory/paroxetine200512.htm

Wilhelm, K., Parker, G., Geerligs, L. & Wedgwood, L. (2008). Women and depression: A 30-year learning curve. *Australian and New Zealand Journal of Psychiatry, 42*(1), 3–12.

Willman, D. (2000, December 20). How a new policy led to seven deadly drugs. *Los Angeles Times.* Retrieved August 22, 2008, from: www.drugawareness.org/ Archives/Miscellaneous/122002Howanew.html

Woloshin, S., Schwartz, L.M., Tremmel, J. & Welch, H.G. (2001). Direct-to-consumer advertisements for prescription drugs: What are Americans being sold? *Lancet, 358,* 1141–1146.

Writing Group for the Women's Health Initiative Investigators. (2002). Risks and benefits of estrogen plus progestin in healthy postmenopausal women: Principal results from the Women's Health Initiative randomized controlled trial. *JAMA, 288*(3), 321–333.

Chapter 3

Alliance for Human Research Protection. (2000). *Re: High-risk experiment with children who have no medical diagnosis.* Letter from Vera Hassner Sharav, president, AHRP (formerly CIRCARE), to Gary Ellis, director, and Michael A. Carome, M.D., Office of Protection from Research Risks. Retrieved October 29, 2008, from: www.ahrp.org/Initiatives/YaleComplaint.php

Barlow, M. & May, E. (2000). *Frederick Street: Life and death on Canada's Love Canal.* Toronto: HarperCollins.

Bean, G.R., Kimler, B.F. & Seewaldt, V.L. (2006). Correspondence: Long-term raloxifene in a woman at high risk for breast cancer. *New England Journal of Medicine, 355*, 1620–1622.

Bureau of Women's Health and Gender Analysis (BWHGA). (2005). *Determinants of health and identity: Perspectives on genetic and social markers.* Report of a Health Canada Symposium on Emerging Policy Issues Organized by the Bureau of Women's Health and Gender Analysis and the Health Sciences Policy Division, Health Canada, Ottawa, March 22, 2005. Ottawa: Health Canada.

Canadian Cancer Research Alliance. (2007). *Cancer research investment in Canada 2005: The Canadian Cancer Research Alliance's survey of government and voluntary sector investment in Cancer Research 2005.* Toronto: Author. Retrieved July 21, 2008, from: www.ccra-acrc.ca/PDF%20Files/CCRA_E_978-0-9784157-0-9.pdf

Centers for Disease Control. (1999, April 2). Ten great public health achievements, United States, 1900–1999. *Morbidity and Mortality Weekly Report (MMWR), 48*(12), 241.

Colborn, T., Dumanoski, D. & Myers, J.P. (1996). *Our stolen future.* New York: Dutton.

Commission on the Future of Health Care in Canada. (2002). *Building on values: The future of health care in Canada. Final report of the Commission on the Future of Health Care in Canada* (Romanow report). Ottawa: Government of Canada.

Courchene, T.J. (2003, October). Medicare as a moral enterprise: The Romanow and Kirby perspectives. *Policy Matters/Enjeux publics, 4*(1). Montreal: Institute for Research on Public Policy.

Cummings, S.R., Eckert, S., Krueger, K.A., Grady, D., Powles, T.J., Cauley, J.A. et al. (1999). The effect of raloxifene on risk of breast cancer in postmenopausal women: Results from the MORE randomized trial. *JAMA, 281*(23), 2189–2197.

Daubs, K. (2008, May 28). Asbestos report "misused": Scientists. *Ottawa Citizen*. Retrieved October 29, 2008, from: www.canada.com/ottawacitizen/news/story. html?id=4c342ebe-2633-4ea4-bc06-34797b8ed932

Davis, D.L. (2007). *The secret history of the war on cancer.* New York: Basic Books.

Environment Canada. (2001). *A Canadian perspective on the precautionary approach/ principle.* Retrieved July 25, 2008, from: www.ec.gc.ca/econom/pamphlet_ e.htm

Epp, J. (1986). *Achieving health for all: A framework for health promotion.* Ottawa: Health Canada. Retrieved August 21, 2008, from: www.hc-sc.gc.ca/hcs-sss/pubs/ system-regime/1986-frame-plan-promotion/index-eng.php

Ford, L. (1995). Point/counterpoint: PRO Breast Cancer Prevention on trial. *Journal of Women's Health 4*(1), 11–12.

Fugh-Berman, A. (1991, September–October). Tamoxifen in healthy women: Preventive health or preventing health? *The Network News*, 3–4.

Fulton, E.D., Durnil, G.K., Welch, R.S.K., Cleveland, H.P., Lanthier, C. & Goodwin, R.F. (1992). *Sixth biennial report under the Great Lakes Water Quality Agreement of 1978.* Retrieved October 29, 2008, from: www.ijc.org/php/publications/html/ 6bre.html#commissioners

Health Canada. (1998). *Health protection for the 21st century: Renewing the federal health protection legislation.* Ottawa: Author.

Health Canada. (1999, March). *Health Canada's Women's Health Strategy.* Ottawa: Author.

Joint Working Group of the Atomic Energy Control Board. (1998). *Assessment and management of cancer risks from radiological and chemical hazards.* Ottawa: Health Canada. Retrieved August 21, 2008, from: www.hc-sc.gc.ca/ewh-semt/pubs/ radiation/98ehd-dhm216/index-eng.php

Kerlikowske, K., Miglioretti, D.L., Buist, D.S.M., Walker, R. & Carney, P.A. (2007). Declines in invasive breast cancer and use of postmenopausal hormone therapy in a screening mammography population. *Journal of the National Cancer Institute*, *99*, 1335–1339.

Krieger, N., Lowy, I., Aronowitz, R., Bigby, J., Dickersin, K., Garner, E. et al. (2005). Hormone replacement therapy, cancer, controversies, and women's health: Historical, epidemiological, biological, clinical, and advocacy perspectives. *Journal of Epidemiology and Community Health, 59*(9), 740–748.

Lalonde, M. (1974, April). *A new perspective on the health of Canadians: A working document.* Ottawa: Government of Canada. Retrieved August 21, 2008, from: www.hc-sc.gc.ca/hcs-sss/com/fed/lalonde-eng.php

Lippman, A. (1999). Choice as a risk to women's health. *Health, Risk, and Society*, *1*(3), 281.

McKinlay, J.B. & McKinlay, S.M. (1977). The questionable contribution of medical measures to the decline of mortality in the United States in the twentieth century. *Milbank Memorial Fund Quarterly, Health, and Society, 55,* 405–428.

Minister's Advisory Council on Women's Health. (1998). *Report of the Minister's Advisory Council on Women's Health 1996–1998.* Victoria: Ministry of Health and Ministry Responsible for Seniors. Retrieved July 25, 2008, from: www.health. gov.bc.ca/whb/publications/biennial.html

Mintzes, B. (2003, Spring). Direct-to-consumer advertising of prescription drugs— whatever the problem, you can always pop a pill. *Centres of Excellence for Women's Health Research Bulletin, 3*(2), 11–13. Retrieved November 17, 2008, from: www. cewh-cesf.ca/PDF/RB/bulletin-vol3no2EN.pdf

Moynihan, R. & Cassels, A. (2005). *Selling sickness: How the world's biggest pharmaceutical companies are turning us all into patients.* Vancouver: Greystone.

Parson, E.A. (2003). *Protecting the ozone layer: Science and strategy.* New York: Oxford University Press.

Payer, L. (1992). *Disease-mongers: How doctors, drug companies, and insurers are making you feel sick.* Hoboken: John Wiley & Sons.

Proctor, R.N. (1995). *Cancer wars: How politics shapes what we know and don't know about cancer.* New York: Basic Books.

Robillard, L. (2001). *Integrated risk management.* Ottawa: Treasury Board of Canada Secretariat. Retrieved July 25, 2008, from: www.tbs-sct.gc.ca/pubs_pol/dcgpubs/ riskmanagement/rmf-cgr01-1_e.asp#Risk%20Management.

Saunders, P.T. (2000, July 13). Use and abuse of the precautionary principle. *Institute of Science in Society (ISIS) submission to the U.S. Advisory Committee on International Economic Policy (ACIEP) Biotech. Working Group.* Retrieved November 17, 2008, from: www.i-sis.org.uk/prec.php

Science and Environmental Health Network. (1998). *Wingspread Conference on the Precautionary Principle.* Retrieved August 18, 2008, from: www.sehn.org/wing. html.

Semenak, S. (1998, April 6). Breast cancer treatment hailed. *The Gazette* (Montreal), p. A1.

Sherwin, S. (1998). A relational approach to autonomy in health care. In S. Sherwin (Ed.), *The politics of women's health: Exploring agency and autonomy* (pp. 19–47). Philadelphia: Temple University Press.

Shuchman, M. (2000, April 19). Detecting schizophrenia. *Globe and Mail,* p. R7.

Sibbald, B. (1999, September 7). Breast cancer conference marred by questionable presentations, critics charge. *CMAJ, 161*(5), 584.

Standing Committee on Health. (2004, April). *Opening the medicine cabinet: First report on health aspects of prescription drugs.* Ottawa: Parliament of Canada. Retrieved November 17, 2008, from: www2.parl.gc.ca/content/hoc/Committee/373/ HEAL/Reports/RP1282198/healrp01/healrp01-e.pdf

Stein, R. (2006, April 18). A boost for breast cancer prevention. *Washington Post*, p. A1.

Ternes, T.A., Stumpf, M., Mueller, J., Haberer, K., Wilken, R.-D. & Servos, M. (1999). Behavior and occurrence of estrogens in municipal sewage treatment plants—I. Investigations in Germany, Canada, and Brazil. *The Science of the Total Environment, 225*(1–2), 81–90.

Timmermans, S. & Kolker, E. (2004). Evidence-based medicine and the reconfiguration of medical knowledge. *Journal of Health and Social Behavior, 45*(Suppl.), 177–193.

United Nations. (1995). Women and health. In *United Nations Fourth World Conference on Women, Platform for Action*. New York: Author. Retrieved November 17, 2008, from: www.un.org/womenwatch/daw/beijing/platform/health.htm#object1

VanderZwaag, D. (1994). *Reviewing CEPA. The issues #18. CEPA and the precautionary principle/approach*. Ottawa: Environment Canada.

VanderZwaag, D. (1999). The precautionary principle in environmental law and policy: Elusive rhetoric and first embraces. *Journal of Environmental Law and Practice*, 8, 355–375.

Wade, M. (1998). *Human health and exposure to chemicals which disrupt estrogen, androgen, and thryroid hormone physiology*. Ottawa: Environmental and Occupational Toxicology Division, Environmental Health Directorate, Health Protection Branch, Health Canada.

Wald, N.J. & Law, M.R. (2003, 28 June). A strategy to reduce cardiovascular disease by more than 80%. *BMJ, 326*(7404), 1419–1424.

Wang, J., Ho, L., Chen, L., Zhao, Z., Zhao, W., Qian, X. et al. (2007). Valsartan lowers brain β-amyloid protein levels and improves spatial learning in a mouse model of Alzheimer disease. *The Journal of Clinical Investigation, 117*(11), 3393–3402.

Weijer, C. (1995). Our bodies, our science. *The Sciences, 35*(3), 41–45.

Writing Group for the Women's Health Initiative Investigators. (2002). Risk and benefits of estrogen plus progestin in healthy post-menopausal women. Principal results from the women's health initiative randomized controlled trial. *JAMA, 228*(3), 321–333.

Chapter 4

Abraham, C. (2004, September 18). Health talks offer no remedy for disparities in drug policies. *Globe and Mail*, p. A4.

Abraham, J. (2004). Pharmaceuticals, the state, and the global harmonization process. *Australian Health Review, 28*(2), 150–160.

Abraham, J. & Davis, C. (2002). *Mapping the social and political dynamics of drug safety withdrawals in the U.K. and the U.S.: Final report to ESRC*. Sussex: University of Sussex.

Angelmar, R., Angelmar, S. & Kane, L. (2007). Building strong condition brands. *Journal of Medical Marketing, 7*(4), 341–351.

Ball, D.E., Tisoki, K. & Herxheimer, A. (2006). Advertising and disclosure of funding on patient organization websites: A cross-sectional survey. *BMC Public Health, 6,* 201.

Bekelman, J.E., Mphil, Y.L. & Gross, C.P. (2003). Scope and impact of financial conflicts of interest in biomedical research: A systematic review. *JAMA, 289,* 454–465.

Bero, L.A., Glantz, S. & Hong, M.-K. (2005). The limits of competing interest disclosures. *Tobacco Control, 14,* 118–126.

Best Medicines Coalition. (2007). *Statement on funding sources.* Retrieved August 25, 2008, from: www.bestmedicines.org/system/files/BMC_Funding_State_07.pdf

Boyle, T. (1999, April 16). New arthritis drug called "miracle." *Toronto Star,* p. A2.

Bucchi, M. & Neresini, F. (2008). Science and public participation. In E.J. Hackett, O. Amsterdamska, M. Lynch & J. Wajcman (Eds.), *The handbook of science and technology studies* (pp. 449–472). Cambridge: MIT Press.

Canadian Diabetes Association, Clinical Practice Guideline Expert Committee. (2003). Canadian Diabetes Association 2003 clinical practice guidelines for the prevention and management of diabetes in Canada. *Canadian Journal of Diabetes, 27*(Suppl. 2), S1–152.

Canadian Medical Association. (2007). *CMA policy: Guidelines for physicians in interactions with industry.* Ottawa: Author. Retrieved August 25, 2008, from: policybase.cma.ca/dbtw-wpd/Policypdf/PD08-01.pdf

Carpenter, D., Zucker, E.J. & Avorn, J. (2008). Drug-review deadlines and safety problems. *New England Journal of Medicine, 358*(13), 1354–1361.

Cassels, A. (2003, November 28). *Ideas: Manufacturing patients.* Radio broadcast. Toronto: CBC Radio.

Chapman, H. & Rule, E. (1999, April 7). *Strategic alliance between disease-specific non-profit organizations and private sector pharmaceutical companies.* Report presented to the Canadian Institute. Toronto: PricewaterhouseCoopers.

Cohn & Wolfe. (2003). *Partnership report.* Toronto: Cohn & Wolfe. Available from Cohn & Wolfe, 2 Bloor Street E., Suite 1700, Toronto, ON M4W 1A8.

Consumers Health Forum (CHF) of Australia and Medicines Australia. (2005) *Working together, the manual: A guide to relationships between health consumer organisations and pharmaceutical companies.* Canberra: Consumer's Health Forum of Australia and Medicines Australia.

Cossman, B. & Fudge, J. (2002). Conclusion: Privatization, polarization, and policy: Feminism and the future. In B. Cossman & J. Fudge (Eds.), *Privatization, law, and the challenge to feminism* (pp. 403–420). Toronto: University of Toronto Press.

Dana, J. & Loewenstein, G. (2003). A social science perspective on gifts to physicians from industry. *JAMA, 290*(2), 252–255.

Delaney, M. (2005). AIDS activism and the pharmaceutical industry. In M.A. Sontoro & T.M. Gorry (Eds.), *Ethics and the pharmaceutical industry* (pp. 300–325). New York: Cambridge University Press.

Elliott, C. (2001, September 24). Pharma buys a conscience. *The American Prospect, 12*(17), 16–20. Retrieved August 25, 2008, from: www.mindfully.org/GE/GE3/Pharma-Buys-Conscience.htm

Elliott, C. (2004). Six problems with pharma-funded bioethics. *Studies in History and Philosophy of Biological and Biomedical Sciences, 23*, 125–129.

Elliott, R. (2003). *Controlling drug costs for people living with HIV/AIDS: Federal regulation of pharmaceutical prices in Canada.* Montreal: Canadian HIV/AIDS Legal Network. Retrieved August 25, 2008, from: www.aidslaw.ca/publications/publicationsdocEN.php?ref=333

Epstein, S. (1996). *Impure science: AIDS activism and the politics of knowledge.* Berkeley: University of California Press.

Epstein, S. (2008). Patient groups and health movements. In E.J. Hackett, O. Amsterdamska, M. Lynch & J. Wajcman (Eds.), *The handbook of science and technology studies* (pp. 499–539). Cambridge: MIT Press.

Ford, A. (1998). *A different prescription: Considerations for women's health groups contemplating funding from the pharmaceutical industry.* Toronto: Institute for Feminist Legal Studies at Osgoode Hall, York University. Retrieved August 25, 2008, from: www.whp-apsf.ca/en/documents/diff_prescrip.html

Goozner, M. (2004, July). *Unrevealed: Non-disclosure of conflicts of interest in four leading medical and scientific journals.* Washington: Centre for Science in the Public Interest. Retrieved August 25, 2008, from: www.cspinet.org/new/pdf/unrevealed_final.pdf

Harvie, B.A. (2002). *Let charities speak: Report of the charities and advocacy dialogue.* Vancouver: Institute for Media, Policy, and Civil Society.

Health Canada. (2000). *The policy toolkit for public involvement in decision making.* Ottawa: Author. Retrieved August 25, 2008, from: www.hc-sc.gc.ca/ahc-asc/pubs/_public-consult/2000decision/index-eng.php

Health Canada. (2005). HPFB policy on voluntary statement of information for public involvement. Ottawa: Author. Retrieved August 25, 2008, from: www.hc-sc.gc.ca/ahc-asc/pubs/cons-pub/vsi_pvi_intro_e.html.

Health Products and Food Branch. (2007). *Cost recovery framework: Official notice of fee proposal for human drugs and medical devices.* Ottawa: Health Canada.

Herxheimer, A. (2003). Relationships between the pharmaceutical industry and patients' organisations. *BMJ, 326*(7400), 1208–1210.

Hilts, P.J. (2003). *Protecting America's health: The FDA, business, and one hundred years of regulation.* New York: Knopf.

Inter Pares. (2004, November). *Rethinking development: Promoting global justice into the 21st Century.* Occasional Paper no. 6. Ottawa: Author. Retrieved November 9, 2008, from: www.interpares.ca/en/publications/pdf/rethinking_development. pdf

Jensen, J. & Phillips, S. (1996). Regime shift: New citizenship practices in Canada. *International Journal of Canadian Studies, 14,* 113–135.

Johnson, E. (2000, November 14). *CBC marketplace: Promoting drugs through patient advocacy groups.* Radio broadcast. Toronto: CBC Radio.

Katz, D., Merz, J. & Caplan, A. (2003). All gifts large and small: Toward an understanding of pharmaceutical industry gift-giving. *The American Journal of Bioethics, 3*(3), 39–46.

Kelly, P. (2002). *Begging your pardon: Exploring the impacts of pharmaceutical industry funding of non-profit organizations.* Unpublished master's thesis, Royal Roads University, Victoria.

Kent, A. (2007, May 5). Should patient groups accept funding from the pharmaceutical industry? Yes. *BMJ, 334*(7600), 934.

Krimsky, S. (2003). Small gifts, conflicts of interest, and the zero-tolerance threshold in medicine. *The American Journal of Bioethics, 3*(3), 50–52.

Laforest, R. (2004). Governance and the voluntary sector: Rethinking the contours of advocacy. *International Journal of Canadian Studies, 31,* 185–203.

Landzelius, K. (2006). Introduction: Patient organization movements and new metamorphoses in patienthood. *Social Science and Medicine, 62*(3), 529–537.

Lazaruk, S. (2005, February 17). Long-lasting new insulin now available in Canada. *The Province* (Vancouver).

Lofgren, H. (2004). Pharmaceuticals and the consumer movement: The ambivalences of "patient power." *Australian Health Review, 28*(2), 228–237.

Lurie, P. & Wolfe, S.M. (1998). *FDA medical officers report lower standards permit dangerous drug approvals.* Washington: Public Citizen. Retrieved August 25, 2008, from: www.citizen.org/publications/release.cfm?ID=7104

Mauss, M. ([1923–1924] 1967). *The gift: Forms and functions of exchange in archaic societies* (Ian Cunnison, Trans.). New York: Norton.

Mintzes, B. (1998). *Blurring the boundaries: New trends in drug promotion.* Amsterdam: HAI-Europe. Retrieved August 25, 2008, from: www.haiweb.org/pubs/blurring/ blurring.intro.html

Mintzes, B. (2007, May 5). Should patient groups accept funding from drug companies? No. *BMJ, 334*(7600), 935.

Mundy, A. (2003, January–February). Hot flash, cold cash. *The Washington Monthly.* Retrieved August 25, 2008, from: www.washingtonmonthly.com/ features/2001/0301.mundy.html

Nebenzahl, D. (2003, April 9). Do drug firms call the tune? *The Gazette* (Montreal), pp. D1, D4.

O'Donovan, O. (2007). Corporate colonization of health activism? Irish health advocacy organizations' modes of engagement with pharmaceutical corporations. *International Journal of Health Services, 37*(4), 711–733.

Office of Consumer and Public Involvement (OCAPI) & Best Medicines Coalition. (2003). *Consultation workshop report on patient involvement strategy.* Ottawa: Health Canada. Retrieved August 25, 2008, from: www.hc-sc.gc.ca/ahc-asc/alt_formats/hpfb-dgpsa/pdf/pubs/best_med_coa-meilleurs-eng.pdf

Office of Inspector General. (2003, March). *FDA's review process for new drug applications: A management review.* Washington: Department of Health and Human Services. Retrieved August 25, 2008, from: oig.hhs.gov/oei/reports/oei-01-01-00590.pdf

Oldani, M.J. (2004). Thick prescriptions: Toward an interpretation of pharmaceutical sales practices. *Medical Anthropology Quarterly, 18*, 328–356.

Olson, M.K. (2002, October). Pharmaceutical policy change and the safety of new drugs. *Journal of Law and Economics, 45*(2, pt. 2), 615–642.

Orlowski, J. & Wateska, L. (1992). The effects of pharmaceutical firm enticements on physician prescribing patterns. *Chest,* 102, 270–273.

Patient View. (2004, April). Health campaigners, fundraising, and industry involvement. *HSCNews: News for Health and Social Campaigners, 6,* 10.

Picard, A. (2001, January 4). Charities "thank God" for drug firms' money. *Globe and Mail,* p. A8.

Prescrire International. (2007). A look back at pharmaceuticals in 2006: Aggressive advertising cannot hide the absence of therapeutic advances. *Prescrire International, 16*(88), 80–86.

Pross, P. (1992). *Group politics and public policy* (2nd ed.). Toronto: Oxford University Press.

Ruzek, S.B. & Becker, J. (1999). The women's health movement in the United States: From grass roots activism to professional agendas. *Journal of the American Medical Women's Association, 54*(1), 4–9.

Schafer, A. (2004). Biomedical conflicts of interest: A defence of the sequestration thesis—learning from the cases of Nancy Olivieri and David Healy. *Journal of Medical Ethics, 30,* 8–24.

Seaman, B. ([1969] 1995). *The doctors' case against the pill.* Alameda: Hunter House.

Smith, R. (1998, August 1). Beyond conflict of interest: Transparency is the key. *BMJ, 317*(7154), 291–292.

Somerville, M. (2000, Fall). Do we have a legal right to the best cancer treatments? *Cancer Care in Canada, 6.* Toronto: Cancer Advocacy Coalition of Canada.

Special authority coverage of insulin glargine (Lantus). (2007, August 2). *BC Pharmacare Newsletter, 07*-005, 4.

Steinman, M.A., Shlipak, M.G. & McPhee, S.J. (2001). Of principles and pens: Attitudes of medicine house staff towards pharmaceutical industry promotions. *American Journal of Medicine, 110*(7), 551–557.

Taylor, P. (2008, April 26). Health care, under the influence. *Globe and Mail*, pp. A10–A11.

Weeks, C. (2007, January 22). Critics raise red flags as drug giant backs anti-smoking guide. *Ottawa Citizen*, p. A1.

Weiss, R. (2004, August 4). NIH to set stiff restrictions on outside consulting. *Washington Post*, p. A1. Retrieved August 25, 2008, from: www.washingtonpost. com/wp-dyn/articles/A37841-2004Aug3.html

Wibulpolprasert, S., Moosa, S., Satyanarayana, K., Samarage, S. & Tangcharoensathien, V. (2007, November 24). WHO's web-based public hearings: Hijacked by pharma? *Lancet, 370*(9601), 1754.

Wong-Reiger, D. (2003, August 18). A case for regulated direct-to-consumer promotion of prescription drugs. Toronto: Advocare (Consumer Advocare Network). Retrieved November 28, 2004, from: www.consumeradvocare.org/ index.php/ca/content/view/full/57/

Chapter 5

American College of Obstetricians and Gynecologists (ACOG). (2007). Research involving women. ACOG Committee Opinion no. 377. *Obstetrics & Gynecology, 110*(3), 731–736.

American Medical Association, Council on Scientific Affairs. (2004). *Influence of funding source on outcome, validity, and reliability of pharmaceutical research.* Report 10-A-04. Retrieved August 28, 2008, from: www.ama-assn.org/ama/pub/ category/14314.html

Association of Clinical Research Associations (ACRO). (n.d.). *CRO industry at a glance.* Retrieved November 9, 2008, from: www.acrohealth.org/industry- ataglance.php

Aulakh, A.K. & Anand, S.S. (2007). Sex and gender subgroup analyses of randomized trials: The need to proceed with caution. *Women's Health Issues, 17*(6), 342–350.

Avorn, J. & Shrank, W. (2008, April 26). Adverse drug reactions in elderly people: A substantial cause of preventable illness. *BMJ, 336*, 956–957.

Baird, K.L. (1999). The New NIH and FDA medical research policies: Targeting gender, promoting justice. *Journal of Health Politics, Policy, and Law, 24*(3), 531– 565.

Ballantyne, A.J. & Rogers, W.A., on behalf of the Australian Gender Equity in Health Research Group. (2008, June 2). Fair inclusion of men and women in Australian clinical research: Views from ethics committee chairs. *Medical Journal of Australia, 188*(11), 653–656.

Canadian Institutes of Health Research (CIHR). (2007). *Chair: GlaxoSmithKline partnered (2005–2006)*. Retrieved August 31, 2008, from: www.cihr-irsc.gc.ca/e/16173.html

Canadian Institutes of Health Research (CIHR), National Sciences and Engineering Research Council of Canada (NSERC) & Social Sciences and Humanities Research Council of Canada (SSHRC). (2005). *Tri-Council policy statement: Ethical conduct for research involving humans (TCPS)*. Ottawa: Public Works and Government Services Canada. Retrieved November 9, 2008, from: www.pre. ethics.gc.ca/english/pdf/TCPSintroductione.pdf

Caron, J. (2003). *Report on governmental health research policies promoting gender or sex differences sensitivity*. Prepared for the Institute of Gender and Health. Retrieved August 28, 2008, from: www.cihr-irsc.gc.ca/e/pdf_25502.htm

Council of Canadians. (n.d.). *The SPP and public safety: How regulatory harmonization threatens our health and the environment*. Retrieved August 28, 2008, from: www.canadians.org/integratethis/backgrounders/guide/safety.pdf

Day, M. (2006). U.K. drug companies must disclose funding of patients' groups. *BMJ, 332*, 69.

DeAngelis, C.D., Drazen, J.M., Frizelle, F.A., Haug, C., Hoey, J. et al. (2004). Clinical trial registration: A statement from the International Committee of Medical Journal Editors. *JAMA, 292*, 1363–1364.

Downie, J. (2006). Grasping the nettle: Confronting competing issues and obligations in health research policy. In C. Flood (Ed.), *Just medicare: What's in, what's out, how we decide* (pp. 427–448). Toronto: University of Toronto Press.

Downie, J., Munden, L.M. & Butler, L. (2003). Women and clinical trials: A review of unacceptable research practices. *Clinical Researcher, 3*(10), 16–20.

EDICT. (2008). *Major deficiencies in the design and funding of clinical trials: A report to the nation improving on how human studies are conducted*. Houston: Baylor College of Medicine, Chronic Disease Prevention and Control Research Center. Retrieved August 28, 2008, from: www.bcm.edu/edict/PDF/EDICT_Project_White_Paper.pdf

Edison, R.J. & Muenke, M. (2004). Mechanistic and epidemiological considerations in the evaluation of adverse birth outcomes following gestational exposure to statins. *American Journal of Medical Genetics, 131*(3), 287–298.

Einarson, A., Pistelli, A., DeSantis, M., Malm, H., Paulus, W.D., Panchaud, A. et al. (2008). Evaluation of the risk of congenital cardiovascular defects associated with use of paroxetine during pregnancy. *American Journal of Psychiatry, 165*, 749–752.

Epstein, S. (2004). Bodily differences and collective identities: The politics of gender and race in biomedical research in the United States. *Body & Society, 10*(2–3), 183–203.

European Medicines Agency. (2005, January). *Gender considerations in the conduct of clinical trials* (EMEA/CHMP/3916/2005). London: European Medicines Agency.

Fox, D. (2008, March–April). The regulation of biotechnologies: Four recommendations. *Hastings Center Report, 38*(2), 1 page following 56.

Getz, K. & Zisson, S. (2003). Clinical grants market decelerates. *Centerwatch, 10*(4), 4–5.

Ghersi, D. & Pang, T. (2008). En route to international clinical trial transparency. *Lancet 372*(9649), 1531–1532.

Hankivsky, O. (2007). Gender-based analysis and health policy: The need to rethink outdated strategies. In M. Morrow, O. Hankivsky & C. Varcoe (Eds.), *Women's health in Canada: Critical perspectives on theory and policy* (pp. 143–168). Toronto: University of Toronto Press.

Health Action International (HAI) Europe. (2005, July 14). *Does the European Patients' Forum represent patient or industry interests? A case study in the need for mandatory financial disclosure.* Amsterdam: HAI Europe. Retrieved November 9, 2008, from: www.epha.org/IMG/pdf/EPF_paper_final.pdf

Health Canada. (1997). *Therapeutic Products Programme guidelines: Inclusion of women in clinical trials.* Ottawa: Therapeutics Directorate. Retrieved August 28, 2008, from: www.hc-sc.gc.ca/dhp-mps/prodpharma/applic-demande/guide-ld/clini/womct_femec-eng.php

Health Canada. (2008, July 14). *Government of Canada announces post-market Drug Safety and Effectiveness Network.* News release. Retrieved November 9, 2008, from: www.hc-sc.gc.ca/ahc-asc/media/nr-cp/_2008/2008_110-eng.php

Healy, D. (2005). *Manufacturing consensus.* Unpublished paper for a talk, Toronto, April 28.

James Lind Alliance & the Association of Medical Research Charities (AMRC). (2007, September 17). *James Lind Alliance/AMRC Conference (Should patients tell researchers what to do? If so, how?) Afternoon discussion groups.* London: Authors. Retrieved November 9, 2008, from: www.lindalliance.org/pdfs/Summary%20of%20JLA_AMRC%20PM%20discussions.pdf

Kannel, W.B. (1976). The role of cholesterol in coronary atherogenisis. *Medical Clinics of North America, 58*, 363–379.

Krimsky, S. (2003). *Science in the private interest: Has the lure of profits corrupted biomedical research?* Boston: Rowman & Littlefield.

Lewis, S.J., Sacks, F.M., Mitchell, J.S., East, C., Glasser, S., Kell, S. et al. (1998). Effect of pravastatin on cardiovascular events in women after myocardial infarction: The cholesterol and recurrent events (CARE) trial. *Journal of the American College of Cardiology, 32*(1), 140–146.

Lewis, T.R., Reichman, J.H. & So, A.D. (2007, January). The case for public funding and public oversight of clinical trials. *Economists' Voice, 4*(1), article 3. Retrieved August 28, 2008, from: www.bepress.com/ev/vol4/iss1/art3

Lexchin, J.R. (2005). Implications of pharmaceutical industry funding on clinical research. *The Annals of Pharmacotherapy, 39*(1), 194–197.

Lippman, A. (2005). Letter to the editor: Adherence to medications. *New England Journal of Medicine, 353*, 1972–1974.

Mastroianni, A.C., Faden, R. & Federman, D. (Eds.), for the Committee on Ethical and Legal Issues Relating to the Inclusion of Women in Clinical Studies, Institute of Medicine. (1994). *Women and health research: Ethical and legal issues of including women in clinical studies* (vol. 1). Washington: National Academies Press.

Mastroianni, A.C., Faden, R. & Federman, D. (Eds.), for the Committee on Ethical and Legal Issues Relating to the Inclusion of Women in Clinical Studies, Institute of Medicine. (1999). *Women and health research: Ethical and legal issues of including women in clinical studies: Workshop and commissioned papers* (vol. 2). Washington: National Academies Press.

McMurdo, M.E.T., Witham, M.D. & Gillespie, N.D. (2005). Including older people in clinical research: Benefits shown in trials in younger people may not apply to older people. *BMJ, 331*, 1036–1037.

Merkatz, R.B. (1998). Inclusion of women in clinical trials: A historical overview of scientific, ethical, and legal issues. *Journal of Obstetric, Gynecologic, and Neonatal Nursing, 27*(1), 78–84.

Mintzes, B. (2004). *Drug regulatory failure in Canada: The case of Diane-35*. Toronto: Women and Health Protection. Retrieved August 28, 2008, from: www.whp-apsf.ca/en/documents/diane35.html

National Institutes of Health. (2001). *NIH Policy and guidelines on the inclusion of women and minorities as subjects in clinical research amended.* Retrieved August 28, 2008, from: grants.nih.gov/grants/funding/women_min/guidelines_amended_10_2001.htm

Oakley, A. (1990). Who's afraid of the randomized clinical trial? In H. Roberts (Ed.), *Women's health counts* (pp. 167–194). London: Routledge.

Oberlander, T.F., Warburton, W., Misri, S., Aghajanian, J. & Hertzman, C. (2006). Neonatal outcomes after prenatal exposure to selective serotonin reuptake inhibitor antidepressants and maternal depression using population-based linked health data. *Archives of General Psychiatry, 63*, 898–906.

Perell, P., Miranda, J.J., Ortiz, Z. & Casas, J.P. (2008, February). Relation between the global burden of disease and randomized clinical trials conducted in Latin America published in the five leading medical journals. *PloS One, 3*(2), e1696. Retrieved January 26, 2009, from www.pubmedcentral.nih.gov/articlereader. fcgi?artid=2246037.

Petryna, A. (2007). Clinical trials offshored: On private sector science and public health. *BioSocieties, 2*, 21–40.

Pharmaceutical Research and Manufacturers of America (PhRMA). (2007, March). *Pharmaceutical industry profile 2007.* Washington: Author. Retrieved August 28, 2008, from: www.phrma.org/files/Profile%202007.pdf

Prout, M.N. & Fish, S.S. (2001). Participation of women in clinical trials of drug therapies: A context for the controversies. *Medscape Women's Health, 6*(5), 1.

Rochon, P.A., Clark, J.P., Binns, M.., Patel, V. & Gurwitz, J.H. (1998). Reporting of gender-related information in clinical trials of drug therapy for myocardial infarction. *CMAJ, 159*(4), 321–327.

Rootman, I. & Gordon-El-bihbety, D. (2008). *A vision for a health literate Canada: Report of the Expert Panel on Health Literacy.* Ottawa: Canadian Public Health Association. Retrieved August 28, 2008, from: www.cpha.ca/uploads/portals/h-l/report_e.pdf

Schipper, I. & Weyzig, F. (2008). *Ethics for drug testing in low and middle income countries: Considerations for European market authorisation.* Amsterdam: SOMO (Centre for Research on Multinational Corporations).

Shepherd, J., Blauw, G.J., Murphy, M.B., Bollen, E.L., Buckley, B.M. et al. (2002). Pravastatin in elderly individuals at risk of vascular disease (PROSPER): A randomized controlled trial. *The Lancet, 360*(23), 1623–1630.

Shuchman, M. (2008). Clinical trials regulation—how Canada compares. *CMAJ, 179*(9), 635–638.

Simon, V.R., Hai, T., Williams, S.K., Adams, E., Ricchetti, K. & Marts, S.A. (2005). *National Institutes of Health: Intramural and extramural support for research in sex differences 2000–2003.* Scientific report series: Understanding the biology of sex differences. Washington: Society for Women's Health Research. Retrieved August 28, 2008, from: www.womenshealthresearch.org/press/CRISPreport.pdf

Statistics Canada. (2006). *Women in Canada: A gender-based statistical report* (5th ed.). Ottawa: Author.

Stead, M., Eadie, D., Gordon, D. & Angus, K. (2005). "Hello, hello—it's English I speak!": A qualitative exploration of patients' understanding of the science of clinical trials. *Journal of Medical Ethics, 31*, 664–669.

Stevens, P.E. & Pletsch, P.K. (2002). Informed consent and the history of inclusion of women in clinical research. *Health Care for Women International, 23*(8), 809–819.

Therapeutics Initiative. (2003). Do statins have a role in primary prevention? *Therapeutics Letter, 48*. Retrieved August 28, 2008, from: www.ti.ubc.ca/PDF/48.pdf

Walsh, J.M.E. & Pignone, M. (2004). Drug treatment of hyperlipidemia in women. *JAMA, 291*(18), 2243–2252.

Wenger, N.K., Lewis, S.J., Welty, F.K., Herrington, D.M. & Bittner, V. on behalf of the TNT Steering Committee and Investigators. (2008). Beneficial effects of aggressive low-density lipoprotein cholesterol lowering in women with stable coronary heart disease in the Treating to New Targets (TNT) study. *Heart, 94,* 434–439.

Wizemann, T.M. & Pardue, M.-L. (Eds.). (2001). *Exploring the biological contributions to human health: Does sex matter?* Washington: National Academies Press.

World Medical Association. (2008, October). *Declaration of Helsinki: Ethical principles for medical research involving human subjects.* Retrieved November 9, 2008, from: www.wma.net/e/policy/b3.htm

Yerman, T., Gan, W.Q. & Sin, D.D. (2007). The influence of gender on the effects of Aspirin in preventing myocardial infarction. *BMC Medicine 5*(29). Retrieved January 26, 2008, from www.pubmedcentral.nih.gov/picrender.fcgi?artid=2131 749&blobtype=pdf.

Zarin, D.A., Tse, T. & Ide, N.C. (2005). Trial registration at ClinicalTrials.gov between May and October 2005. *New England Journal of Medicine, 353*(26), 2779–2787.

Chapter 6

Baird, P. (2003, May 13). Getting it right: Industry sponsorship and medical research. *CMAJ, 168*(10), 1267–1269.

Berenson, A. (2005, April 24). Evidence in Vioxx suits shows intervention by Merck officials. *New York Times,* p. 1.

Berenson, A. (2007, November 9). Merck agrees to pay $4.85 billion in Vioxx claims. *New York Times.*

Bill C-51: An Act to Amend the Food and Drugs Act and to make consequential other amendments to other Acts. Retrieved November 15, 2008, from: www.parl.gc.ca/common/bills_ls.asp?lang=E&ls=c51&source=library_prb&Parl=39&Ses=2

Bongers, A. (2004, September 22). Drugs gone bad. *Hamilton Spectator,* p. GO5.

Canadian Association of Journalists. (2004, May 9). Code of silence award press release. Retrieved February 8, 2004, from micro.newswire.ca/release.cgi?rkey=12 05090757&view=42015-0&Start=0

Canadian Broadcasting Corporation. (2005). *Sharp increase in children hurt by prescription drugs.* Radio broadcast, February 17, 2004. Retrieved February 6, 2006, from www.cbc.ca/news/adr

Canadian Institute for Health Information. (2008). *Drug expenditure in Canada, 1985 to 2007.* Ottawa: Author. Retrieved November 13, 2008, from: secure.cihi.ca/cihiweb/products/Drug_Expenditure_in_Canada_1985_2007_e.pdf

Center for Science in the Public Interest. (2004, September 23). *Cholesterol recommendations questioned.* Retrieved August 31, 2008, from: www.cspinet.org/integrity/press/200409231.html

Chaudhuri, A.K., Division of Endocrinology, Metabolism and Allergy, Health Canada. (1993, November 29). *Review of new drug submission. Diane-35 (Berlex Canada Inc.).* Memo to Dr. Claire Franklin, director, Bureau of Human Prescription Drugs. 9427-B0074/1-38.

Chaudhuri, A.K. & Leroux A.-M., Division of Endocrinology, Metabolism, and Allergy, Health Canada. (1996, September 5). *Review of new drug submission.* Memo to M. Carman, director, Bureau of Pharmaceutical Assessment. 9427-B74/1-38.

Compendium of Pharmaceuticals and Specialties (e-CPS), Canada. Drug Monograph. Diane-35 (cyproterone acetate and ethinyl estradiol). Canada. Bayer. Prepared: September 11, 1997; Latest update February 27, 2007. Retrieved November 5, 2008, from: www.e-therapeutics.ca/wps/myportal/!ut/p/_s.7_0_A/7_0_2UM/.cmd/acd/.ar/sa.DisplayContent/.c/6_0_2KM/.ce/7_0_2US/.p/5_0_281/.d/1?PC_7_0_2US_searchTerm=&PC_7_0_2US_value=m162500&PC_7_0_2US_title=Diane-35#m162500n00013

Currie, J. (2005). *The marketization of depression: The prescribing of SSRI antidepressants to women.* Toronto: Women and Health Protection.

Dosanjh, U. (2004, September 29). *Address to the Leaders' Forum for Health Research in Canada, Ottawa.* Retrieved February 6, 2006, from: www.hc-sc.gc.ca/ahc-asc/minist/health-sante/speeches-discours/2004_10_01_e.html

Douglas, S. et al. (2004, January 28). *Open letter to Prime Minister Paul Martin.* Ottawa: Canadian Health Coalition. Retrieved November 15, 2008, from: www.healthcoalition.ca/english-openletter.pdf

Eggerston, L. (2005, February 1). Drug approval system questioned in U.S. and Canada. *CMAJ, 172*(3), 317–318.

Farley, T.M.M., Meirik, O., Chang, C.L., Marmot, M.G. & Poulter, N.R. (1995). Effect of different progestagens in low oestrogen oral contraceptives on venous thromboembolic disease. WHO collaborative study of cardiovascular disease and steroid hormone contraception. *Lancet, 346*(8990), 1582–1588.

Garattini, S. & Bertele, V. (2007, October 20). How can we regulate medicines better? *BMJ, 335,* 803–805.

Garland, E.J. (2004). Facing the evidence: Antidepressant treatment in children and adolescents. *CMAJ, 170*(4), 489–491.

Germany's cyproterone warning. (1995). *Lancet, 345*(8955), 979.

Health Action International. (1996). *Statement of the International Working Group on Transparency and Accountability in Drug Regulation.* Ottawa: Author. Retrieved August 31, 2008, from: www.haiweb.org/pubs/sec-sta.html

Health Canada. (2003, June 18). *Legislative renewal issue paper: Confidential commercial information.* Ottawa: Author. Retrieved July 26, 2004, from: www2.itssti.hc-sc.gc.ca/HPCB/Policy/LegislativeRenewal.nsf/vwBgDocsE/9FF96063E13B9E0A

Health Canada. (2004, June 3). *Advisory: Health Canada advises Canadians of stronger warnings for SSRIs and other newer anti-depressants.* Ottawa: Author. Retrieved August 31, 2008, from: www.hc-sc.gc.ca/ahc-asc/media/advisories-avis/_2004/2004_31-eng.php

Health Canada. (2007a). *Revisions to Notice of Compliance with Conditions (NOC/c) guidance and NOC/c policy.* Retrieved November 5, 2008, from: www.hc-sc.gc.ca/dhp-mps/prodpharma/applic-demande/pol/noccrev_acrev_pol-eng.php

Health Canada. (2007b). *Notice—Registration and disclosure of clinical trial information.* Retrieved November 4, 2008, from: www.hc-sc.gc.ca/dhp-mps/prodpharma/activit/proj/enreg-clini-info/notice_ctreg_avis_ecenr-eng.php

Health Canada. (2008a). *Frequently asked questions: Product monographs posted to the Health Canada website.* Retrieved August 31, 2008, from: www.hc-sc.gc.ca/dhp-mps/prodpharma/activit/proj/monograph-rev/pm_qa_mp_qr-eng.php

Health Canada. (2008b). *Notice of Compliance listings.* Retrieved November 14, 2008, from: www.hc-sc.gc.ca/dhp-mps/prodpharma/notices-avis/list/index-eng.php#WeeklyUpdates

Health Products and Food Branch. (2007, July). *2007–08 Business plan: Our key priorities and activities.* Ottawa: Health Canada. Retrieved August 31, 2008, from: www.hc-sc.gc.ca/ahc-asc/pubs/hpfb-dgpsa/businessplan_2007-2008_plan dactivites-eng.php

Heinemann, L.A.J., DoMinh, T., Guggenmoos-Holzmann, C., Thie, E., Garbe, A.R., Feinstein, D. et al. (1997). Oral contraceptives and liver cancer: Results of the Multicentre International Liver Tumor Study (MILTS). *Contraception, 56*(5), 275–284.

Herxheimer, A. & Mintzes, B. (2004, February 17). Antidepressants and adverse effects in young patients: Uncovering the evidence. *CMAJ, 170*(4), 487–489.

International Society of Drug Bulletins (ISDB). (1998, June). ISBD assessment of nine European Public Assessment Reports published by the European Medicines Evaluation Agency (EMEA). Paris: Author.

Kirsch, I., Deacon, B.J., Huedo-Medina, T.B., Scoboria, A., Moore, T.J. et al. (2008). Initial severity and antidepressant benefits: A meta-analysis of data submitted to the Food and Drug Administration. *PLoS Medicine, 5*(2), 0260–0268.

Knight Ridder Newspapers. (2003, November 2). *Knight Ridder exclusive: Off-label drug prescriptions skyrocket in U.S. Thousands became ill last year after taking nation's most popular drugs off-label.* Media release. Retrieved from Factiva database.

Levy, M. (2000). Advertisement for Relenza: Glaxo Wellcome responds. *CMAJ, 162*(12), 1663.

Lexchin, J. (2007, May). Pharmaceutical secrecy endangers our health. *The Monitor.* Retrieved November 10, 2008, from the Canadian Centre for Policy Alternatives: www.policyalternatives.ca/MonitorIssues/2007/05/MonitorIssue1638/

Lexchin, J. & Mintzes, B. (2004). Transparency in drug regulation: Mirage or oasis? *CMAJ, 171*(11), 1363–1365.

Medical News Today. (2004, June 18). *Cross border drug sales from Canada to the USA.* Reprint of article from Health Canada. Retrieved November 5, 2008, from: www.medicalnewstoday.com/articles/9640.php

Melander, H., Ahlqvist-Rastad, J., Meijer, G. & Beermann, B. (2003, May 31). Evidence b(i)ased medicine: Selective reporting from studies sponsored by pharmaceutical industry: review of studies in new drug applications. *BMJ, 326*(7400), 1171–1173.

Office of the Information Commissioner of Canada. (2002). *Annual report 2001– 2002.* Ottawa: Author. Retrieved September 1, 2008, from: www.infocom.gc.ca/reports/section_display-e.asp?intSectionId=229

Office of the Inspector General, Department of Health and Human Services. (2003, March). *FDA's Review Process for New Drug Applications: A Management Review.* Washington: Author. Retrieved September 1, 2008, from: www.oig.hhs.gov/oei/reports/oei-01-01-00590.pdf.

Pharmaceutical Advertising Advisory Board (PAAB). (2000, April). *PAAB update.* Retrieved November 4, 2007, from: www.paab.ca/local/files/en/newsletter//qtrpt00_1_en.pdf

Pini, M., Scoditti, U., Caliumi, F., Manotti, C., Quintavalla, R., Pattacini, C. et al. (1996). Risk of venous thromboembolism and stroke associated with oral contraceptives. Role of congenital thrombophilias. *Recenti Progressi in Medicina, 87*(7–8), 331–337.

Reid, J.M. (2002, September). Information Commissioner of Canada. *Response to the report of the Access to Information Review Task Force.* Appendix A, Part B—Legislative Tune-up. Ottawa: Office of the Information Commissioner of Canada.

Science Advisory Board to Health Canada. (2000, February). *Report of the Committee on the Drug Review Process.* Ottawa: Health Canada.

Seaman, B. (2003). *The greatest experiment ever performed on women: Exploding the estrogen myth.* New York: Hyperion Books.

Seaman, H.E., de Vries, C.S. & Farmer, R.D.T. (2003). Venous thromboembolism associated with cyproterone acetate in combination with ethinyloestradiol (Dianette): Observational studies using the U.K. General Practice Research Database. *Pharmacoepidemiology and Drug Safety, 13*(7), 427–436.

Standing Committee on Health. (2004, April). *Opening the medicine cabinet: First report on health aspects of prescription drugs.* Report of the Standing Committee on Health. Ottawa: House of Commons.

Sztuke-Fournier, A. (2006). *Affidavit. Ontario Superior Court of Justice. CanWest MediaWorks vs. Attorney General of Canada.* Respondent's record, vol. 1. Court

File no.: 05-CV-303001PD2. Retrieved September 1, 2008, from: www.whp-apsf.ca/en/documents/charter.html

Therapeutic Products Directorate. (2000). *Expert Advisory Committee on HIV Therapies. Minutes of meeting March 17, 2000.* Retrieved November 15, 2008, from: www.hc-sc.gc.ca/dhp-mps/prodpharma/activit/sci-com/hiv-vih/sachivt_rop_ccstavih_crd_2000-03-17-eng.php

Therapeutic Products Directorate. (2002). *Notice of Compliance with Conditions— NOC/c (Therapeutic products).* Retrieved November 15, 2008, from: www.hc-sc.gc.ca/dhp-mps/prodpharma/activit/fs-fi/noccfs_accfd-eng.php

Therapeutics Initiative. (2004, April/May/June). Antidepressant medications in children and adolescents. *Therapeutics Letter, 52.*

Tuana, N. (2006). The speculum of ignorance: The women's health movement and epistemologies of ignorance. *Hypatia, 21*(3), 1–19.

Vasilakis-Scaramozza, C. & Jick, H. (2001). Risk of venous thromboembolism with cyproterone or levonorgestrel contraceptives. *Lancet, 358*(9291), 1427–1429.

Vitry, A., Lexchin, J., Sasich, L., Dupin-Spriet, T., Reed, T., Bertele, V. et al. (2008). Provision of information on regulatory authorities' websites. *Internal Medicine Journal, 38*(7), 559–567.

Walsh, J.M.E. & Pignone, M. (2004, May 12). Drug treatment of hyperlipidemia in women. *JAMA, 291*(18), 2243–2252.

Whittington, C.J., Kendall, T., Fonagy, P., Cottrell, D., Cotgrove, A. et al. (2004). Selective serotonin reuptake inhibitors in childhood depression: Systematic review of published versus unpublished data. *Lancet, 353*(9418), 1341–1345.

Chapter 7

Abraham, C. & Taylor, P. (1998, April 15). Drug reactions kill thousands: Researchers. *Globe and Mail.* Retrieved from Lexis Nexis database.

Adverse drug reaction reporting—1998. (1999). *Canadian Adverse Reaction Newsletter (CARN), 9*(2), 5–6. Retrieved October 26, 2008, from: www.hc-sc.gc.ca/dhp-mps/alt_formats/hpfb-dgpsa/pdf/medeff/carn-bcei_v9n2_e.pdf

Adverse reaction reporting—2006. (2007). *Canadian Adverse Reaction Newsletter (CARN), 17*(2), 3–4. Retrieved September 9, 2008, from: www.hc-sc.gc.ca/dhp-mps/alt_formats/hpfb-dgpsa/pdf/medeff/carn-bcei_v17n2_e.pdf

Appel, W.C. (2002, April 2). Adverse drug reaction reporting controversy. *CMAJ, 166*(7), 884–885.

Auditor General of Canada. (2004, March). *Report of the Auditor General of Canada to the House of Commons.* Ottawa: Author. Retrieved September 9, 2008, from: www.oag-bvg.gc.ca/internet/docs/20040300ce.pdf

Bains, N. & Hunter, D. (1999). Adverse reporting on adverse reactions. *CMAJ, 160*(3), 350–351.

Baker, G.R., Norton, P.G., Flintoft, V., Blais, R., Brown, A., Cox, J. et al. (2004, May 25). The Canadian Adverse Events Study: The incidence of adverse events among hospital patients in Canada. *CMAJ, 170*(11), 1678–1686.

Blenkinsopp, A., Wilkie, P., Wang, M. & Routledge, P.A. (2006). Patient reporting of suspected adverse drug reactions: A review of published literature and international experience. *British Journal of Clinical Pharmacology, 73*(2), 148–156.

Bouvy, M.L., van Berkel, J., De Roos-Huisman, C.M. & Meijboom, R.H.B. (2002). Patients' drug-information needs: A brief view on questions asked by telephone and on the Internet. *Pharmacy World and Science, 24*(2), 43–45.

Canadian Treatment Action Council (CTAC). (2007, October). *Ensuring greater involvement of consumers in post-approval surveillance system: Where we are and recommendations for moving forward.* Summary report of a symposium held March 8–9, 2007, Toronto. Toronto: Author.

Danish Medicines Agency. (2004, October 13). *One year with ADR consumer reports.* Retrieved August 15, 2008, from: www.dkma.dk/1024/visUKLSArtikel.asp?artikelID=4710

Decima Research. (2003, December). *Public opinion survey on key issues pertaining to post-market surveillance of marketed health products in Canada, final report to Health Canada.* Ottawa: Author.

Editorial, Lessons from cisapride. (2001, May 1). *CMAJ, 164*(9), 1269.

Editorial, Postmarketing drug surveillance: What it would take to make it work. (2001, November 13). *CMAJ, 165*(10), 1293.

Editorial, Vioxx: Lessons for Health Canada and the FDA. (2005, January 4). *CMAJ, 172*(1), 5.

Figueiras, A., Tato, F., Fonatinas, F. & Gestal-Otero, J.J. (1999, August). Influence of physicians' attitudes on reporting adverse drug events: A case-control study. *Medical Care, 37*(8), 809–814.

Finer, D., Albinson, J., Westin, L. & Dukes, G. (2000). Consumer reports on medicines—CRM: Policy and Practice. *International Journal of Risk & Safety in Medicine, 13*(2–3), 117–127.

Gabriel, S.E., Woods, J.E., O'Fallon, W.M., Beard, C.M., Kurland, L.T. & Melton III, L.J. (1997). Complications leading to surgery after breast implantation. *New England Journal of Medicine, 336*(10), 677–682.

Gandhi, M., Aweeka, F., Greenblatt, R.M. & Blaschke, T. (2004). Sex differences in pharmacokinetics and pharmacodynamics. *Annual Review of Pharmacology and Toxicology, 44*, 499–523.

Garcia, J., Study Group 2, Global Harmonization Task Force. (2007, October). Post market surveillance status report. Symonston: Therapeutic Goods Administration, Department of Health and Aging, Australian Government.

General Accounting Office (GAO). (2000, January). Report to congressional requesters. Adverse drug events: The magnitude of health risk is uncertain because of limited incidence data. Washington: GAO. Retrieved September 7, 2008, from: ascpcampaign2011.org/advocacy/briefing/upload/adegaoreport.pdf

Gorman, D. (2002, April 2). *HPFB announces a new organisation: Marketed Health Products Directorate (MHPD), Letter to stakeholders.* Ottawa: Health Canada. Retrieved September 1, 2008, from: www.hc-sc.gc.ca/ahc-asc/branch-dirgen/hpfb-dgpsa/mhpd-dpsc/mhpd-adm_ltr-eng.php

Greener, M. (2008). First do no harm. Improving drug safety through legislation and independent research. *EMBO Reports, 9*(3), 221–224.

Halliwell, J.E., Smith, W. & Walmsley, M. (1999a). *Science in government decision-making: The Canadian experience.* Ottawa: Council of Science and Technology Advisors. Retrieved September 1, 2008, from: www.csta-cest.ca/index.php?ID=92&Lang=En

Halliwell, J.E., Smith, W. & Walmsley, M. (1999b). Science in government decision-making: The Canadian experience, Appendix 1, Departmental profiles: Health Canada. Ottawa: Council of Science and Technology Advisors. Retrieved September 1, 2008, from: www.csta-cest.ca/index.php?ID=92&Lang=En

Hazell, L. & Shakir, S.A.W. (2006). Under-reporting of adverse drug reactions: A systematic review. *Drug Safety, 29*(5), 385–396.

HDP Group. (1999, March 19). *Functional review of post-approval drug assessment operational activities for Therapeutic Products Programme, Bureau of Drug Surveillance.* Prepared for the Continuing Assessment Division, Bureau of Drug Surveillance by the HDP Group Inc. Ottawa: Author.

Health Canada. (1999). *Women's health strategy.* Ottawa: Author. Retrieved August 16, 2008, from: www.hc-sc.gc.ca/ahc-asc/pubs/strateg-women-femmes/strateg-eng.php

Health Canada. (2006, October). *Blueprint for renewal: Transforming Canada's approach to regulating health products and food. Annex 2, Strengthening post-market safety and effectiveness, Discussion paper.* Ottawa: Health Products and Food Branch, Health Canada. Retrieved September 1, 2008, from: www.hc-sc.gc.ca/ahc-asc/branch-dirgen/hpfb-dgpsa/blueprint-plan/blueprint-plan-eng.php

Health Canada. (2007). History of cost recovery. Retrieved September 1, 2008, from: www.hc-sc.gc.ca/dhp-mps/finance/costs-couts/passe-present/hist_e.html

Hunter, D. & Bains, N. (1999). Rates of adverse events among hospital admissions and day surgeries in Ontario from 1992 to 1997. *CMAJ, 160*(11), 1585–1586.

Kaitin, K.I. (2002, April–June). Regulatory reform at a crossroads. *Drug Information Journal, 36*(2), 245–246.

Katzin, W. et al., (2005). Pathology of lymph nodes from patients with implants: A histologic and spectroscopic evaluation. *American Journal of Surgical Pathology, 29*(4), 510.

Lazarou, J., Pomeranz, B.H. & Corey, P.N. (1998, April 15). Incidence of adverse drug reactions in hospitalized patients: A meta-analysis of prospective studies. *JAMA, 279*(15), 1200–1205.

Leape, L.L. (2002, November 14). Reporting of adverse events. *New England Journal of Medicine, 347*(20), 1633–1638.

Lexchin, J. (1991, January). Adverse drug reactions: Review of the Canadian literature. *Canadian Family Physician, 37*, 109–118.

Lexchin, J. (1999). Rethinking the numbers on adverse drug reactions. *CMAJ, 160*(10), 1432.

Lexchin, J. (2002, September). New drugs with novel therapeutic characteristics: Have they been subject to randomized clinical trials? *Canadian Family Physician, 48*, 1487–1492.

Lexchin, J. (2004, August 3). New directions in drug approval. *CMAJ, 171*(3), 229–230.

Manzer, J. (2006, December 22). Canada's drug safety system, part IV: Damage control: It's on the market, so now what? *Ottawa Citizen*, p. A6.

Marketed Health Products Directorate (MHPD). (2005). *Canadian Adverse Drug Reaction Monitoring Program (CADRMP) guidelines for the voluntary reporting of suspected adverse reactions to health products by health professionals and consumers.* Ottawa: The Author. Retrieved October 26, 2008, from: www.napra.ca/pdfs/cadr/adr_guideline_e.pdf

Martin, R.M., Biswas, P.N., Freemantle, S.N., Pearce, G.L. & Mann, R.D. (1998). Age and sex distribution of suspected adverse drug reactions to newly marketed drugs in general practice in England: Analysis of 48 cohort studies. *British Journal of Clinical Pharmacology, 46*(5), 505–511.

Medawar, C. & Herxheimer, A. (2003/2004). A comparison of adverse drug reaction reports from professionals and users, relating to risk of dependence and suicidal behaviour with paroxetine. *International Journal of Risk & Safety in Medicine, 16*, 5–19.

Medawar, C., Herxheimer, A., Bell, A. & Jofre, S. (2002). Paroxetine, Panorama, and user reporting of ADRs: Consumer intelligence matters in clinical practice and post-marketing drug surveillance. *International Journal of Risk & Safety in Medicine, 15*, 161–169.

Miller, M.A. (2001). Gender-based differences in the toxicity of pharmaceuticals—the Food and Drug Administration's perspective. *International Journal of Toxicology, 20*(3), 149–152.

Mittman, N., Liu, B.A., Iskedjian, M., Bradley, C.A., Pless, R., Shear, N.H. et al. (1997). Drug-related mortality in Canada (1984–1994). *Pharmacoepidemiology and Drug Safety, 6*(3), 157–168.

Motl, S., Timpe, E. & Eichner, S. (2004, September 1). Proposal to improve MedWatch: Decentralized, regional surveillance of adverse drug reactions. *American Journal of Health-System Pharmacy, 61*(17), 1840–1842.

Murtagh, M.J. & Hepworth, J. (2003). Feminist ethics and menopause: Autonomy and decision-making in primary medical care. *Social Science & Medicine, 56*(8), 1643–1652.

Organisation for Economic Co-operation and Development (OECD), Trade Directorate, Trade Committee. (1999, January 28). *Regulatory reform and international standardisation.* TD/TC/WP(98)36/Final. Paris: Author.

Pandolfini, C. & Bonati, M. (2005). A literature review on off-label drug use in children. *European Journal of Pediatrics, 164*(9), 552–558.

Pederson, A. & Tweed, A. (2003). *Registering the impact of breast implants.* Vancouver: British Columbia Centre of Excellence for Women's Health.

Progestic International Inc. (2004, May). *Final report for the financial models project.* Ottawa: Health Canada.

Quarterly index: Adverse drug reactions. (2002/2003). *Hospital Quarterly, 6*(2), 95–96.

Rademaker, M. (2001, June 1). Do women have more adverse drug reactions? *American Journal of Clinical Dermatology, 2*(6), 349–351.

Reynolds, E. (2006, June). *A national network to promote consumer ADR reporting.* Report to the Public Health Agency of Canada by DES Action, PharmaWatch, and the Canadian Women's Health Network (Project #6785-15-2005/4340161). Vancouver: DES Action.

Robinson, J. (2001). *Prescription games: Money, ego, and power inside the global pharmaceutical industry.* Toronto: McClelland & Stewart.

Rosenbloom, D. & Wynne, C. (1999, August 10). Detecting adverse drug reactions. *CMAJ, 161*(3), 247.

Sibbald, B. (2001, November 13). Cisapride, before and after: Still waiting for ADE-reporting reform. *CMAJ, 165*(10), 1370.

Sismondo, S. (2008). Pharmaceutical company funding and its consequences: A qualitative systematic review. *Contemporary Clinical Trials, 29*, 109–113.

Thalidomide Victims Association of Canada. *What is thalidomide?* Retrieved May 24, 2002, from: www.thalidomide.ca/english/wit.html

The War Amputations of Canada. (1989). *Report of the Thalidomide Task Force to the Minister of National Health and Welfare* (vol. I). Ottawa: Author. Retrieved September 9, 2008, from: www.waramps.ca/news/thalid/

Tran, C., Knowles, S.R., Liu, B.A. & Shear, N.H. (1998, November). Gender differences in adverse drug reactions. *Journal of Clinical Pharmacology, 38*(11), 1003–1009.

Tweed, A. (2003). *Health care utilization among women who have undergone breast implant surgery*. Vancouver: British Columbia Centre of Excellence for Women's Health.

V.A. Center for Medication Safety. (2006, November). *Adverse drug events, adverse drug reactions, and medication errors: Frequently asked questions*. Washington: Author. Retrieved August 15, 2008, from: www.pbm.va.gov/vamedsafe/Advers e%20Drug%20Reaction.pdf

Van Grootheest, K., de Graaf, L. & de Jong-van den Berg, L.T.W. (2003). Consumer adverse drug reaction reporting: A new step in pharmacovigilance? *Drug Safety, 26*(4), 211–217.

Chapter 8

Abraham, J. & Davis, C. (2005). A comparative analysis of drug safety withdrawals in the U.K. and the U.S. (1971–1992): Implications for current regulatory thinking and policy. *Social Science and Medicine, 61*(5), 881–892.

Auditor General of Canada. (2000, December). Chapter 24, Federal health and safety regulatory programs. In *2000 Report of the Auditor General of Canada*. Ottawa: Office of the Auditor General. Retrieved November 12, 2008, from: www.oag-bvg.gc.ca/internet/English/parl_oag_200012_24_e_11211.html

Brill-Edwards, M. (1999). Canada's Health Protection Branch: Whose health, what protection? In M.L. Barer, K. McGrail, K. Cardiff, L. Wood & C.J. Green (Eds.), *Tales from the other drug wars (Papers from the 12th Annual Health Policy Conference held in Vancouver, BC, November 26, 1999)* (pp. 39–54). Vancouver: Centre for Health Services and Policy Research, University of British Columbia.

Canadian Environmental Law Association (CELA). (2002). *Implementing precaution: An NGO response to the Government of Canada's discussion document "A Canadian perspective on the precautionary approach/principle."* Toronto: Author. Retrieved August 17, 2008, from: www.cela.ca/publications/cardfile.shtml?x=1002

Canadian Environmental Law Association (CELA). (2004a, March). *Health protection legislative renewal: Analysis and recommendations*. Prepared for the Canadian Environment Network. Retrieved August 17, 2008, from: cela.ca/uploads/f8e04 c51a8e04041f6f7faa046b03a7c/ENGO_Subm_on_CHPA.pdf

Canadian Environmental Law Association (CELA). (2004b, April). *Submission to the External Advisory Committee on Smart Regulation*. Retrieved November 11, 2008, from: cela.ca/uploads/f8e04c51a8e04041f6f7faa046b03a7c/469smartreg.pdf

Carpenter, D., Zucker, E.J. & Avorn, J. (2008, March 27). Drug-review deadlines and safety problems. *New England Journal of Medicine, 358*(13), 1354–1361.

External Working Group. (2004, January). *Section 3 and Schedule A of the Food and Drugs Act. Final report of the External Working Group*. Ottawa: Health Canada.

Health Canada. (1998a). *Health protection for the 21st century: Renewing the Federal Health Protection Program*. Ottawa: Author. Retrieved August 31, 2008, from: www.hc-sc.gc.ca/ahc-asc/pubs/cons-pub/health-protect-sante-21c-cp-pc-eng. php

Health Canada. (1998b, July). *Shared Responsibilities, Shared Vision: Renewing the Federal Health Protection Legislation*. Ottawa: Author.

Health Canada. (2000, April 17). *Health Canada realigns its activities*. News release. Ottawa: Author.

Health Canada. (2003). *Improving Canada's regulatory process for therapeutic products: Building the action plan*. PowerPoint presentation to the multi-stakeholder session of the Public Policy Forum consultation, Improving Canada's Regulatory Process for Therapeutic Products, November 2–3, 2003. Ottawa: Public Policy Forum.

Health Canada. (2006a, October). *The Role of the General Safety Requirement in Canada's Protection Regime*. Ottawa: Author. Retrieved February 4, 2009, from www.hc-sc.gc.ca/sr-sr/finance/hprp-prpms/results-resultats/2007-benidickson-eng.php.

Health Canada. (2006b, November 22). *The Progressive Licensing Framework: Concept paper for discussion*. Ottawa: Author. Retrieved August 18, 2008, from: www.hc-sc.gc.ca/dhp-mps/homologation-licensing/develop/proglic_homprog_concept-eng.php

Health Products and Food Branch (HPFB). (2006, October). *Blueprint for renewal: Transforming Canada's approach to regulating health products and food*. Ottawa: Health Canada. Retrieved August 17, 2008, from: www.hc-sc.gc.ca/ahc-asc/branch-dirgen/hpfb-dgpsa/blueprint-plan/index-eng.php

Health Products and Food Branch (HPFB). (2007). *Health Products and Food Branch review of regulated products: Policy on public input*. Ottawa: Health Canada. Retrieved August 17, 2008, from: www.hc-sc.gc.ca/ahc-asc/branch-dirgen/hpfb-dgpsa/public-rev-exam/index_e.html

Industry Canada. (1994). *Building a more innovative economy (Summary)*. Ottawa: Author.

Krever, H. (1997, November). *Final report: Commission of Inquiry on the Blood System in Canada*. Ottawa: The Commission.

Lexchin, J. (2006). Relationship between pharmaceutical company user fees and drug approvals in Canada and Australia: A hypothesis-generating study. *Annals of Pharmacotherapy, 40*(12), 2216–2222.

Lexchin, J. & Mintzes, B. (2004). Transparency in drug regulation: Mirage or oasis? *CMAJ, 171*(11), 1363–1365.

McKie, D. (2008, June 17). *Off limits, in depth: A CBC news investigation into the increasing use of atypical antipsychotics among the elderly*. Toronto: CBC News. Retrieved January 8, 2008, from: www.cbc.ca/news/background/seniorsdrugs/off-limits.html

Michols, D.M. (1997). *Drugs and medical devices program quality initiative bulletin,* no. 2. Ottawa: Health Protection Branch, Health Canada.

National Forum on Health. (1997). *Canada health action: Building on the legacy. Volume II: Synthesis reports and issues papers.* Ottawa: Minister of Public Works and Government Services. Retrieved August 17, 2008, from: www.hc-sc.gc.ca/hcs-sss/pubs/renewal-renouv/1997-nfoh-fnss-v2/index-eng.php

Privy Council Office. (2006). *Summary report of the public workshops on the draft Government Directive on Regulating. Summary of what was heard at the workshops.* Retrieved August 17, 2008, from: www.regulation.gc.ca/consultation/summary-sommaire/summary-sommaire00-eng.asp

Progestic International, Inc. (2004, May). *Final report for the Financial Models Project.* Prepared for the Health Products and Food Branch. Ottawa: Health Canada.

Sherwin, S. (1998, October). *Health protection for the 21st century? A response from the Maritime Centre of Excellence for Women's Health on Health Protection Branch discussion papers.* Gender and Health Policy series discussion paper no. 2. Halifax: MCEWH.

Sismondo, S. (2008). Pharmaceutical company funding and its consequences: A qualitative systematic review. *Contemporary Clinical Trials, 29,* 109–113.

Standing Committee on Health. (2003). *37th Parliament, 2nd Session, Standing Committee on Health, Evidence/Content, Wednesday, October 29.* Retrieved August 17, 2008, from: cmte.parl.gc.ca/cmte/CommitteePublication.aspx?SourceId=67157

Standing Committee on Health. (2004, April). *Opening the medicine cabinet: First report on health aspects of prescription drugs.* Ottawa: Parliament of Canada. Retrieved November 17, 2008, from: www2.parl.gc.ca/content/hoc/Committee/373/HEAL/Reports/RP1282198/healrp01/healrp01-e.pdf

Therapeutic Products Directorate (TPD). (2004). Business transformation strategy. In *Business transformation progress report 2003–2004.* Ottawa: Health Canada. Retrieved November 11, 2008, from: www.hc-sc.gc.ca/dhp-mps/prodpharma/applic-demande/docs/bt_rep_to_rap_2003_2004-eng.php

Women and Health Protection (WHP). (1998, September). *To do no harm: Why women are concerned about the dismantling of health protection legislation in Canada.* Toronto: Author. Retrieved August 17, 2008, from: www.whp-apsf.ca/en/documents/no_harm.html

Women and Health Protection (WHP). (2000, August). *Recommendations respecting the HPB transition and legislative renewal.* Submitted to Mario Simard, legal counsel to the Health Protection Branch, Health Canada. Toronto: Author.

Women and Health Protection (WHP). (2006, November). *Submission from WHP to Health Canada in response to "Blueprint for Renewal: Transforming Canada's Approach to Regulating Health Products and Food."* Toronto: Author. Retrieved August 17, 2008, from: www.whp-apsf.ca/en/documents/blueprint.html

Chapter 9

Andersen, L., Goto-Kazeto, R., Trant, J.M., Nash, J.P., Korsgaard, B. & Bjerregaard, P. (2006, March 10). Short-term exposure to low concentrations of the synthetic androgen methyltestosterone affects vitellogenin and steroid levels in adult male zebrafish (*Danio rerio*). *Aquatic Toxicology, 76*(3–4), 343–352.

Berenson, A. (2008, March 15). Eli Lilly e-mail discussed unapproved use of drug. *New York Times*. Online edition.

Boivin, M. (1997, May). The cost of medication waste. *Canadian Pharmacists Journal, 130*(4), 32–39. Retrieved August 17, 2008, from: www.napra.org/practice/toolkits/toolkit9/wastecost.pdf

Brian, J.V., Harris, C.A., Scholze, M., Backhaus, T., Booy, P., Lamoree, M. et al. (2005). Prediction of the response of freshwater fish to a mixture of estrogenic chemicals. *Environmental Health Perspectives, 113*(6), 721–728.

Buser, H., Müller, M.D. & Theobald, N. (1998). Occurrence of the pharmaceutical drug clofibric acid and the herbicide mecoprop in various Swiss lakes and the North Sea. *Environmental Science and Technology, 32*(1), 188–192.

Campbell, J. (2007, January). Drugs on tap: Pharmaceuticals in our drinking water. *Pharmacy Practice*, 27–29.

Canadian Partnership for Children's Health and the Environment. (2007, June 15). *A Father's Day report: Men, boys, and environmental health threats*. Ottawa & Toronto: Author. Retrieved March 9, 2008, from: www.healthyenvironmentforkids.ca/img_upload/13297cd6a147585a24c1c6233d8d96d8/father_s_day_report.pdf

Carson, R. (1962). *Silent spring*. Boston: Houghton Mifflin.

Colburn, T., Dumanoski, D. & Meyers, J.P. (1996). *Our stolen future*. New York: Dutton.

Collier, A.C. (2007). Pharmaceutical contaminants in potable water: Potential concerns for pregnant women and children. *EcoHealth, 4*(2), 164–171.

Daughton, C.G. (2003a, March). Environmental stewardship of pharmaceuticals: The green pharmacy. In *Proceedings of the 3rd International Conference on Pharmaceuticals and Endocrine Disrupting Chemicals in Water, National Groundwater Association, 19–21 March, Minneapolis, MN*. Retrieved September 13, 2008, from: www.bioud.com/Documents/ngwa2003.pdf

Daughton, C.G. (2003b). Cradle-to-cradle stewardship of drugs for minimizing their environmental disposition while promoting human health. I. Rationale for and avenues toward a green pharmacy. *Environmental Health Perspectives, 111*(5), 757–774.

Daughton, C.G. (2003c). Cradle-to-cradle stewardship of drugs for minimizing their environmental disposition while promoting human health. II. Drug disposal, waste reduction, and future directions. *Environmental Health Perspectives, 111*(5), 775–785.

Daughton C.G. (2006, March). *Origins and fate of PPCPs in the environment.* Illustrated poster. Las Vegas: U.S. Environmental Protection Agency. (Updated from an original work published in February 2001.) Retrieved September 14, 2008, from: www.epa.gov/ppcp/pdf/drawing.pdf

Davis, D.L. (2007). *The secret history of the war on cancer.* New York: Basic Books.

D'Eaubonne, F. (1974). *Le Féminisme ou la mort.* Paris: Pierre Horay.

DeBruin, L.S., Pawliszyn, J.B. & Josephy, P.D. (1999). Detection of monocyclic aromatic amines, possible mammary carcinogens, in human milk. *Chemical Research in Toxicology, 12*(1), 78–82.

DES Action Canada. (2001). *Hormonal pollution alert: Protecting our long-term health, protecting the environment.* Montreal: DES Action.

Desbrow, C., Routledge, E.J., Brighty, G.C., Sumpter, J.P. & Waldock, M. (1998). Identification of estrogenic chemicals in STW effluent. 1. Chemical fractionation and in vitro biological screening. *Environmental Science & Technology, 32*(11), 1549–1558.

Donn, J., Mendoza, M. & Pritchard, J. (2008a, March 9). Drugs found in U.S. drinking water. *Time.* Retrieved March 11, 2008, from: www.time.com/time/nation/article/0,8599,1720758,00.html

Donn, J., Mendoza, M. & Pritchard, J. (2008b, March 11). Pharmawater III: No standards to handle pharmaceuticals in water. *Washington Post.* Retrieved January 29, 2009, from: hosted.ap.org/specials/interactives/pharmawater_site/day3_01.html.

Environmental Commissioner of Ontario. (2005). Human pharmaceuticals in the aquatic environment: An emerging issue. In *Planning our landscape: 2004–2005 annual report* (pp. 179–185). Toronto: Ontario Ministry of the Environment. Retrieved March 11, 2008, from: www.eco.on.ca/eng/uploads/eng_pdfs/ar2004.pdf

Gagné, F., Blaise, C. & André, C. (2006). Occurrence of pharmaceutical products in a municipal effluent and toxicity to rainbow trout (*Oncorhynchus mykiss*) hepatocytes. *Ecotoxicology and Environmental Safety, 64*(3), 329–336.

Gerhardt, A., de Bisthoven, L.J., Mo, Z., Wang, C., Yang, M. & Wang, Z. (2002). Short-term responses of *Oryzias latipes* (*Pices Adrianichthyidae*) *Macrobrachium nipponense* (*Crustacea: Palaemonidae*) to municipal and pharmaceutical waste water in Beijing, China: Survival, behaviour, biochemical biomarkers. *Chemosphere, 47*(1), 35–47.

Halling-Sørensen, B., Nors Nielsen, N.S., Lanzky, P.F., Ingerslev, F., Holten Lützhøft, H.C. & Jørgensen, S.E. (1998). Occurrence, fate, and effects of pharmaceutical substances in the environment: A review. *Chemosphere, 36*(2), 357–393.

Health Canada. (2001, September 1). Environmental assessment regulations, notice of intent. *Canada Gazette,* Part 1. Retrieved September 13, 2008, from: www.hc-sc.gc.ca/ewh-semt/contaminants/person/impact/200109_noi-adi-eng.php

Health Canada. (2002a). Workshop conclusions. In the PowerPoint presentation, *EAR: Science and Research,* presented at the EAR consultation session, Ottawa, May 3, 2003.

Health Canada. (2002b). *F&DA Environmental Assessment Regulations Project benchmark survey,* Appendix 1. Retrieved August 18, 2008, from: www.hc-sc.gc. ca/ewh-semt/contaminants/person/impact/por-02-13-eng.php#demographic

Health Canada. (2002c, Spring). Notice of intent: Consultation report. *EAR Newsletter, 1*(1), 2.

Health Canada. (2003). *Issue identification paper: Environmental assessment regulations:* Ottawa: Author. Retrieved October 31, 2008, from: www.hc-sc.gc.ca/ewh-semt/ alt_formats/hpfb-dgpsa/pdf/contaminants/iip-dde-eng.pdf

Health Canada. (2006, February 23). *Options analysis paper feedback analysis report.* Ottawa: Author. Retrieved March 22, 2008, from: www.hc-sc.gc.ca/ewh-semt/ contaminants/person/impact/consultation/oap_feedback_dao_retroaction_ e.html

Health Canada. (2007). *Environmental impact initiative.* Retrieved June 9, 2008, from: www.hc-sc.gc.ca/ewh-semt/contaminants/person/impact/index-eng.php

Heberer, T. & Stan, H.-J. (1997). Determination of clofibric acid and N(phenylsulfonyl)-sarcosine in sewage, river, and drinking water. *International Journal of Environmental Analytic Chemistry, 67*(1), 113–124.

Heinrich, J. (2001). *Drug safety: Most drugs withdrawn in recent years had greater health risks for women.* Washington: United States General Accounting Office, GOA 01-286R. Retrieved August 18, 2008, from: www.gao.gov/new.items/d01286r.pdf

Hignite, C. & Azarnoff, D.L. (1977, January 15). Drugs and drug metabolites as contaminants: Chlorophenoxyisobutyrate and salicyclic acid in sewage water effluent. *Life Sciences, 20*(2), 337–341.

Holtz, S. (2006). *There is no "away." Pharmaceuticals, personal care products and endocrine-disrupting substances: Emerging contaminants detected in water.* Toronto: Canadian Institute for Environmental Law and Policy.

Houlihan, J., Brody, C. & Schwan, B. (2002, July 8). *Not too pretty: Phthalates, beauty products & the FDA.* Washington: Environmental Working Group. Retrieved August 18, 2008, from www.safecosmetics.org/docUploads/NotTooPretty_r51. pdf

Jobling, S. & Tyler, C.R. (2003). Endocrine disruption in wild freshwater fish. *Pure and Applied Chemistry, 75*(11–12), 2219–2234.

Jordan, A. & O'Riordan, T. (1999). The precautionary principle in contemporary environmental policy and politics. In C. Raffensperger & J.A. Tickner (Eds.), *Protecting public health and the environment: Implementing the precautionary principle* (pp. 15–35). Washington & Covelo: Island Press.

Jørgensen, S.E. & Halling-Sørensen, B. (2000). Editorial: Drugs in the environment. *Chemosphere, 40*(7), 691–699.

Kavanagh, R.J., Balch, G.C., Kiparissis, Y., Niimi, A.J., Sherry, J., Tinson, C. et al. (2004, June). Endocrine disruption and altered gonadal development in white perch (*Morone americana*) from the lower Great Lakes region. *Environmental Health Perspectives, 112*(8), 898–902.

Kidd, K.A., Blanchfield, P.J., Mills, K.H., Palace, V.P., Evans, R.E., Lazorchak, J.M. et al. (2007). Collapse of a fish population after exposure to synthetic estrogen. *Proceedings of the National Academy of Sciences, 104*(21), 8897–8901.

Lyssimachou, A. & Arukwe, A. (2007). Alteration of brain and interrenal StAR protein P450scc, and Cyp11β and mRNA levels in Atlantic salmon after nominal waterborne exposure to the synthetic pharmaceutical estrogen ethynylestradiol. *Journal of Toxicology and Environmental Health*, Part A, *70*(7), 606–613.

Markman, S., Leitner, S., Catchpole, C., Barnsley, S., Müller, C.T., Pascoe, D. et al. (2008). Pollutants increase song complexity and the volume of the brain area HVC in a songbird. *PLoS ONE, 3*(2), e1074. Retrieved October 7, 2008, from: doi:10.1371/journal.pone.0001674

Mies, M. & Shiva,V. (1993). *Ecofeminism.* London: Zed Books.

Mittelstaedt, M. (2003, February 10). Drug traces found in cities' water. *Globe and Mail*, p. A1.

Montague, P. (1998, September 2). Drugs in the water. *Rachel's Environmental and Health News*, 614. Retrieved September 14, 2008, from: www.rachel.org/en/node/3819

Oaks, J.L., Gilbert, M., Virani, M.Z., Watson, R.T., Meteyer, C.U., Rideout, B.A. et al. (2004). Diclofenac residues as the cause of vulture population decline in Pakistan. *Nature, 427*, 630–633.

O'Brien, M. (2000). *Making better environmental decisions: An alternative to risk assessment.* Cambridge: MIT Press.

Post-consumer Pharmaceutical Stewardship Association (PCPSA). (2008). *Medications Return Program*. Retrieved March 22, 2008, from: www.medicationsreturn.ca/home_en.php

Prakash, V., Pain, D.J., Cunningham, A.A., Donald, P.F., Prakash, N., Verma, A. et al. (2003). Catastrophic collapse of Indian white-backed *Gyps bengalensis* and long-billed *Gyps indicus* vulture populations. *Biological Conservation, 109*(3), 381–390.

Schultz, I.R., Skillman, A., Nicolas, J.M., Cyr, D.G. & Nagler, J.J. (2003). Short-term exposure to 17-alpha ethynylestradiol decreases the fertility of sexually maturing male rainbow trout (*Oncorhynchus mykiss*). *Environmental Toxicology and Chemistry, 22*(6), 1272–1280.

Seager, J. (1993). *Earth follies: Coming to feminist terms with the global environmental crisis.* New York: Routledge.

Steingraber, S. (1997). *Living downstream: An ecologist looks at cancer and the environment*. Reading: Addison-Wesley.

Steingraber, S. (1999). Research commentary: Human milk contamination. *The Ribbon, 4*(3). Retrieved August 18, 2008, from: envirocancer.cornell.edu/Newsletter/articles/v4rc.milk.cfm

Steingraber, S. (2001). *Having faith: An ecologist's journey to motherhood*. Cambridge: Perseus Publishing.

Steingraber, S. (2007). *The falling age of puberty in U.S. girls: What we know, what we need to know*. San Francisco: The Breast Cancer Fund. Retrieved March 9, 2008, from: www.breastcancerfund.org/site/pp.asp?c=kwKXLdPaE&b=3291891

Stevenson, M. (2002, October 21). Tests find drug taint in water. *Globe and Mail*, p. A1.

Swan, G.E., Cuthbert, R., Quevedo, M., Green, R., Pain, D.J., Bartels, P. et al. (2006). Toxicity of diclofenac to *Gyps* vultures. *Biology Letters, 2*(2), 279–282.

Ternes, T.A. (1998). Occurrence of drugs in German sewage treatment plants and rivers. *Water Research, 32*(11), 3245–3260.

U.S. Environmental Protection Agency. (2007, December). *Pharmaceuticals and personal care products: Frequent questions*. Retrieved March 11, 2008, from: www.epa.gov/ppcp/faq.html

U.S. Environmental Protection Agency. (2008). Pharmaceuticals and personal care products (PPCPs): Home page. Retrieved July 16, 2008, from: www.epa.gov/ppcp/

U.S. Geological Survey. (2008). *Emerging contaminants in the environment*. Retrieved March 9, 2008, from: toxics.usgs.gov/regional/emc/

Vaidyanath, S. (2008, February 6). Scientists, politicians aim to tackle drugs in the water supply. *The Epoch Times*. Retrieved March 9, 2008, from: en.epochtimes.com/news/8-2-6/65506.html

Van Esterik, P. (2002). *Risks, rights, and regulations: Communicating about risks and infant feeding*. Toronto: National Network on Environments and Women's Health. Retrieved August 18, 2008, from: www.yorku.ca/nnewh

Van Larebeke, N.A., Sasco, A.J., Brophy, J.T., Keith, M.M., Gilbertson, M. & Watterson, A. (2008, April–June). Sex ratio changes as sentinel health events of endocrine disruption. *International Journal of Occupational and Environmental Health, 14*(2), 138–143.

Warren, K.J. (2000). *Ecofeminist philosophy: A Western perspective on what it is and why it matters*. Lanham: Rowman and Littlefield.

Webb, S., Ternes, T., Gibert, M. & Olejniczak, K. (2003) Indirect human exposure to pharmaceuticals via drinking water. *Toxicology Letters, 142*(3), 157–167.

Wyman, M. (1999). Introduction. In M. Wyman (Ed.), *Sweeping the earth: Women taking action for a healthy planet* (pp. 16–25). Charlottetown: Gynergy Books.

Chapter 10

Food and Drug Administration (FDA), Vaccine and Related Biological Products Advisory Committee (VRBPAC). (2006). *VRBPAC background document, Gardasil™ HPV quadrivalent vaccine, May 18, 2006 VRBPAC meeting.* Retrieved October 27, 2008, from: www.fda.gov/ohrms/dockets/ac/06/briefing/2006-4222B3.pdf

Frisby, W., Blair, F., Dorer, T., Hill, L., Fenton, J. & Kopelow, B. (2001). *Taking action: Mobilizing communities to provide recreation for women on low incomes.* Vancouver: British Columbia Centre of Excellence for Women's Health.

Kerlikowske, K., Miglioretti, D.L., Buist, D.S., Walker, R. & Carney, P.A. for the National Cancer Institute-Sponsored Breast Cancer Surveillance Consortium. (2007, September 5). Declines in invasive breast cancer and use of postmenopausal hormone therapy in a screening mammography population. *Journal of the National Cancer Institute, 99*(17), 1335–1339. Erratum (2007, October 3). *Journal of the National Cancer Institute, 99*(19), 1493.

World Health Organization (WHO). (2008). *Closing the gap in a generation: Health equity through action on the social determinants of health: Final report of the Commission on Social Determinants of Health.* Geneva: Author. Retrieved September 22, 2008, from: whqlibdoc.who.int/publications/2008/9789241563 703_eng.pdf

Copyright
Acknowledgements

Front cover and chapter opening photo ©istockphoto.com/stock-photo-6801944-holding-pills

Figure 3.1: From McKinlay, J.B., and McKinlay, S.M. (Summer 1977). The questionable contribution of medical measures to the decline of mortality in the United States in the twentieth century. *The Milbank Memorial Fund Quarterly. Health and Society*, Vol. 55, No. 3, 405–428.

Table 4.1: From "A Look Back at Pharmaceuticals in 2006: Aggressive Advertising Cannot Hide the Absence of Therapeutic Advances," *Prescrire International* 16, no. 88 (2007): 80–86.

Figure 6.1: From Lexchin, J. (2007, May). Pharmaceutical secrecy endangers our health. *The Monitor*. Retrieved November 10, 2008, from the Canadian Centre for Policy Alternatives: www.policyalternatives.ca/MonitorIssues/2007/05/MonitorIssue1638/

Box 7.1: Food and Drugs Act: Food and Drug Regulations (Schedule No. 844), November 7, 1995

Table 7.1: Adverse drug reaction reporting—1998. (1999). Canadian Adverse Reaction Newsletter (CARN), 9(2), 5–6. Retrieved October 26, 2008, from www.hc-sc.gc.ca/dhp-mps/alt_formats/hpfb-dgpsa/pdf/medeff/carn-bcei_v9n2_e.pdf. Adverse reaction reporting—2006. (2007). Canadian Adverse Reaction Newsletter (CARN), 17(2), 3–4. Retrieved September 9, 2008, from www.hc-sc.gc.ca/dhp-mps/alt_formats/hpfb-dgpsa/pdf/medeff/carn-bcei_v17n2_e.pdf

Figure 7.1: Adverse drug reactions (Winter 2002/03). Quarterly Index, Hospital Quarterly (now Healthcare Quarterly) 6(2), 95-96.

Table 8.1: From Health Canada (2003). Improving Canada's regulatory process for therapeutic products: Building the action plan. PowerPoint presentation to the multi-stakeholder session of the Public Policy Forum consultation, Improving Canada's Regulatory Process for Therapeutic Products, November 2–3, 2003. Ottawa: Public Policy Forum.

Box 8.1: From Brill-Edwards, M. (1999). Canada's Health Protection Branch: Whose health, what protection? In M.L. Barer, K. McGrail, K. Cardiff, L. Wood, & C.J. Green, (Eds.), *Tales from the other drug wars. Papers from the 12th Annual Health Policy Conference held in Vancouver, BC, Nov 26, 1999*. Vancouver: Centre for Health Services and Policy Research, University of British Columbia, pp. 39–54.

Figure 8.1: From Lexchin, J. (2006). Relationship between pharmaceutical company user fees and drug approvals in Canada and Australia: A hypothesis-generating study. *Annals of Pharmacotherapy, 40*(12), 2216–2222.

Box 8.3: Excerpted from Standing Committee on Health, 2003. 37th Parliament, 2nd Session, Standing Committee on Health, Evidence /Content, Wednesday, October 29. Retrieved August 17, 2008, from: http://cmte.parl.gc.ca/cmte/CommitteePublication. aspx?SourceId=67157

Figure 9.1: Illustration (modified) from: Daughton, C.G. "Pharmaceuticals in the Environment: Sources and Their Management," Chapter 1, 1–58, in *Analysis, Fate and Removal of Pharmaceuticals in the Water Cycle* (M. Petrovic and D. Barcelo, Eds.), Wilson & Wilson's Comprehensive Analytical Chemistry series (D. Barcelo, Ed.), Volume 50, Elsevier Science, 2007.

Figure 10.1: Heather Walters for the Side Effects project. Side Effects, a play on women and pharmaceuticals, was originally developed and produced by Inter Pares and the Great Canadian Theatre Company for Women's Health Interaction.

Index

Aamjiwnaang (Ontario), birth rates in, 192
abacavir sulfate, 128
ability, as determinant of health, 9, 100
Aboriginal women, 7–8, 214
abortion, 13n1, 214
abusive relationships, mental illness and, 43
Access to Information (ATI), 30, 121, 123, 129–31
Access to Information Act, 129–30, 132
accountability, 166
acid reflux, 22
acne, 125–27
activism, 2–5, 56, 85, 158, 210–15;
    AIDS, 68, 169
adjustment disorder, 45
adverse drug event, 141, 142
adverse drug reactions (ADRs), 80, 139–59, 170;
    consumer reporting of, 154–59;
    current issues in, 149–52;
    data collection, 144–45;
    deaths from, 150–51;
    definition of, 141, 142;
    gender and, 156;
    physicians and, 145;
    regional monitoring centres, 149;
    reports of by type, 155;
    serious, 142;
    under-reporting of, 150–52;
    women and, 153–56, 159
adverse effect, 141
Adverse Effects: Women and the Pharmaceutical Industry, 214
advertising:
    consequences of, 18, 19–20;

direct-to-consumer, 17–46, 52, 80–81, 82, 126, 166, 170, 176–77, 197, 204, 209, 211;
    "disease-oriented," 18, 28;
    "help-seeking," 28;
    illegality of prescription drug, 18–19, 21, 32, 80–81, 82;
    increasing effectiveness of, 22;
    "made-in-Canada," 18;
    in medical journals, 32;
    negative stereotypes in, 20;
    vs. public health message, 36;
    "reminder," 18;
    targeting of women in, 19, 22, 24–26, 30–32, 120.
    See also marketing.
advocacy groups. *See* patient advocacy groups.
age:
    adverse drug reactions and, 156;
    in clinical trials, 98, 108;
    as determinant of health, 9
Agriculture and Agri-Food Canada, 167
AIDS, 33, 64, 68, 84, 127;
    activism, 68, 169
ALARA (as low as reasonably achievable) principle, 60
Alberta, take-back program in, 196
alcohol, 64, 193;
    addiction to, 7
Alesse (levonorgestrel/estradiol), 25, 36, 38
Alzheimer's disease, 49–50, 73–74
Alzheimer Society of Canada (ASC), 73–74
Ambien (zolpidem), 22